2nd Edition

Applied Paramedic

LAW, ETHICS AND PROFESSIONALISM

AUSTRALIA AND NEW ZEALAND

2nd Edition

Applied Paramedic

LAW, ETHICS AND PROFESSIONALISM

AUSTRALIA AND NEW ZEALAND

Ruth **Townsend** & Morgan **Luck**

ELSEVIER

ELSEVIER

Elsevier Australia. ACN 001 002 357
(a division of Reed International Books Australia Pty Ltd)
Tower 1, 475 Victoria Avenue, Chatswood, NSW 2067

This edition © 2020 Elsevier Australia. 1st Edition © 2013 Elsevier Australia. Reprinted 2015.

ISBN: 978-0-7295-4308-8

Notice

Practitioners and researchers must always rely on their own experience and knowledge in evaluating and using any information, methods, compounds or experiments described herein. Because of rapid advances in the medical sciences, in particular, independent verification of diagnoses and drug dosages should be made. To the fullest extent of the law, no responsibility is assumed by Elsevier, authors, editors or contributors for any injury and/or damage to persons or property as a matter of products liability, negligence or otherwise, or from any use or operation of any methods, products, instructions, or ideas contained in the material herein.

National Library of Australia Cataloguing-in-Publication Data

A catalogue record for this
book is available from the
National Library of Australia

Content Strategist: Rachel Simone Ford
Content Project Manager: Shruti Raj
Edited by Kate Stone
Proofread by Katie Millar
Permissions Editing and Photo Research: Regina Lavanya Remigius
Cover and internal design by Lisa Petroff
Index by Innodata Indexing
Typeset by Toppan Best-set Premedia Limited
Printed in China by 1010 Printing International Limited

Last digit is the print number: 9   8   7   6   5   4   3   2   1

Contents

Acknowledgements

I would like to thank my co-editor, Morgan, whose counsel and wisdom helped make this project run so smoothly. I would also like to thank all the contributors for their marvellous efforts in compiling the material for this text, and to all those other paramedic colleagues I have worked with over the years for their passion and commitment to their work. You were the inspiration for this book. Thanks to my parents for instilling in me a strong sense of social justice and encouraging me into the noble and rewarding areas of both healthcare and law. And, finally, I would like to thank my boys, Andrew, Tom and Will, for their unending love and support. RT

I would like to thank: my co-editor, Ruth, for the time and energy she put into this project; my father, Malcolm Luck, for helping me with many of the cases within this book (and for impressing upon me, at an early age, the importance of reason); and, lastly, Daniel Cohen for his work in this area, which partly inspired this collection. ML

Foreword

The paramedic profession has seen monumental change in practice over recent decades, and now has a comprehensive range of skills and technologies to provide world-class services to Australian communities. Regulation of the paramedicine profession and the registration of paramedics will ensure that our communities can be confident that those practising as paramedic healthcare professionals meet expected national standards, and comply with the Code of Conduct and guidelines set by the Paramedicine Board of Australia under the Health Practitioner Regulation National Law.

But what exactly does it mean to be a paramedic healthcare professional? And what does it mean for individual paramedics to work as part of a nationally regulated profession?

Paramedics in Australia have been professionalising slowly over time, and national regulation is an important step in the journey towards professionalisation of paramedicine in Australia. The Paramedicine Board of Australia is authorised to establish education and accreditation standards alongside behavioural standards, thus contributing to the development of professionalism within the profession.

This book will introduce student paramedics and those already working as paramedics to the new regulatory arrangements, which will apply to the profession of paramedicine now that they are regulated nationally as the fifteenth registered health profession in Australia. It will set out the key elements of the national standards for education and practice, the national Code of Conduct and other behavioural standards regulated under the national regulatory scheme. It will also introduce readers to key principles that apply to all healthcare professionals, particularly with regards to ethics and ethical practice, and provide paramedics with the non-clinical knowledge they need to deal with complex ethico-legal cases in a way that is expected of healthcare professionals. The importance of learning and applying these standards and principles is critical to the continuing professional development of paramedics, and their duty to act in the best interests of their patients.

New Zealand is progressing towards the adoption of a similar regulatory process. Key ethical and legal principles that apply to New Zealand paramedics are covered in this text.

Paramedicine is a unique and specialised profession that occupies a special place in the Australian and New Zealand communities. The profession is made up of people who are committed to providing high-quality out-of-hospital care, and this book will contribute to ensuring that future generations of paramedics are prepared, and continue, to meet the high standards expected of a registered health practitioner in Australia and New Zealand.

Stephen Gough ASM
Chair Paramedicine Board of Australia

Contributors

Bruce Baer Arnold JD, PhD, GCTE
Assistant Professor, Canberra Law School, University of Canberra, ACT, Australia

Stephen Bartlett LLB, LLM
Lecturer, Queensland University of Technology, Qld, Australia

Bronwyn Betts ASM, LLM, LLB, BAppSc (Nursing), RN
Senior Educator, Queensland Ambulance Service, Qld, Australia

Wendy Bonython BSc(Hons) PhD, JD, GDLP, GCTE
Associate Professor, School of Law and Justice, University of Canberra, ACT, Australia

Kate Diesfeld BA, JD
Professor, Health Law, AUT University, New Zealand

Philip Groves BA, LLB, GDLP, PhD
Managing Director, JOPL, NSW, Australia

Alisha Hensby BA, Bed
Lecturer, Paramedic Discipline, Charles Sturt University
Co-chair of the Education Committee, Australian and New Zealand College of Paramedicine, NSW, Australia

Peter Jurkovsky LLM, LLB(Hons), Grad Cert Legal Practice, Grad Cert Higher Education, DipParaSc(Ambulance)
Honorary President of Paramedics Australasia

Peter Lang BHlthSc(PreHospCare), BNurs, DipParaSc, MACAP, AdvDipParaSc, FANZCP
Intensive Care Paramedic, Ambulance Service of NSW, NSW, Australia

Morgan Luck BA, BComm, BA(Hons), MA, PGCE, PhD
Associate Professor, School of Humanities and Social Science, Charles Sturt University, NSW, Australia

Contributors

Ramon Z. Shaban BSc(Med), BN, GradCertInfCon, PGDipPH&TM, MEd, MCommHealthPrac(Hons1), PhD, RN, FCENA, FACN, CICP-E
Professor and Clinical Chair, Infection Prevention and Disease Control, Susan Wakil School of Nursing and Midwifery and the Marie Bashir Institute for Infectious Diseases and Biosecurity, Faculty of Medicine and Health, University of Sydney, NSW, Australia

Brian Steer BA(Hons), ThA, DipEd, BParamedStudies
Ambulance Paramedic, Ambulance Victoria, Vic, Australia

Ruth Townsend BN, LLB, LLM, GradDipLegalPrac, GradCertVET, DipParaSc PhD
Senior Lecturer, Paramedicine, Charles Sturt University, NSW, Australia
Solicitor of the Supreme Court of NSW, NSW, Australia

Reviewers

Miriam Dayhew, LLB MBA MEd
University Ombudsman, Office of Governance and Corporate Affairs, Charles Sturt University, NSW, Australia

Peter O'Meara, FPA
Adjunct Professor, Department of Community Emergency Health and Paramedic Practice, Monash University, Vic, Australia

Lauren Saling, PhD
Lecturer, School of Health and Biomedical Sciences, RMIT University, Vic, Australia

Craig Taylor, PhD
Lecturer
Community Emergency Health and Paramedics, Monash University, Vic, Australia

Chapter 1
Paramedic professionalism

Ruth Townsend and Morgan Luck

Learning objectives

After reading this chapter, you should:
- understand why it is necessary for paramedics to learn about the law and ethics
- have an introductory-level understanding of the development of paramedicine as a profession
- have an awareness of the broad nature of the topics to be discussed in this book
- be informed of how law and ethics are broadly applied in paramedic practice.

Definitions

Ethics The study of what it means for something to be morally right or wrong.

Law 'The system of rules which a particular country or community recognises as regulating the actions of its members and which it may enforce by the imposition of penalties.'[1]

Profession 'An occupation whose core element is work, based on the mastery of a complex body of knowledge and skills. It is a vocation in which knowledge of some department of science or learning, or the practice of an art founded on it, is used in the service of others. Its members profess a commitment to competence, integrity, morality, altruism, and the promotion of the public good within their domain. These commitments form the basis of a social contract between a profession and society.'[2]

An introductory case

A competent refusal of care

A paramedic is called to an elderly man's home by a family member who is concerned for his welfare. The man tells the paramedic that he is terminally ill, and, although he is in some discomfort (which could be remedied were he taken to hospital), he would rather remain at home to die. The paramedic assesses the patient's competence and his clinical needs. They determine that the patient is competent, but decide to call a doctor (an Australian senior medical officer) for advice about his clinical needs. The doctor advises the paramedic to transport the patient to the hospital, despite the patient having been determined as competent and having objected to transportation.

This chapter will provide you with some context in which to consider and reflect on this case.

Introduction

To begin to understand the notion of paramedic professionalism, it is useful to consider the origins of medical professionalism more generally. Around the turn of the 20th century, Abraham Flexner, the now well-recognised father of medical education, wrote a series of reports regarding medical education in universities in response to a 'revolution in understanding about the scientific foundations of clinical medicine'.[3] Flexner made links between science, tertiary education and medicine, and famously attempted to list the traits of a profession in his paper on social work and professionalism.[4] He identified one of the key traits of a profession as 'an increasingly altruistic motivation'.

The fostering of the virtue of altruism in professionals is based on the idea that they have power and privilege derived from their position that others do not. The most obvious of these is professional knowledge. Professionals have knowledge that others do not have, and, as such, this makes those without the knowledge dependent on those who have it. In the case of paramedics, this knowledge places the paramedic in a position of power over their patient. The recognition of this power imbalance in the therapeutic relationship was recognised by medicine millennia ago.

To promote the role of the doctor, to foster trust that members of this profession would not abuse their power, and to outline the principles that the profession would adopt to mitigate such abuse, doctors adopted the Hippocratic Oath and its modern variant, the Declaration of Geneva, to set out their responsibilities to their patients. This included a commitment to put their patient's interests above their own—a nod to altruism. For example, the Declaration of Geneva pronounces that: 'The health of my patient shall be my first consideration.'[5] Other virtues required of a clinician are also referred to; for example, courage ('I will not use my medical knowledge to violate human rights and civil liberties, even under threat') and compassion ('I will remember that there is art to medicine as well as science, and that warmth, sympathy, and understanding may outweigh the surgeon's knife or the chemist's drug'). These responsibilities are replicated in today's health practitioner codes of conduct and form the basis for standards of professionalism. But what exactly is professionalism? We shall consider this question next.

Defining 'professionalism'

The term '**professionalism**' carries different meanings in different contexts. There is no single, universally accepted definition. However, for the purposes of this chapter the term 'professionalism' means 'to act within a set of norms, principles and standards of conduct and competency'.[6] To be a professional is to work as part of a profession within these 'norms, principles and standards' (i.e. with professionalism). These 'norms, principles and standards', as we shall discover, play a crucial role in *regulating* the paramedic profession.

In September 2018, Australian paramedics began being placed on the national register of health practitioners regulated by the *Health Practitioner Regulation National Law Act 2009 (Qld)*; also known in the abbreviated form as 'the National Law'.[7] Once they commence practising as registered paramedics they will be required to work in accordance with the principles of this law. The primary purpose of this law is patient safety. A large component of the legislation contains principles and objectives that are consistent with the notion of 'professionalism'. We can therefore refer to the health practitioner regulation's legal jurisdiction as a 'professionalism jurisdiction'. Regulation by professionalism involves consistently demonstrating a set of identifiable positive professional attributes, values and behaviours, and being held to these standards by your professional peer group and others.

One question that paramedics and the profession of paramedicine must now consider is: what is it about self-regulation as a profession that makes it distinct from the regulation that applied to paramedics before the national regulation scheme? Historically paramedics in Australia have predominantly been employed by state-based ambulance services, and so have been regulated by an employer–employee relationship. This relationship remains, but regulation as part of a profession that regulates itself (and does so within the framework a professional code) adds an additional layer of regulation to the governance of paramedics that has not previously existed.

So what is the 'goverance of paramedics'? One good way to start thinking about it is in terms of circles of control. The innermost circle is a small circle that represents you. Clustered around you are other small circles that represent your professional colleagues. By working together to form a professional association, you create a larger circle that contains you and your colleagues. There are lots of advantages to forming an association, not least of which is that it can help govern the behaviour of its members—both toward one another and toward the public (who are outside the circle). The largest circle, encompassing you, your colleagues, your association and the wider public, is the law. The law governs both personal and professional interactions in lots of ways; for example, laws govern marriage, births, deaths, pet ownership, conscription and real estate transactions, and the professional duty of care.[8] So we have overlapping circles of governance relating to: how you govern yourself; how your profession governs its members; and how the law governs everyone. To help professions govern their members, the law provides them with professionalism regulation, and it is to this regulation that we now turn.

To better enable the governance of paramedicine 'professionalism', laws are in place that allow for the establishment of a paramedicine board to set the standards of education, competence and conduct for the entire paramedic profession, separate from employer standards.[9] Professionalism regulation includes the following functions and aspects.

- The protection of the title of a 'paramedic' so that only those suitably qualified can use it.
- The profession is allowed to determine its own standards for entry into the profession, allowing it to set its own eligibility requirements in terms of distinct expertise, practice, knowledge and skills.
- The regulations establish not only standards for entry into the profession, but also the standards of conduct expected of paramedics. These standards reflect the values and identity of the profession. (Interestingly, these professional values may conflict with those of the paramedic's employer. However, this does not relieve paramedics of their professional duty to act in accordance with professional values. In other words, a professional's obligation to their professional values trumps any obligation they may have to their employer's values.)
- The regulations also provide a process for the profession to sanction those members who do not meet the required standard of competence or conduct (regardless of whether an employer judges the paramedic to be fit to practise).

In addition to these new powers and protections, professionalism regulation also imposes a new form of professional autonomy and associated responsibility on paramedics that they have not previously had to consider. And one such responsibility, which is key, is the requirement to work as a professional.

In order to meet the requirements of working as a professional, it is critical that paramedics learn (and be supported to learn) how to navigate any conflicts—as mentioned above—that may arise. They must understand the power that they wield as professionals, and the responsibilities associated with the exercising of that power. This is particularly so as paramedics begin to work more autonomously both within, and outside of, their current employment arrangements. The primary focus of professional regulation is the provision of high-quality patient care; care that requires paramedics to put the interests of their patients first, even if this results in a conflict with their employer. This is because the 'ideology of professionalism asserts above all else, devotion to the use of [a] discipline's knowledge and skill for the public good'.[10] This ideology is also evident in the interim code of conduct for registered health practitioners (released by the Paramedicine Board of Australia in 2018), which states that 'Practitioners have a duty to make the care of patients or clients their first concern' and that the underpinning of the code is the 'assumption that practitioners will exercise their professional judgement to deliver the best possible outcome for their patients'.[11]

The unique and important nature of the work of paramedics, in dealing commonly with people who are at their most vulnerable, means that paramedics must understand and apply principles of professionalism to their work. Professionalism extends beyond accountability as set out in the National Law, to also include professional responsibility as set out in the code of conduct. So, what is a code of conduct?

Paramedics are now included under the National Registration Accreditation Scheme (NRAS); making paramedicine the 15th registered health profession in Australia. A core element of accreditation is setting professional standards—the most important of which is the profession's code of conduct. This code works to establish a culture that can be disseminated through education and clinical leadership,[12] and makes known the expected standards of professional behaviour and values of the group. The code of conduct relevant to paramedics is the *Code of Conduct*.[13] The purpose of the code is 'to assist and support registered health practitioners to deliver effective regulated health services within an ethical framework'.[14] As a member of the profession it is incumbent upon you to understand this framework and be guided by it—this is a professional obligation.

A distinguishing feature between professionals and non-professionals is the *obligation* on professionals to act with professionalism; key to which is practitioners putting the patient's interests first. This eliminates, in principle, conflicts of interest for professionals between their own interests and those of the patient (or the interests of another party that may conflict with those of the patient). This requirement is not something that the gaining of legal professional status alone will confer; rather, it is established in conjunction with the ethos of professionalism. Indeed, for paramedics as emerging health professionals, their status as professionals (holding expert knowledge and skills, having peer-to-peer governance, and having the power to self-regulate) provides them with an independence that allows, and may at times *requires,* them to judge, criticise or disobey 'employers, patrons and the laws the state'.[15]

Putting a patient's interests ahead of personal and employer interests is an essential aspect of being a professional. Freidson argues that professions, as a powerful and collegial body, can, and should, provide a strong voice in broad policy-making forums, especially in situations where services are not being provided to those who may benefit from them. Townsend points out that an example of this professional advocacy can be seen in the actions of Doctors for Refugees, a group of health professionals who have challenged a government policy that restricted their role as patient advocates at a detention centre. In 2015 the federal government attempted to introduce legislation that would limit the right of health professionals to raise concerns about patients who were refugees. It was, in effect, a provision that would gag healthcare staff from speaking out on the effects of the detention regime on their patients; the provision indicated that speaking up might result in the health professional's employment being terminated for misconduct, or their being imprisoned for up to two years.[16]

Doctors for Refugees prepared a High Court challenge, which argued that the gag provisions breached the constitutional freedom of health professionals to engage in political communication, and to 'determine whether doctors and nurses are allowed to advocate in the interests of their patients'.[17] The healthcare staff at the detention centre argued that they would continue to advocate for their patients 'despite the threats of imprisonment' because they had a professional obligation to do so.[18] Healthcare staff were faced with the prospect of potentially breaking the law to protect their patients, or, alternatively, complying with the law and abrogating their professional obligation to put their patients' interests first.

Not only should professional paramedics put the care of their patients above their own interests, the interests of their government, or those of their employer, they should also put it above the interests of other healthcare professionals. An example from paramedic practice where such patient advocacy is required may be where a paramedic must assess the competency of a patient to determine their treatment and transport choice.[19]

Reconsider the introductory case (entitled 'A competent refusal of care') given at the start of this chapter. In this case, the paramedic is faced with a terminally ill patient who wishes to die at home, even though they may receive some benefit from care in hospital. Clinical practice guidelines include contingencies for situations like these. They allow paramedics to make assessments of both a patient's competence[20] and their clinical needs. If necessary, paramedics can contact another clinical specialist, for example a doctor (an Australian senior medical officer), to ask for further advice. If, however, the doctor advises that the paramedics should transport the patient to the hospital, despite the patient being determined competent and objecting to transportation, then the paramedics could find themselves in breach of their professional responsibilities if they follow the doctor's advice, instead of following the patient's wishes. Potentially they could be committing battery, and thus be engaging in behaviour that is both unethical and unlawful.[21] As independent health professionals, paramedics are required to make an assessment of the action that is in the patient's best interest: a defence of 'just following doctor's orders' will not be available to paramedics with regard to their responsibilities as registered paramedics under the National Law.

Nevertheless, there may be some risk to paramedics who refuse to abide by a doctor's advice; for example, their employer might sanction them for not following employer guidelines. However, the point of having guidelines rather than prescriptive protocols is to allow for practitioner discretion in making treatment decisions. This discretion recognises the paramedic's professional status, and—combined with the imperative under the National Law to act with professionalism (and so in the patient's interest)—can allow paramedics to make a decision that upholds the patient's rights to remain at home. Legally, employees are only required to obey the 'reasonable' direction of an employer. The direction to commit a crime—for example, committing a battery—would not be considered 'reasonable'.[22]

It could be argued that this is simply a situation where strong legal regulation will give the patient the most rights; but the reality is that, in the grainy detail of daily encounters, it is a culture of commitment to ethical values that determines the quality and safety of the care provided. Just as Australian paramedics have not previously been regulated in a nationally standardised way, they also have not had any experience of this form of professional advocacy. It is therefore imperative that paramedics build a solid understanding of their professional, legal and ethical obligations both through education and practice.

Professionalism as ethical practice: codes of conduct

The essence of professionalism regulation is that it requires practitioners to develop not only professional competence, but also professional character, which together create a professional conscience. Freidson called this the 'soul of professionalism'.[23] Professional codes of conduct, and associated policies that embody elements of professionalism, play an important role in establishing, coordinating and making known the expected standards of professional behaviour and values of a group. But what is a code of conduct?

Codes of conduct have been with us for millennia, and are strongly associated with the strictest of laws. One example of such a code from ancient history is the *Code of Hammurabi* (1870 BCE), a legal codification of the laws governing most aspects of life in the Babylonian empire, which were carved in black granite blocks placed as boundary markers. The Byzantine equivalent was the *Code of Justinian* (565 CE), another collection of the civil and criminal laws of the empire.

Although modern professional codes do not have the same imperative force as these old imperial codes, governments and professional groups do see their modern codes as stronger than mere guidelines. Codes, in the modern sense, are a form of conceptual coherence—the attempt to align values and aspirations to virtuous actions. Professional codes in this modern sense attempt to capture a principled and coherent way of life that is core to a professional's very identity: the Japanese samurai code—the way of the warrior—is an excellent example of this sense of a code).[24]

As previously mentioned, the code of conduct relevant to paramedics is the Registered Health Practitioners Code of Conduct. This code was developed by the Paramedicine Board of Australia, a group established under the Health Practitioner Regulation National Law to 'regulate paramedics in Australia under the National Registration and Accreditation Scheme'.[25] The purpose of the Registered Health Practitioners Code of Conduct is 'to assist and support registered health practitioners to deliver effective regulated health services within an ethical framework'.[26] Adhering to this ethical framework is a professional obligation. However, being professional does not merely consist of adhering to such standards. It can go much deeper than mere adherence; some professionals identify with these standards—they are an important part of their self-conception. As Freidson suggests, some professionals 'do not merely exercise a complex skill, but identify themselves with it'.[27]

For some professionals their professional conscience is developed over time, but for others it is the core to their very being. It is 'being, thinking and acting as a professional' and 'knowing what one stands for because knowing what one stands for clarifies … making judgements and decisions and taking responsibility for these judgements and decisions'.[28] This notion of professionalism, as something beyond codes and policies, is likely more related to the notion of professional conscience. Codes of conduct and other behavioural standard-setting documents may be able to be used, in conjunction with other teaching and mentoring, to stimulate the development of health professional character and conscience over time.[29] However, as Faunce argues, that professional ethos (like one's individual character) springs from the accretion of virtues themselves, maintained by the consistent application of altruistically-focused principles.[30]

The Australian health practitioner regulatory system seeks to promote professionalism both as an element of an individual's professional conscience[31] (as shaped by codes, universal ethical norms, policies, professional identity and role, purpose, specialised knowledge and skills), and as legal rules and procedures. The National Law is therefore an example of an 'integrated' professional regulatory system that provides for a coherence between the regulation of the profession's specialised knowledge and skills (and the power that is associated with it), and the profession's conscience and character (as developed by culture and education). All of these elements work together for the public good and in the public's interest—which is the very heart of professionalism.

There is no doubt that healthcare is a complex system that can present health practitioners with numerous legal, ethical and professional dilemmas. In attempting to best deal with these, paramedics should have the benefit of some knowledge that will allow them to better navigate such situations. It is understood that we live in a society that is strongly regulated both morally and legally. Those practising in healthcare delivery are subject to those regulations and are required to comply with them and, as discussed above, to be a professional requires an understanding of the virtues of altruism, empathy, compassion, courage and the keeping of confidences. It is necessary, therefore, for a paramedic to understand what those rules and regulations are, when to weigh them against each other, and how to apply them to their practice.

Why teach law and ethics to paramedics?

The purpose of applying these rules and regulations, both legal and moral, is not just to ensure compliance for the benefit of the paramedic, the profession or the employer—this would be a very crude view. A deeper justification for the teaching of law and ethics reveals itself when we consider why people typically want to become paramedics, because it is largely a virtuous profession. Paramedics demonstrate the virtues of compassion, altruism, self-development, interdisciplinary teamwork and integrity on a daily basis. It is these traits that have led to paramedics being considered the most 'trusted profession', and on which their 'moral contract' with the public is based.

Pellegrino argues that the necessity for teaching clinical ethics exists because health practitioners not only apply clinical science to solve a clinical problem, but will be confronted by, and therefore will be required to solve, ethical problems that will necessitate a reliance on an equally technical process of deliberation to arrive at a morally and legally defensible position.[32]

It is fortunate in some ways that the professionalisation of paramedicine has come after the professionalisation of medicine and nursing, because, although each profession has its own unique body of knowledge, in the broad schema of healthcare delivery there are many elements that are common to many healthcare disciplines. This allows paramedics to build on the work already done by those groups. For example, the Paramedicine Board of Australia has introduced an Interim Code of Conduct for paramedics that is based on the 'Good Medical Practice' Code established first by medicine, because the conduct of healthcare practitioners, regardless of the specialty, shares the same principles.[33]

In this book, you will be exposed to the theories and principles used by other healthcare professionals, not only to recognise and deal with legal and ethical problems encountered in the field, but to 'communicate and justify these decisions to others in a consistent manner'.[34] The professional health practitioner should understand that acting ethically does not just mean helping people or following the law. To be a professional requires a practitioner to not dismiss difficult decision-making by relativising the situation and applying a 'well, as long as you're happy then everything is OK' approach.[35] Being a professional requires the practitioner to be able to approach ethical problems by:

- correctly identifying the underlying ethical problem
- gathering information to properly contextualise the problem
- considering the relevant ethical principles
- considering the relevant professional code of conduct
- considering alternative solutions to the problem
- considering the relevant legal regulations, and
- evaluating possible solutions, making a justified decision, and then reflecting on it.[36]

Further to this, an understanding of the purpose of the law and how and when it applies to paramedic practice is a necessary tool in the health professional's armoury, not only spelling out the practitioner's responsibilities, but also establishing boundaries and expectations that provide safety and support for patients, their families and practitioners.

The approach taken in teaching paramedics about ethics is a mixed one, but in this text it is largely via the use of real and hypothetical cases and a discussion of key concepts and narratives. These methods are used to demonstrate, for example, how knowledge of a relevant code of conduct may help paramedics to first conceive of and then develop the tools to act effectively in ethically and legally challenging situations.[37] Knowledge of ethics, law and a code of conduct provides paramedics with an insight into how these normative value systems intersect.

Although laws are not universalisable, they nevertheless make up an essential component of a professional's knowledge, which enables them to make more informed and justifiable decisions. For example, understanding the legal and ethical concepts of consent allows paramedics to involve patients in their own healthcare decision-making. By empowering patients with the knowledge of the professional, the patient and others gain a number of benefits, including being better able to:

- engage with the process of healthcare decision-making on this occasion and in the future
- manage their own health
- act as a conduit to the community to assist in the dissemination of healthcare information to others, and
- act as an additional 'safety net' for their own and the practitioner's protection against adverse events.[38]

In this way the practitioner is acting ethically and promoting the autonomy of the patient, acting to benefit the patient in both the short term and the long term, and limiting the risk of harm to the patient. It also arguably provides an avenue of justice, in that offering the patient the opportunity to be involved in their healthcare presents them with an opportunity to be involved in decisions regarding, for example, the allocation of healthcare resources.

There are challenges with involving patients in healthcare decision-making in the emergency care setting. It would, however, be inadvisable for paramedics seeking to be recognised as professionals to avoid involving patients. Attempts by paramedics to involve patients (or their surrogate decision-makers) in healthcare decision-making are not only fundamental to applying an ethical standard of practice, but equally essential to applying a legal standard of care.

In the challenging areas of end-of-life decision-making and mental healthcare, the paramedic must be able to identify the moral and legal dilemmas that will inevitably arise, and be equipped with the knowledge and skills to deal most effectively with them in order to promote the best care for the patient. Understanding these issues also empowers the paramedic to contribute to local, national and international discussions on these difficult and contentious issues. These are issues that account for an increasing proportion of the paramedic workload,[39] and, as such, it should be expected that professional paramedics make a significant contribution to such policy debates.

The ultimate purpose of improving decision-making is to increase patient safety. Paramedics can do this by either making 'care' decisions that impact directly on the patient, or making broader, more indirect decisions that ultimately shape policy and regulations that work towards the same end. This latter point is supported by Olick, who argues that professional values can play an important role in 'shaping public policy in the legislature, before the judiciary and in the court of public opinion'.[40]

Conclusion

As members of a profession, it is necessary for paramedics to develop broad professional leadership skills, which include taking part in research to advance knowledge, honing the ability to effectively convey information to a range of audiences, and productively participating in debates and advocacy on professional and general health issues of national and international importance. A solid grounding in law, ethics and professional codes of conduct provides paramedics with the tools and knowledge to present good arguments in those powerful forums—arguments that could reshape the Australian healthcare landscape and assist in the improvement of future patient services.

Review Questions

1   What is one of the traits Flexner identified as being necessary to have in order to be considered a profession?
2   What is a virtue? What virtues do you have? Why are they important?
3   What does it mean to you to be a 'professional'? Does this concur with the definition of a profession?
4   Why is it important to involve patients in healthcare decision-making? Can you think of other benefits not listed here?
5   How do law and ethics intersect with the notion of being a professional?

Endnotes

1 Simpson, J. (ed.) (2012) *Oxford English Dictionary*. Oxford: Oxford University Press. Online. Available: http://oxforddictionaries.com/definition/law (accessed 27 November 2018).

2 Cruess, S.R., Johnston, S. and Cruess, R.L. (2004) Profession: a working definition for medical educators. *Teaching and Learning in Medicine* 16(1), 74–76; Cruess, S.R., Johnston, S. and Cruess, R.L. (2002) Professionalism for medicine: opportunities and obligations. *Medical Journal of Australia 177*, 208–211.

3 Faunce, T. and Gatenby, P. (2005) Flexner's ethical oversight reprised? Contemporary medical education and the health impacts of corporate globalisation. *Medical Education* 39(10), 1066–1074.

4 Flexner, A. (1915) Is social work a profession? *School and Society* 1, 904.

5 General Assembly of the World Medical Association. *Declaration of Geneva*. Online. Available: https://www.wma.net/policies-post/wma-declaration-of-geneva (accessed 27 November 2018).

6 Evetts, J. (2014) The concept of professionalism: professional work, professional practice and learning. In: S. Billett, C. Harteis and H. Gruber (eds), *International Handbook of Research in Professional and Practice-based Learning* (pp. 29–56). Dordrecht, The Netherlands: Springer International.

7 The law is an example of cooperative federalism, and has been copied or adopted with amendments by all of the other states and territories: *Health Practitioner Regulation National Law 2010* (ACT); *Health Practitioner Regulation National Law 2009* (NSW); *Health Practitioner Regulation National Law (National Uniform Legislation) Act 2009* (NT); *Health Practitioner Regulation National Law (South Australia) Act 2010* (SA), sch 2; *Health Practitioner Regulation National Law (Tasmania) 2010* (Tas); *Health Practitioner Regulation National Law 2009* (Vic); *Health Practitioner Regulation National Law 2010* (WA).

8 Stofell, B. (2013) The ethical governance of paramedic practice. In: R. Townsend and M. Luck (eds), *Applied Paramedic Law and Ethics*, 1st ed. (pp. 48–66). Sydney: Elsevier.

9 *Health Practitioner Regulation National Law Act 2009* (Qld), Pt 5.

10 Freidson, E. (2001) *Professionalism: The Third Logic*. Cambridge: Polity Press, at p. 217.

11 Paramedicine Board of Australia. (2018) *Interim Code of Conduct for Registered Health Practitioners*. Melbourne: Australian Health Practitioner Regulation Agency. Online. Available: https://www.paramedicineboard.gov.au/professional-standards/codes-guidelines-and-policies/code-of-conduct.aspx (accessed 3 December 2018).

12 First, S., Tomlins, L. and Swinburn, A. (2012) From trade to profession—the professionalisation of the paramedic workforce. *Journal of Paramedic Practice* 4(7), 378–381.

13 Paramedicine Board of Australia, *Interim Code of Conduct for Registered Health Practitioners*.

14 Ibid.

15 Freidson, E. (2001) *Professionalism*, at p. 221.

16 Townsend, R. (2017) The role of the law in the professionalisation of paramedicine in Australia. (PhD thesis, Canberra, Australian National University). *Border Force Act 2015* (Cth), s 42.

17 NSW Nurses and Midwives Association. (2015, 5 December) Brave stand leads to back down on *Border Force Act*. Online. Available: http://www.nswnma.asn.au/brave-stand-leads-to-back-down-on-border-force-act/ (accessed 27 November 2018).

18 Various (2015, 30 June) Open letter regarding the *Border Force Act 2015*. *The Guardian*. Online. Available: <https://www.theguardian.com/australia-news/2015/jul/01/open-letter-on-the-border-force-act-we-challenge-the-department-to-prosecute> (accessed 14 February 2019).

19 Townsend, R. (2017) The role of the law in the professionalisation of paramedicine in Australia.

20 *In Re C (Adult: Refusal of Treatment)* [1994] 1 WLR 290.

21 *Rogers v Whitaker* (1992) 175 CLR 479, Mason CJ at [14]: 'except in cases of emergency or necessity, all medical treatment is preceded by the patient's choice to undergo it'; and on necessity, *In Re F* [1990] 2

AC 1 found: 'officious intervention cannot be justified by the principle of necessity. So intervention cannot be justified when … it is contrary to the known wishes of the assisted person, to the extent that he is capable of rationally forming such a wish.' Beauchamp T.L. and Childress, J.F. (2103) *Principles of Biomedical Ethics,* 7th ed. New York: Oxford University Press.

22   Eburn, M. (2017, 16 August) Ambulance transport against patient's will. *Australian Emergency Law.* Online. Available: https://emergencylaw.wordpress.com/2017/08/16/ambulance-transport-against-patients-will/ (accessed 28 November 2018).

23   Freidson, *Professionalism,* at p. 217.

24   Daidōji, Y. and Sadler, A.L. (1988) *The Code of the Samurai.* Rutland, Vt: C.E. Tuttle.

25   Paramedicine Board of Australia. (2018) About [the Paramedicine Board of Australia]. Online. Available: https://www.paramedicineboard.gov.au/About.aspx (accessed 3 December 2018).

26   Paramedicine Board of Australia. (2018) *Professional capabilities for registered paramedics.* Online. Available: https://www.paramedicineboard.gov.au/professional-standards/professional-capabilities-for-registered-paramedics.aspx (accessed 3 February 2019).

27   Freidson, E. (1994) *Professionalism Reborn: Theory, Prophecy and Policy.* Cambridge: Polity Press, at p. 200.

28   Trede F. and McEwen, C. (2012) Developing a critical professional identity. In: J. Higgs, R. Barnett, S. Billett et al. (eds), *Practice-based Education: Perspectives and Strategies* (pp. 27–40). Rotterdam: SensePublishers, at p. 27.

29   Faunce, T. (2007) *Who Owns Our Health?* Sydney: UNSW Press, at p. 244; First, et al., From trade to profession, at p. 378.

30   Faunce, ibid., at p. 244.

31   As distinct from personal conscience, often referred to as 'individual morals'.

32   Pellegrino, E.D. (1989) Teaching medical ethics: some persistent questions and some responses. *Academic Medicine* 64, 701–703.

33   Paramedicine Board of Australia, *Interim Code of Conduct.*

34   Luck, M. (2013) An introduction to ethics for paramedics. In: R. Townsend and M. Luck (eds), *Applied Paramedic Law and Ethics,* 2nd ed. (pp. 8–32). Sydney: Elsevier, at p. 9.

35   Olick, R.S. (2001) It's ethical, but is it legal? Teaching ethics and law in the medical school curriculum. *Anatomical Record* 265(1), 5–9.

36   Luck, M., Steer, B. and Townsend, R. (2013) PRECARE—an ethical decision-making model for paramedics. In: R. Townsend and M. Luck (eds), *Applied Paramedic Law and Ethics,* 2nd ed. (pp. 37–51). Sydney: Elsevier, at p. 37.

37   Stofell, The ethical governance of paramedic practice, at p. 48.

38   This final point is particularly relevant to the area of medication administration. See Leape, L., Bates, D.W., Cullen, D.J. et al. (1995) Systems analysis of adverse drug events. ADE Prevention Study Group. *Journal of the American Medical Association* 274(1), 35–43.

39   Roberts, L. and Henderson, J. (2009) Paramedic perceptions of their role, education, training and working relationships when attending cases of mental illness. *Journal of Emergency Primary Health Care* 7(3), 1–16.

40   Olick, It's ethical, but is it legal?, at p. 9.

Chapter 2
Paramedic ethics

Morgan Luck

Learning objectives

After reading this chapter, you should be able to:

- give a broad account of ethics
- dispel some common misunderstandings regarding ethics
- give an account of three major ethical theories
- offer some objections to each of the major ethical theories
- give an account of the four principles of bioethics
- apply the four principles of bioethics to an ethical case.

Definitions

Consequentialist ethics The view that holds that an action is ethical if, as a consequence of the action, the maximum overall amount of good results (e.g. happiness).

Deontological ethics The view that holds that an action is ethical if it is guided by a set of universal moral rules.

Virtue ethics The view that holds that an action is ethical if it is motivated by virtue.

Also outlined is a method of determining the ethical course of action that is widely used within the healthcare profession today—a method known as the 'four principles of bioethics':

The four principles of bioethics The view that holds that an action is ethical if it is the action that best upholds the principles of autonomy, non-maleficence, beneficence and justice.

An introductory case

Multiple patient overdose

A paramedic is called to the scene of a New Year's Eve party where a multiple patient overdose is suspected to have taken place. On arriving at the scene, the paramedic discovers four people unconscious and suffering respiratory depression, indicating a potentially life-threatening overdose. The paramedic is told that they collapsed after trying a new party drug, which is quickly determined to be an opiate. Because it is New Year's Eve, emergency services are stretched and back-up may not arrive in time.

The paramedic might normally administer the drug naloxone in these circumstances. Typically, a paramedic would only carry two doses of naloxone. One full dose would be needed to properly treat one person suffering from a narcotic overdose. Half a dose may have a beneficial effect on a single patient, but may not be enough to successfully counter the respiratory depression.

This chapter will introduce you to some of the tools used, not simply to make ethical judgements about what a paramedic should do in cases such as this one, but to communicate and justify these decisions to others in a consistent manner.

Introduction

It is common to hear people say things such as 'Rob is a good person', 'Abortion is wrong' or 'The decision to fire the foreman was immoral.' It is also common to hear people justify such judgements by offering reasons. For example, someone might say, 'Rob is a good person *because* he does lots of voluntary work', 'Abortion is wrong *because* it is the same as murder' or 'The decision to fire the foreman was immoral *because* he did nothing wrong.' In each case, a justification for an ethical judgement is being offered. The aim of this chapter is to introduce some of the main tools used not simply to make ethical judgements, but to communicate and justify these decisions to others in a consistent manner.

It is also worth noting that the Paramedic Professional Competency Standards (version 2) clearly state that paramedics must practise 'within the legal and ethical boundaries of their profession'.[1] This chapter hopes to introduce ethics to help paramedics see these ethical boundaries and operate as professionals in their field.

However, before we proceed it is useful to consider the notion of an ethical decision more broadly.

What is ethics? And what isn't it?

Ethics is the study of what it means for something to be morally right or wrong. In other words, it is the study of what you 'ought' to do. Here we do not mean what you *legally* ought to do, but what you should do in order to be a moral person. This may seem like a perfectly straightforward area of enquiry; however, it often gives rise to a number of misunderstandings. In this section, we will address the following common *misunderstandings*:

- Acting ethically just means helping people.
- Acting ethically just means following the law.
- Acting ethically is only something to worry about in difficult cases.
- Acting ethically is about avoiding moral dilemmas.
- Acting ethically is relative.

We shall examine each of these misunderstandings, and work to resolve the confusion.

Misunderstanding: 'Acting ethically just means helping people'

Some people might think that, so long as they are helping other people, they are acting ethically. However, such a simplistic view does not bear up under close scrutiny. To demonstrate this, consider Case 2.1.

Case 2.1 The embarrassed paramedic

A paramedic arrives on scene to find a 50-year-old male patient having severe chest pains. The paramedic determines that a glyceryl trinitrate (GTN) spray should be used to lower the patient's blood pressure and reduce the strain on his heart.

However, before administering this drug, the paramedic realises that she should ask the patient whether he has taken any erectile dysfunction drugs (such as Viagra) in the previous 24 hours; if he has, the GTN spray may drop his blood pressure to a dangerously low level.

The paramedic decides not to enquire, as she is embarrassed to ask. By chance, it turns out that the patient had not taken erectile dysfunction drugs, so the administration of the GTN spray did, indeed, help the patient recover from the chest pains.

Here we can see that, although the paramedic performed an action that helped the patient, we would not want to say that she acted ethically. In fact, it seems likely that she acted unethically, as she potentially endangered the patient's life simply because she did not want to endure the embarrassment of asking about the possible use of an erectile dysfunction drug.

This example demonstrates that, in some situations, our intuitions about what constitutes an ethical decision are more closely linked with people's motivations or reasons for performing the actions they do, rather than the actions themselves. In other words, to act ethically as a paramedic, it is not enough to incidentally help the patient; you must also act with the patient's best interests at heart. Studying ethics helps to further an awareness of your own reasons for action, or motivations. Such awareness should in turn assist you in determining whether you are acting with the patient's best interests at heart.

Misunderstanding: 'Acting ethically just means following the law'

Some people fall into the trap of thinking that, so long as they do not break the law, their actions will be ethical. As Kenneth De Ville points out:

> When ethical issues arise in emergency medicine, they frequently entail legal issues. The commonest and often the first question asked by physicians in an ethical dilemma is: 'What does the law say?' If that question is answered (and it cannot always be), they are many times content to end the analysis there. Adhering to the law does not guarantee a morally correct outcome, however.[2]

To illustrate this point, consider Case 2.2, provided by Derse.[3]

Although Derse reports that it was lawful for the emergency staff not to retrieve the patient, it is less clear whether such an action was ethical. We can often be sure of the legality of an action, while being unsure of its ethical status (and vice versa), and this points to the fact that the two notions *can* be distinct. In other words, what is ethical might not be legal, and what is legal might not be ethical.

Case 2.2 The death of Christopher Sercye

On May 16, 1998, an event occurred that outraged many and presented an emergency department's physicians and nurses with an ethical and legal dilemma. Christopher Sercye, a 15-year-old boy, was shot and wounded. His friends carried him to within 50 feet of Chicago's Ravenswood Hospital, put him down, and left. Hospital staff saw Christopher lying there but did not go out to help him because hospital policy did not allow staff to leave the hospital premises to render emergency care. Should the doctors and nurses have violated hospital policy and left the patients for whom they were caring to assist this injured boy?

The policy was crafted to prevent hospital liability for actions taken by staff off the premises, as well as to circumscribe the duties of the hospital's personnel. The policy was also designed to protect personnel from injury. Violation of hospital policy was grounds for reprimand or dismissal. Ravenswood was not a Level 1 trauma center, so that if its doctors and nurses intervened before paramedics arrived, they might have delayed the process of getting the patient to an appropriate level of care. It was also possible that the victim's assailants would return and put staff at risk. After a frustrated police officer finally commandeered a wheelchair and brought the boy in by himself, it was too late. The boy died of a gunshot wound to the aorta. In retrospect, immediate action might have saved his life.

Although public outrage was considerable, the hospital personnel had done nothing illegal. They violated no laws by waiting until the patient was brought to the emergency department (ED).[4]

Another example, which will be expanded on in Chapter 9, concerns frisking. Paramedics have the legal right to frisk some patients. However, this legal right does not necessarily constitute an ethical right. A patient's right to bodily autonomy—the right to self-govern one's own body—must be weighed against the legal right a paramedic has to frisk a patient. And sometimes the moral weight of a patient's autonomy will outweigh other concerns.

Of course, what is legal and what is ethical often overlap, and indeed this is no coincidence, for the two domains are closely linked. For example, the principle of justice motivates both legal reform and many of our own ethical intuitions. In addition, since it is often difficult to determine the correct ethical course of action (especially in emergencies), it is entirely prudent to defer to the law in many cases. However, as De Ville quite rightly states:

> Medical professionals must recognize the limited goals and insights of the law and legal thought. As a rule, legal standards are unreliable guides to ethical conduct and should never be allowed to substitute for, or dominate, ethical analysis.[5]

In addition, paramedics who rely too heavily on the law run the risk of developing what Megan-Jane Johnstone refers to as moral blindness, as 'someone who, upon encountering a moral problem, simply does not see it as a moral problem. Instead, they may perceive it as either a clinical or a technical problem'.[6] The danger here is that a paramedic whose actions are primarily being guided by legal, technical or clinical concerns may gradually become insensitive to ethical considerations.

What is more, even if people believed that by following the letter of the law their actions were guaranteed to be ethical, they would still have to have an independent sense of what is ethical before they could know this to be true.

To sum up, although law is an invaluable means of determining the correct course of action, this should not be to the exclusion of ethical considerations. As professionals, paramedics are obliged to develop both their legal and their ethical compasses, and apply them together to the situations they encounter.

Misunderstanding: 'Acting ethically is only something to worry about in difficult cases'

Some people make the mistake of thinking that ethical considerations only come into play when they are faced with a difficult decision. For example, consider Case 2.3.

In this case ethical questions seem to abound, such as 'Is it ethical to let someone die if it is in your power to save them?' and 'Is it ethical to save someone if they wish to be left to die?' Yet ethical considerations do not just come into play when decision-making becomes hard. For example, consider a much easier case (Case 2.4).

It may seem obvious that the paramedic should not stop for a burger. But this is not simply because it is the paramedic's job to respond as quickly as possible to an emergency. It is also because stopping for this reason while lives are at risk would be unethical.

In short, ethical considerations do not pop up only when hard decisions need to be made. Rather, they are ever-present. In order to cultivate a consistent professional attitude,

Case 2.3 'Do Not Resuscitate' tattoo

A paramedic is called to the scene of a suspected heart attack. On arriving at the scene, it is determined that the patient, an 88-year-old man, is unconscious and not breathing.

While preparing to resuscitate the patient, the paramedic discovers the words 'Do not resuscitate' tattooed on the patient's chest.

Case 2.4 Burger stop

A paramedic is called to the scene of a car crash. However, she is a little hungry and there is a fast-food restaurant en route to the crash where she can stop to get a burger.

Case 2.5 Jehovah's Witness car crash

An intensive care paramedic arrives on the scene of a car crash to find a patient conscious but severely haemorrhaging. After slowing the bleeding and providing the patient with a saline solution, the patient's blood pressure continues to drop, and she becomes unconscious. The paramedic is worried that the patient may die before reaching the hospital.

One promising course of action open to the paramedic is to administer packed red blood cells, which should help stabilise the patient.

However, the patient informed the paramedic before falling unconscious that she is a Jehovah's Witness and did not want to be given a blood transfusion.

you should not *choose* to think ethically in particular situations, but instead consider the ethical dimension in all instances of professional decision-making.

Misunderstanding: 'Acting ethically is about avoiding moral dilemmas'

In this instance, the misunderstanding is less about what constitutes ethical thinking and more about how best to develop a stronger ethical foundation. Throughout this book a variety of ethical cases will be introduced, some of which will appear to entail dilemmas. It can be said that a case involves a dilemma if, in responding to the case, you are faced with making a choice between equally unfavourable options. For example, consider Case 2.5.

This case may entail a dilemma, as the paramedic is forced to choose between letting the patient die of blood loss or disregarding her religious beliefs. When faced with such a dilemma, there are three ways paramedics might generally respond: they might ignore the dilemma, avoid it or resolve it. Let us examine all three responses.

A paramedic ignores a dilemma by not taking the ethical aspects of the case seriously, or even by being completely blind to them. Such a paramedic would respond to dilemmas in a mechanical and unconsidered manner, typically by considering only the law. This type of response is not consistent with best practice, as paramedics should not be guided solely by legal, technical or clinical concerns, but also by the ethical issues at play. A case in point here is the Nuremberg defence; a defence famously used by Nazi war criminals during the Nuremberg Trials: 'I was only following orders.' Although this is a rather extreme example, history has taught us that we should never turn off our own moral compass and just mechanically do what we are told. However, although it is bad to ignore dilemmas in this fashion, it is perfectly acceptable to attempt to avoid them.

A dilemma is avoided when you attempt to find a way out of the situation without taking either of the hard options. For example, when considering the ethical course of action in Case 2.5 (the Jehovah's Witness car crash case), you might think to yourself, 'I would use a non-human blood substitute to treat the patient, as this substitute is approved by their religion.' This course of action, if available, avoids the dilemma, as it allows the paramedic to both save the patient and respect her religious commitments. This type of avoidance is good, and is obviously preferable when you are in the field. However, while it is good to avoid dilemmas in this way, you will not be able to do so in all cases. It is therefore important that paramedics also consider how to resolve, rather than avoid, ethical dilemmas.

Paramedics resolve a dilemma when they consider the ethical problems and legal issues involved in the case and, after due consideration, choose one of the hard options posed by the dilemma. Often these ethical problems are best highlighted by questions, which in the case of the Jehovah's Witness car crash case might be:

- Do patients have the right to refuse treatment?
- Is it ever ethical to let someone die when you are able to save them?

Identifying and thinking about these central ethical problems should help you to form justifiable reasons for action. (Chapter 3 will involve picking out such ethical problems from case studies.) It is by taking a stance on these issues and acting in line with your convictions that you will resolve the dilemma. For example, if after due consideration the paramedic decided that the Jehovah's Witness does have the right to refuse treatment, and as a result does not administer the packed red blood cells, this would be an example of a paramedic attempting to resolve the dilemma.

When *studying* ethics you should resist the temptation to always avoid dilemmas rather than resolve them. Although avoiding a dilemma is desirable in the field, you will learn little about difficult ethical cases, and how to resolve them, if you are constantly thinking of ways to avoid them. While *studying* ethics it is therefore better—even if you know of an ingenious way to avoid the dilemma (which is preferable in practice)—to embrace the underlying problem that each case is designed to highlight.

In short, even though it is best to avoid dilemmas when you can in practice, in many cases this will not be possible, and in such cases acting ethically will require you to take a stand on quite hard issues. In order to strengthen your ability to do this, you should take the opportunity to resolve, rather than avoid, the ethical dilemmas presented in this book.

Misunderstanding: 'Acting ethically is relative'

It is common to hear people say, 'Beauty is in the eye of the beholder', the thought being that it is legitimate for two people to look at the same thing, such as a painting, and one of them think it is beautiful and the other think it is not. Some people think ethics is like beauty in this respect. In other words, whether or not an action is ethical depends on who you ask—it is relative to individuals. We can call this *individual relativism*. A related position is *cultural relativism*, where ethical standards are taken to be relative to cultures rather than individuals. Both individual and cultural relativism are types of *ethical relativism*. Ethical relativists, as Shafer-Landau explains, believe that something is ethical simply:

> … because a person, or a society, is deeply committed to it. That means that the standards that are appropriate for some people may not be appropriate for others. There are no objective, universal moral principles that form an eternal blueprint to guide us through life. Morality is a 'human construct'—we make it up, and like the law, or like standards of taste, there is no uniquely correct set of rules to follow.[7]

To help illustrate ethical relativism, consider Case 2.6.

Most paramedics in our culture would be inclined to believe female genital mutilation is unethical. However, if they were a cultural relativist they would have to concede that this procedure *is* ethical relative to a culture where it is permitted.

Some people find ethical relativism attractive because it seems quite a tolerant position to take. For example, rather than saying 'Abortion is wrong and that's that', relativists

---

Case 2.6 The tribal procedure

A paramedic decides to volunteer her services to an overseas aid program, transporting patients from various remote African communities to a medical centre.

One day the paramedic is asked to transport a young girl to the centre to undergo an operation resulting in female genital mutilation. The girl herself tells the paramedic that she doesn't want to undergo the procedure.

Shocked by this request, the paramedic radios the centre en route to find out more about the procedure. She discovers that the procedure is not illegal here, that it is one of the culture's oldest traditions, and that in this culture the daughter has no say in whether or not the procedure should be carried out.

would be more inclined to say 'Although abortion is unethical relative to my culture, I appreciate that it is ethical relative to yours.' However, being tolerant in this manner has its drawbacks. For example, the relativist will be committed to saying: 'Although the attempted genocide of the Jews by the Nazis was unethical relative to the Jews, it was ethical relative to the Nazis.' Note the relativist is not simply pointing out that the Nazis *believed* that their actions were ethical, but rather that the Holocaust *was* ethical relative to the Nazis. In other words, there is a very real sense in which the Holocaust was *actually* ethical. To many people this conclusion would be quite unacceptable.

It may seem to follow from ethical relativism that it is wrong for one group to impose their ethical standards on another. And, again, this seems like quite a tolerant position to take in a multicultural society. However, if this is the case, ethical relativists cannot attempt to stop one group from imposing their ethical standards on another. This is because, if they did, they would be imposing their *own* ethical standards onto another group. Therefore, this type of tolerance is, in this limited respect, impotent. For example, I may think it is wrong for religious groups to indoctrinate children because no person should impose their beliefs on another. However, if I step in and stop this from happening, I am imposing my belief that indoctrination in this religious group is wrong.

Many people are drawn to ethical relativism because of the realisation that different cultures and individuals do in fact have different ethical standards. This understanding has led some to mount the following argument, as captured by Rachels and Rachels:

1 Different cultures have different moral codes.
2 Therefore, there is no objective 'truth' in morality. Right and wrong are only matters of opinion, and opinions vary from culture to culture.[8]

Putting aside the fact that there are also considerable similarities between the ethical standards of different cultures, it does not follow from there being disagreement about what is ethical that there is no fact of the matter. For example, if during a primary-school maths quiz one student claims $5 + 3 = 8$, and another claims $5 + 3 = 9$, this should not lead us to conclude that there is no fact of the matter.

Some relativists may disagree with this analogy, for in the maths quiz example there is a maths teacher who is acknowledged as an authority. Ethics, the relativist may argue, is not like this—there is no agreement on who has the final say. This point is often underlined by posing the question: 'Who are you to say what is right or wrong?' However, even if there is no single person or method that can definitely tell us what is, or is not, ethical, should we really conclude that there is no fact of the matter? For example, there is presently no authority figure who can tell me exactly where my cat went last night. But should I really conclude there is no fact of the matter? Surely not.

Some may worry that the rejection of ethical relativism, and the adoption of ethical objectivism, will permit people to be intolerant of different ethical beliefs. In response to this, note first of all that sometimes intolerance is appropriate: if I am in a position to stop a rape, then I should do so, even if the attempted rapist thinks that there is nothing wrong with what he is doing. Setting aside cases like this, it may still be of concern that ethical objectivism might permit an *inappropriate* intolerance of different ethical beliefs. But this need not be the case. Here are a few reasons why.

First, just because someone believes in an objective ethical standard, this does not mean they know what the standard is. There may still be good reason to be humble and remain open to alternative ideas and approaches, for such alternatives may turn out to be objectively correct. For example, if someone believes that abortion is wrong but does not *know* that it is wrong, then that is good reason for them to tolerate people who believe otherwise.

Second, even if we know we are right, it may be that we are ethically required to be tolerant of people with different beliefs. If so, then we are not permitted to be intolerant (even if we know we are right). For example, even if we know it is wrong to shout at our own children, it may still be wrong to interfere with parents who choose to shout at theirs.

Lastly, there is nothing stopping ethical relativism from also permitting intolerance. For a relativist might say, 'I know that being tolerant is ethical relative to your culture, but relative to my culture it is ethical to be intolerant.' And, indeed, there are examples of this. Consider the following quote by the founder of the Italian National Fascist Party, Benito Mussolini:

> Everything I have said and done in these last years is relativism, by intuition. From the fact that all ideologies are of equal value, that all ideologies are mere fictions, the modern relativist infers that everybody has the right to create for himself his own ideology, and to attempt to enforce it with all the energy of which he is capable. If relativism signifies contempt for fixed categories, and men who claim to be the bearers of an objective immortal truth, then there is nothing more relativistic than fascism.[9]

In short, a paramedic who rejects ethical relativism is no more in danger of becoming intolerant of other ethical beliefs than a paramedic who does not.

So you should not conclude that there is no objective ethical standard because (a) there is disagreement about what is ethical or (b) there is no single ethical authority. This does not mean that there is no good argument for relativism—just that these two arguments are not among them. In addition, ethical relativists seem committed to claiming that atrocities such as the Holocaust are actually *ethical*, in a particular sense. Now it may turn out that this is right, but it would be very surprising. So, in the absence of better arguments for ethical relativism, we should be wary of it. And lastly, just because someone rejects ethical relativism does not mean that they are permitted to be intolerant of different ethical beliefs.

The three main ethical theories

Now that we have considered some misunderstandings about ethical decision-making, let us turn our attention to the different ethical theories by which such decisions are often justified. An ethical theory, broadly speaking, is any systematic attempt to classify actions as either morally right or morally wrong, in an objective sense. That is, it is a theory about what makes something ethical.

The three most influential ethical theories are consequentialist ethics, deontological ethics and virtue ethics. In this section we shall provide a brief introduction to each of these ethical theories, and look at some objections often levelled against each of them.

Case 2.7 Multiple patient overdose

A paramedic is called to the scene of a New Year's Eve party where a multiple patient overdose is suspected to have taken place. On arriving at the scene, the paramedic discovers four people unconscious and suffering respiratory depression (indicating a potentially life-threatening overdose). The paramedic is told that they collapsed after trying a new party drug, which is quickly determined to be an opiate. Because it is New Year's Eve, emergency services are stretched and back-up may not arrive in time.

The paramedic might normally administer the drug naloxone in these circumstances. Typically, a paramedic would only carry two doses of naloxone. One full dose would be needed to properly treat one person suffering from a narcotic overdose. Half a dose may have a beneficial effect on a single patient, but may not be enough to successfully counter the respiratory depression.

Consequentialist ethics

Consequentialists believe that you should always try to perform the action that is likely to lead to the best possible consequences. The emphasis here is on the consequences of the action, rather than the action itself.

To illustrate this theory, consider the multiple patient overdose in Case 2.7.

Paramedics influenced by consequentialist ethics might choose to administer a full dose to just two patients, rather than four half-doses to all four patients, if they felt that the half-doses would probably not be enough to save anyone's life. This is because, all things being equal, the high likelihood of saving two lives might seem to be a better outcome than probably not saving anyone's life.

This view may seem almost too obvious to be a useful theory. You may wonder how it could be possible for an action to be ethical if it did not result in the best consequences. However, this theory is not at all as self-evident as it first seems. This is because without defining what the 'best' is, it can be quite difficult to determine what is ethical.

Some people believe that the best outcome is the outcome that produces the most happiness. This view is known as *hedonism*. According to hedonism, in order to make an ethical choice you must determine which option will cause the most happiness. For example, in the case of the multiple patient overdose, probably saving two lives (rather than probably not saving anyone's life) seems like the better option, because, all things being equal, the more lives saved the happier people will be. This is the type of justification that a consequentialist would offer for this decision. We might refer to this type of consequentialism as *hedonistic consequentialism*; and although there are many other types of consequentialism, such as *preference consequentialism* (where an action is ethical if it maximally satisfies people's preferences), we shall focus on hedonistic consequentialism for the sake of simplicity.

We understand consequentialism as follows:

Consequentialist ethics The view that holds that an action is ethical if, as a consequence of the action, the maximum overall amount of good results (e.g. happiness).

Note that consequentialist ethics is sometimes also referred to as *utilitarianism* or *teleological ethics*.

Despite this theory often delivering intuitively correct results, there are objections to its wholesale adoption.

Objection: does consequentialist ethics demand too much from us?

On first glance, the idea that an ethical action is an action that causes the most happiness might seem uncontroversial—however, it is in fact deeply radical. To understand why, consider Case 2.8.

Commonsense morality (what most people intuitively consider to be moral) says that giving money to charity is admirable—that it is the kind of thing that good people do. However, commonsense morality does not say that giving to charity is morally obligatory. Yet consequentialist ethics does suggest that we act unethically every time we do not donate our lunch money. This is because saving lives usually causes more happiness than having lunch. So our ethical obligations, according to consequentialist ethics, are far more demanding than we normally take them to be.

Consequentialist ethics not only demands that we give up our money, but it also demands we be impartial in our efforts to maximise happiness, in a manner not usually expected of us (see Case 2.9).

Commonsense morality says that we have special obligations to our friends and family. Therefore, it might suggest that we would not act wrongly in saving our own child, even when we could have saved two strangers instead. Again, consequentialist ethics disagrees. Given that we would produce an outcome that is twice as happy, all things being equal, by saving two children rather than one, consequentialist ethics implies that we are obligated to save two. If we save only one child (even if it is our own), we act wrongly.

Objection: should we always try to maximise happiness?

In some situations, maximising happiness does not seem quite fair. To illustrate this point, consider Case 2.10.

Case 2.8 Medical treatments in Ethiopia

In the hospital cafeteria there is a donation box for a charity organisation that helps to pay for medical treatments for children in Ethiopia.

Every day a paramedic brings $5 to work to pay for lunch. It is true that if the paramedic went without lunch every day he would be very hungry by dinner-time. However, it is also true that if the paramedic gave $5 to this charity every day, the money would help to save lives.

Case 2.9 The blood relative

A paramedic arrives on the scene of a road accident. A truck has hit a school bus and three children are in a critical condition.

If they are left untreated, all three children have only around 20 minutes to live. The first child can be stabilised in about 10 minutes. So, too, can the second child. However, the third child will take 15 minutes to stabilise.

To the paramedic's horror, she also discovers that the third child is her own.

Case 2.10 The sporting celebrity

A paramedic arrives at the scene of a car crash, where she finds three patients in a critical condition and in equal need of immediate attention.

The paramedic recognises that one of the patients is a popular sporting celebrity. The two other patients are an unknown man and an unknown 10-year-old child.

The paramedic is unable to stabilise more than one person, and back-up is too far away to be of help.

In this case there is a very strong possibility that thousands of people will become unhappy if the sporting celebrity were to die. The same cannot be definitely said of the unknown man and the 10-year-old child. Therefore, in this case consequentialism would suggest we save the celebrity, for by doing so we maximise happiness.

Choosing to save the celebrity's life in this case, just because she is popular, may for many people seem unfair. The thought is that popularity should not be playing such a major role in determining who lives and who dies. Yet under consequentialist ethics this is what seems to result. In fact, even if the choice were between the celebrity's life and 10 unknown people, consequentialist ethics would still suggest we save the celebrity, providing this would ultimately cause more happiness.

Consequentialist ethics asserts that whether or not an action is ethical depends on the consequences of the action. However, some believe that there are certain actions that are always unethical, regardless of their consequences. This is because these people take moral rules, rather than human happiness, to be the most important factor in determining what is ethical. It is this view that is upheld by our next ethical theory—deontological ethics.

Case 2.11 The charitable patient

A paramedic is en route to the hospital with a patient suffering from a narcotic overdose. With the real threat of death playing on the patient's mind, he thrusts a large sum of money into the paramedic's lap.

The patient informs the paramedic that he was going to spend this money on illegal drugs, but would now like the paramedic to donate this money to a hospital charity instead.

Before reaching the hospital the patient makes a partial recovery, and, on feeling somewhat better, requests the money be returned to him.

Deontological ethics

According to deontologists, an ethical action is not determined by its consequences. Rather, an ethical action is one that is guided by moral rules.

To illustrate this approach, consider the charitable patient in Case 2.11. A paramedic influenced by deontological ethics would return the money if they believed that there was a fundamental moral rule that stated: 'Paramedics should not accept money from patients—especially if they are in a vulnerable state of mind, such as under the influence of drugs, or believing they are facing death.' However, bear in mind that far less happiness is likely to result from giving back the money. That is, the hospital charity will not receive the money, and the patient who has just suffered a drug overdose will then probably use the money to buy further drugs. However, despite the fact that returning the money may make the world a less happy place, according to deontological ethics this may be the right thing to do. This is because deontological ethics is about following moral rules, or principles, rather than weighing up the happiness of possible outcomes.

Compared to consequentialist ethics, deontological ethics may appear simpler. This is because, rather than considering what actions are likely to result in what consequences and calculating how much happiness will result, deontological ethics requires only that a set of rules be upheld. However, it can often be hard to determine exactly what these rules are.

Many people think moral rules arise from human rights and duties. A right is something we have a moral entitlement to. For every right there is usually a corresponding duty. So, for example, if you have the right not to be murdered, then everyone else has the corresponding duty not to murder you—and from this duty the moral rule 'Do not murder' could be established.

Rights are generally considered to be universal. In other words, they apply to everyone at all times. For example, if we have a right to free healthcare, then it would always be unethical for anyone to deny another such care. Note, however, that although everyone may have rights, their corresponding duties need not concern everyone. Take, for example, the right to patient–doctor confidentiality. Although this right applies to everyone, the duty to uphold such confidentiality concerns only doctors.

Although the notion of rights seems straightforward, there is some disagreement over why people have them.

Some believe that certain rights have been established by God. Within Christianity and Judaism, an example of such rights can be found with the Ten Commandments. For instance, the commandment 'Thou shall not murder' describes our duty not to murder, which in turn reflects our right not to be murdered. Others believe that rights follow from those rules that, if followed by everyone, best ensure we can live together in a civil manner. An example of such a set of rules might be the Universal Declaration of Human Rights.

For our purposes, we shall define deontological ethics as follows:

Deontological ethics The view that holds that an action is ethical if it is guided by a set of universal moral rules.

Note that deontological ethics is sometimes also referred to as *Kantianism* (after one of the major proponents of the view—Immanuel Kant), *duty theory* or *right-based ethics*.

Although many of our ethical decisions seem guided by such moral rules, this theory is not without its critics.

Objection: is deontological ethics too rigid?

One seemingly good point about deontological ethics is that people influenced by this theory should always act consistently. That is, if they always follow the same set of rules, they should always perform the same actions under the same circumstances. Yet where some see consistency, others see problematic rigidness; for example, consider Case 2.12.

Let us imagine that the paramedic is influenced by deontological ethics and believes there is a moral rule that states: 'All patients have the right not to have their medical

Case 2.12 The STD cheater

A paramedic is at the scene of an assault outside a nightclub, bandaging the assailant's fist. The assailant claims that he hit his partner in self-defence. He reports that she flew into a rage after he told her that he was sleeping with another woman. The police have advised the paramedic that no one is pressing charges and the man is free to leave.

In his drunken state, the patient reveals that he has just been diagnosed with a mild and treatable sexually transmitted disease (STD). He is aware of the risks associated with engaging in risky sexual activity; however, he does not intend to abstain from unprotected sex with the numerous partners he has, nor inform them of his condition.

After the paramedic has finished bandaging the man, one of the man's (allegedly many) partners arrives to take him home.

information disclosed to others'; that is to say, patients have the right to privacy. (Such a right may seem appropriate, for if people believed that paramedics might tell others about their medical condition, they might not be comfortable divulging important information to them in more critical situations.)

However, imagine now that, instead of a mild and treatable sexually transmitted disease (STD), the patient reveals he was diagnosed with human immunodeficiency virus (HIV), and he also tells the paramedic that he has over 20 regular sexual partners. Under these conditions, should the paramedic still uphold the patient's moral right to privacy? According to deontological ethics, if there is a moral rule that states that you should not disclose medical information to others, it may never be ethical to do so, no matter what the consequences.

Alternatively, what if the paramedic also holds a rule that states: 'One should protect people from unnecessary harm as much as possible'? It seems that this rule might be in conflict with the earlier rule concerning privacy. For if the paramedic does not break the privacy rule, the rule about protecting people from harm will end up being broken, and vice versa. What is needed are further rules to tell us what to do when such rules conflict.

To many people it seems almost impossible to determine all the moral roles that might guide our behaviour. This has led some to think that, rather than focusing on rules or consequences, perhaps the best ethical compass we have is our own virtue. This is the underlying idea behind the final ethical theory we will be introducing—virtue ethics.

Virtue ethics

According to virtue ethics, an ethical action is not determined by the consequences of the action or whether it is guided by a particular rule. Rather, what is ethical about an action is determined by whether it is guided by a person's virtue. To illustrate this theory, consider Case 2.13.

According to virtue ethics, the paramedic in this case has not acted ethically. This is because his actions were not guided by a virtue, such as sympathy or compassion for the patient, but rather by a vice, in this case lust.

According to virtue ethics, being ethical is less about what type of action you perform and more about what type of person you are. The theory is that a perfectly virtuous person

Case 2.13 The attractive celebrity

Imagine that a paramedic is called to the scene of a heart attack. On discovering that the patient is an attractive movie star, the paramedic does everything in his power to make sure the patient is properly treated.

Importantly, however, he does this not because it is the right thing to do, but because he imagines that if he saves the patient's life, the patient won't be able to say no if, once she has recovered, he asks her out on a date.

would always act ethically. So if you wish to be ethical, your focus should not be on rules or consequences, but instead on your own character.

Thus, if paramedics are serious about acting ethically, they should be equally serious about becoming an ethical person—and to do so they should begin at once to cultivate their own character. For example, they should be mindful of those occasions where they may have acted in anger, and instead train themselves to practise restraint.

This theory can be loosely defined as follows:

Virtue ethics The view that holds that an action is ethical if it is motivated by virtue.

Most ethicists currently consider virtues to be deeply rooted character or personality traits that exemplify a complex and highly moral state of mind. As Hursthouse explains:

> A virtue such as honesty or generosity is not just a tendency to do what is honest or generous, nor is it to be helpfully specified as a 'desirable' or 'morally valuable' character trait. It is, indeed, a character trait—that is, a disposition which is well entrenched in its possessor, something that, as we say, 'goes all the way down', unlike a habit such as being a tea-drinker—but the disposition in question, far from being a single track disposition to do honest actions, or even honest actions for certain reasons, is multi-track. It is concerned with many other actions as well, with emotions and emotional reactions, choices, values, desires, perceptions, attitudes, interests, expectations and sensibilities. To possess a virtue is to be a certain sort of person with a certain complex mindset.[10]

Another central feature of a virtue is its *universal applicability*. In other words, any character trait defined as a virtue should be regarded as a virtue for everyone. According to this view, for example, it is inconsistent to claim that servility and chastity are female virtues, while at the same time suggesting that they are not male virtues.

Examples of virtues include compassion, kindness, empathy, sympathy, altruism, generosity, respectfulness, trustworthiness, personal integrity, forgiveness, friendship, love, wisdom, courage and fairness.

Although this theory enjoys much support among ethicists, it too has its drawbacks.

Objection: what do we do in the meantime?

Although cultivating a virtuous character seems like a good foundation to an ethical life, given that very few of us will ever become perfectly virtuous people (even given our best efforts), it is hard to see how virtue ethics will help us to make good ethical decisions right now. To illustrate this difficulty, reconsider the case of the blood relative (Case 2.9).

In this case it is hard to see what virtuous people might do. Perhaps virtuous people would save their own child, as they are guided by the virtues of loyalty and kinship. However, perhaps they would not save their own child's life, because they are guided by the virtue of selflessness.

So, although it may be true that perfectly virtuous people will always act ethically, this may not help us, as imperfect people, to ultimately determine what course of action is ethical right now.

While we are busy cultivating our virtues, it would be a good idea if we could have a practical system in place to help guide our ethical decisions straightaway. To such an end, the four principles of bioethics have been developed.

The four principles of bioethics

So far we have introduced three different ethical theories typically used by ethicists to justify ethical decision-making. However, it may prove useful to also introduce a more practical method. The method perhaps most widely used amongst healthcare professionals was developed by Beauchamp and Childress,[11] and is known as the *four principles of bioethics*.

The four principles of bioethics are four ethical principles, which, when applied together to an ethical case, should help you to determine the best course of action. The four ethical principles are:

1 autonomy
2 non-maleficence
3 beneficence
4 justice.

Staunton and Chiarella describe the notion of a principle as 'a rule or standard to be applied in a given situation. There is a sense in a principle that it is the right thing to do, that it will guide one's behaviour.'[12] We shall now introduce each of these principles one by one, and then examine how they come together to guide our actions.

The principle of autonomy

The principle of autonomy states that you should ensure that your patient is as able as possible to make free and informed decisions about their treatment, and that you should respect, as far as possible, their decisions.

The principle of autonomy respects the right of self-determination and non-interference of others when making decisions about themselves. It respects the person, and places an obligation on others not to interfere or constrain the person unnecessarily. Furthermore, we are charged with the responsibility to enable the person to exercise their autonomy whenever possible. Autonomy underpins privacy, confidentiality, veracity and consent, and assumes that the individual has the capacity for deliberation.[13]

It is this principle that provides the basis for informed consent.[14] In order to gain informed consent (and so uphold the patient's autonomy), the following three conditions must be satisfied (at the very least):

1 **Liberty** The patient must be free from controlling influences.
2 **Agency** The patient must have the capacity to make a choice.
3 **Understanding** The patient must have the capacity to understand the range of choices and their consequences.

To illustrate these conditions, consider Case 2.14.

In this case, the patient clearly displays signs of agency—that is, he is able to make a choice regarding whether or not he wishes to go to the hospital. However, this alone is not enough to suggest that the patient is able to provide informed consent. There is strong evidence in this case to suggest that the condition of liberty has not been met, for it seems the patient may well be under the controlling influence of morphine. Likewise, there is

Case 2.14 A possible suicide

A 63-year-old man has terminal cancer. He has been receiving palliative care for some time, and is in some pain. To deal with the pain he is able to self-administer morphine.

On Wednesdays, a nurse routinely makes a home visit. During one of these visits, the man asks the nurse how much morphine he would have to administer in order to kill himself. Although the nurse is unsure whether the patient is serious, or indeed whether he has already administered a fatal dose, she decides to call an ambulance just in case.

The paramedics arrive to find the man fully conscious. At first he claims to have administered a dangerously large dose of morphine. However, as soon as the paramedics attempt to transport him to the local hospital, he changes his story, saying he was confused earlier and has not administered a large dose of morphine.

He is adamant that he does not want to be taken to the hospital.[15]

evidence to suggest that the patient lacks the capacity to understand the choice he has made, as he keeps changing his story and is confused.

Paramedics only have a duty to uphold a patient's autonomy as far as it is possible. In this case, because it may be impossible to get the patient's informed consent, the paramedic would not fail in upholding the patient's autonomy were he to choose to take the patient to the hospital against the patient's wishes. We only fail to uphold the principle in those cases where a patient is *able* to provide informed consent for some treatment and does not give it, but we still decide to administer the treatment.

The principle of autonomy is clearly upheld in the Paramedicine Board of Australia's interim Registered Health Practitioners Code of Conduct (the code of conduct relevant to paramedics). It stresses the importance of practitioners working in partnership with their patients, which involves:

- encouraging and supporting patients or clients and, when relevant, their carer/s or family in caring for themselves and managing their health
- encouraging and supporting patients or clients to be well-informed about their health and assisting patients or clients to make informed decisions about their healthcare activities and treatments by providing information and advice to the best of a practitioner's ability and according to the stated needs of patients or clients, and
- respecting the right of the patient or client to choose whether or not they participate in any treatment or accept advice.[16]

Sections within the code are also dedicated to effective communication,[17] informed consent,[18] and working with patients with impaired decision-making capacity.[19] All such considerations are underpinned by the principle of autonomy.

Case 2.15 The broken leg

A paramedic arrives at a sports stadium to find a patient with a badly fractured leg, brought on by a particularly nasty rugby tackle.

The paramedic thinks that it might be worth realigning the leg and placing it in a traction splint before transporting the patient to the hospital.

Realigning the leg in this way will cause the patient further pain initially. However, once in the splint, the pain will normally decrease and there is less chance of further injury to the limb.

The principle of non-maleficence

The principle of non-maleficence states that, as far as possible, you should not harm a patient, either through action or inaction. Failure to protect a patient from needless foreseeable harm is commonly referred to as *negligence*.

This principle seems quite straightforward, and for the most part it is. However, at times its application might seem difficult. Consider Case 2.15.

Although the realignment and traction of the leg will decrease the chance of further injury, it will also cause further initial pain. And since the principle of non-maleficence states that paramedics should not harm their patients, the paramedic would not, in respect to this further pain, be adhering to this principle. However, if by causing harm now a paramedic is able to lessen a greater harm in the future, then causing this lesser harm may be acceptable overall.

The principle of non-maleficence is also upheld in the code of conduct, as it stresses the importance of practitioners minimising risk (i.e. the chances of harm). This involves:

- working in practice and within systems to reduce error and improve the safety of patients or clients and supporting colleagues who raise concerns about the safety of patients or clients, and
- taking all reasonable steps to address the issue if there is reason to think that the safety of patients or clients may be compromised.[20]

Such guidance is underpinned by the principle of non-maleficence.

The code also states that for paramedics to take good care of their patients, they should consider 'the balance of benefit and harm in all clinical management decisions'.[21] To better understand this guidance, it may be helpful to consider the principle of non-maleficence in conjunction with the next principle—the principle of beneficence.

The principle of beneficence

The principle of beneficence states that, as far as it is possible, you should help your patients. Again, this principle is for the most part straightforward. It is only when we come across cases such as the broken leg in Case 2.15 that this principle requires some explaining.

The principles of beneficence and non-maleficence sometimes need to be weighed against one another. For example, in the case of the broken leg, it may be acceptable to harm the patient a little now in order to help them a lot in the future. This process of weighing these two principles against one another is also captured in what is known as the *doctrine of double-effect*.

> **The doctrine of double-effect** It is ethically permissible to cause some unintended harm if this harm is a side-effect of some intended good, providing that this good could not be achieved any other way, and not to cause this good would result in a greater harm.

So, in the case of the broken leg, it may be permissible to cause the patient some pain by realigning the leg, since this harm is an unintended side-effect of the intended good of lessening the chance of further injury to the limb, given that the paramedic could not have done this any other way, and not lessening the chance of further harm would be a greater harm than the temporary pain caused by the realignment.

The principle of beneficence is also upheld in the code of conduct, as it emphasises that 'Care of the patient or client is the primary concern for health professionals in clinical practice',[22] and that the very underpinning of the 'code is the assumption that practitioners will exercise their professional judgement to deliver the best possible outcome for their patients'.[23]

The principle of justice

A good way to think about the principle of justice within the healthcare profession is to first consider how it operates within the legal profession. So far as the law is concerned, justice, it is often said, is blind. This does not mean that legal professionals do not consider the evidence in front of them, but rather that each person, regardless of race, religion or class, should be treated equally. In other words, the law sets out to treat each person fairly. In the same way, the healthcare profession is 'blind'.

The principle of justice states that you should treat your patients fairly. A good way to start thinking about this principle is to consider Case 2.16, in which there is more than one patient to look after.

The principle of justice suggests that the paramedic should give each patient two ampoules of morphine. This is because, all things being equal, treating each patient fairly seems to entail reducing each patient's pain, rather than leaving one patient completely untreated.

Yet we should not mistake the principle of justice as meaning we should treat each patient identically. To understand why, consider a slightly modified version of the previous case—Case 2.17.

If you were to treat both patients identically, you would end up giving both equal amounts of morphine: two ampoules each. Yet, although the second patient would be relieved of all his pain, the first would still be in some discomfort. Such a result seems ridiculous given the alternative (i.e. three ampoules to the first and one to the second).

Case 2.16 Two patients in equal pain

A paramedic has two patients in the ambulance en route to the hospital. Both patients are in considerable amounts of pain after incurring burns to much of their bodies. Unfortunately, the paramedic only has four ampoules of morphine to hand.

If the paramedic were to give one patient four ampoules of morphine, that patient's pain would be completely removed until they reached the hospital. However, the other patient would be in considerable pain for the remainder of the trip.

If the paramedic were to give both patients two ampoules of morphine, their pain would be halved; however, they would still be in some discomfort.

Case 2.17 Two patients in unequal pain

A paramedic has two patients in the ambulance en route to the hospital. The first is in a considerable amount of pain, while the second is in a moderate amount of pain. The paramedic has four ampoules of morphine to hand.

If the paramedic were to give the first patient three ampoules of morphine, his pain would be completely removed until they reached the hospital. The second patient only requires the one remaining ampoule to numb the pain for the remainder of the trip.

Rather than thinking of the principle of justice as just 'treat all patients equally', it might be better understood as 'treat all patients equally according to their needs'.

The principle of justice is also upheld in the code of conduct, as it emphasises that 'Practitioner decisions about access to care need to be free from bias and discrimination.'[24] This involves:

- not prejudicing the care of a patient or client because a practitioner believes that the behaviour of the patient or client has contributed to their condition
- upholding the duty to the patient or client and not discriminating on grounds irrelevant to healthcare, including race, religion, sex, disability or other grounds specified in anti-discrimination legislation, and
- investigating and treating patients or clients on the basis of clinical need and the effectiveness of the proposed investigations or treatment, and not providing unnecessary services or encouraging the indiscriminate or unnecessary use of health services.[25]

Now that all four principles have been introduced, let us consider how they come together into a single method of ethical decision-making.

Applying the four principles

The four principles of bioethics are designed to help healthcare professionals make ethical decisions. The idea is that, even when these principles conflict, we can weigh them against each other in order to determine the course of action that best conforms to the principles *overall*. Given this approach, the method might best be defined as follows:

> **The four principles of bioethics** An action is ethical if it is the action that is best able to uphold the principles of autonomy, non-maleficence, beneficence and justice.

To illustrate how this is achieved, please reconsider the case of the multiple patient overdose (Case 2.7).

Imagine that the two actions the paramedic is considering are:

- Action 1: Administer one full dose to one patient and another full dose to a second, leaving two patients untreated.
- Action 2: Administer half-doses to all four patients, leaving no patient untreated.

Now examine the salient points of each action, in respect to each of the four principles, set out in Table 2.1. The idea is to see which of the two actions best conforms to the four principles overall. To help illustrate this method, let us work through each principle in turn.

With respect to the principle of autonomy, both actions conform equally well. This is because in both cases the patients are unconscious, and so unable to provide informed consent.

With respect to the principle of beneficence, it seems action 1 performs a little better. This is because action 1 is more likely to help a greater number of people, for the paramedic would most likely be saving two lives by performing action 1, rather than risking only a small chance of saving a life if action 2 is performed.

Table 2.1 Applying the four principles of bioethics to the case of multiple patient overdose		
Principle	**Action 1**	**Action 2**
Autonomy	As all of the patients are unconscious, informed consent in this instance is impossible	As all of the patients are unconscious, informed consent in this instance is impossible
Beneficence	There is a high chance that two of the four patients will survive	There is a high chance that none of the four patients will survive
Non-maleficence	There is a high chance that two of the four patients will die	There is a high chance that all four patients will die
Justice	Two patients are being favoured over the others	No patient is being favoured over another

With respect to the principle of non-maleficence, it seems action 1 again performs better. This is because action 1 seems to allow for less harm. The paramedic only allows two people to die by performing action 1, whereas there is a strong chance that all four patients might die if action 2 is performed.

Lastly, with respect to the principle of justice, it seems action 2 on this occasion performs better. This is because, in performing action 2, the paramedic is treating all of the patients equally, rather than favouring just two patients as would be the case by performing action 1.

Action 1 seems to come out best with respect to beneficence and non-maleficence. Action 2 seems to come out best with respect to justice. And the two actions tie with respect to autonomy. Therefore, it seems that action 1 better conforms to the four principles overall, and, as such, is the most ethical course of action.

Conclusion

The aim of this chapter was to introduce some of the main tools used to make ethical judgements, and to communicate and justify these decisions to others in a consistent manner. Before examining these tools, we first attempted to dispel some *common misunderstandings* about ethics. These were:

- Acting ethically just means helping people.
- Acting ethically just means following the law.
- Acting ethically is only something to worry about in difficult cases.
- Acting ethically is about avoiding moral dilemmas.
- Acting ethically is relative.

We then introduced three competing ethical theories, and considered some objections against each of them. The theories outlined were:

Consequentialist ethics The view that holds that an action is ethical if, as a consequence of the action, the maximum overall amount of happiness results.

Deontological ethics The view that holds that an action is ethical if it is guided by a set of universal moral rules.

Virtue ethics The view that holds that an action is ethical if it is motivated by virtue.

These theories were then complemented with a widely used practical method for decision-making: the four principles of bioethics.

The four principles of bioethics An action is ethical if it is the action that is best able to uphold the principles of autonomy, non-maleficence, beneficence and justice.

When reading the remaining chapters in this book, we suggest you attempt to apply the four principles of bioethics and the three ethical theories to the various cases presented.

By repeatedly attempting to apply these tools, you should be in a better position to make more consistent ethical decisions. In addition, by referring to these tools, you should also be able to justify your decisions to others in a more robust manner. Finally, by seriously considering hypothetical cases, you should be better prepared to make ethical decisions out in the field.[26]

Review Questions

1 Why is an ethical action more than just an action that helps people?
2 What is hedonism, and how does it relate to consequentialist ethics?
3 According to deontological ethics, when can a moral rule be broken?
4 What is a virtue?
5 What three conditions must be satisfied in order for a person to provide informed consent?
6 What rule or principle relates beneficence to non-maleficence when you are considering whether to cause some harm in order to advert a greater harm?

Endnotes

1 Council of Ambulance Authorities. (2010) *The (2010) Paramedic Professional Competency Standards*, v. 2. Flinders Park: Council of Ambulance Authorities Inc, at p. 7.

2 De Ville, K. (1994) 'What does the law say?' Law, ethics, and medical decision making. *Western Journal of Medicine* 160(5), 478–480, at p. 478.

3 Derse, A.R. (1999) Law and ethics in emergency medicine. *Emergency Medicine Clinics of North America* 17(2), 307–325, at p. 307.

4 Derse, Law and ethics in emergency medicine, at p. 307.

5 De Ville, 'What does the law say?'.

6 Johnstone, M.-J. (2008) *Bioethics: A Nursing Perspective*. Sydney: Elsevier Health Sciences, at p. 98.

7 Shafer-Landau, R. (2010) *The Fundamentals of Ethics*. New York: Oxford University Press, at pp. 277–278.

8 Rachels, J. and Rachels, S. (2007) *The Elements of Moral Philosophy*. New York: McGraw-Hill, at p. 20.

9 Mussolini, B. (1943) Diuturna. In: H. Kuhn, *Freedom Forgotten and Remembered*. Chapel Hill: University of North Carolina Press, at pp. 17–18.

10 Hursthouse, R. (2007) Virtue ethics. In: E.N. Zalta (ed.), *Stanford Encyclopedia of Philosophy*. Stanford: Stanford University. Online. Available: https://plato.stanford.edu/entries/ethics-virtue/ (accessed 3 December 2018).

11 Beauchamp, T.L. and Childress, J.F. (2013) *Principles of Biomedical Ethics*, 7th ed. New York: Oxford University Press.

12 Staunton, P. and Chiarella, M. (2008) *Nursing and the Law*. Marrickville: Elsevier, at p. 31.

13 Freegard, H. (2012) Making ethical decisions. In: H. Freegard (ed.), *Ethical Practice for Health Professionals,* 2nd ed. (pp. 29–46). Melbourne: Thomson, at p. 37.

14 Please note that further conditions regarding informed consent will be outlined in Chapter 5.

15 My thanks to Brian Steer for a version of this case.

16 Paramedicine Board of Australia (2018) *Interim Code of Conduct for Registered Health Practitioners* (the 'Interim Code'), s 3.2. Online. Available: https://www.paramedicineboard.gov.au/professional-standards/codes-guidelines-and-policies/code-of-conduct.aspx (accessed 3 December 2018).

17 Ibid., s 3.3.

18 Ibid., s 3.5.

19   Ibid., s 3.8.

20   Ibid., s 6.2.

21   Ibid., s 2.2.

22   Ibid., s 2.1.

23   Ibid., Overview.

24   Ibid., s 2.4.

25   Ibid., s 2.4.

26   My thanks to Malcolm Luck, Brian Steer, Catherine Strong, Rachael Fox, Emma Rush, Daniel Cohen, Wylie Breckenridge, John Weckert, Graeme McLean, Brian Stoffell, Lisa Bowerman, Ann Jensen and Anita Van Riet for their input into this chapter.

Chapter 3
PRECARE—an ethical decision-making model for paramedics

Morgan Luck, Brian Steer and Ruth Townsend

Learning objectives

After reading this chapter, you should be able to:

- identify the central problem in a variety of ethical cases
- recognise which facts might be salient in addressing an ethical problem
- consider and apply the four principles of bioethics
- consider and apply the relevant professional code of conduct
- consider an alternative way of resolving the ethical problem
- understand where the law assists in resolving an ethical problem
- evaluate various concerns and your own decisions with regard to ethical decision-making.

Definitions

Alternative argument The best argument you can conceive of for an alternative course of action.

Code of conduct The published basis for the guidance of ethical and professional behaviour.

Ethical dilemma A case that requires you, in responding, to make a choice between seemingly equally unfavourable options.

Reconnaissance The process of going out into the field to gather salient facts in order to make better informed decisions.

The four principles of bioethics The view that holds that an action is ethical if it is the action that best upholds the principles of autonomy, non-maleficence, beneficence and justice.

An introductory case

Speaking up

A crew has been called to a railway station because of an assault. The police are in attendance and have apprehended a young man who is alleged to have struck another. While the injuries are minor, the police have requested both parties be assessed.

The alleged assailant has an open wound to his hand and the victim an open wound to his forehead; neither injury is considered to require hospital treatment. The police inform the paramedics that the assailant voluntarily disclosed to them that he was hepatitis C positive, but this information has not been communicated to the victim.

Sensing the need for the victim to be medically assessed and treated due to the risk of cross-infection, the paramedics urge the victim to attend hospital, as a standard universally applied precaution for anyone at risk of contamination (without explicitly mentioning hepatitis C). However, the patient repeatedly declines to do so as his wound is minor.

This chapter will introduce an ethical decision-making model designed to help paramedics make considered decisions in difficult cases such as this one.

Introduction

Chapter 2 introduced some of the main theories used to ground ethical judgements. In this chapter, we shall explain how these theories, together with the law and a professional code of conduct, might be brought together into a single applied ethical decision-making model.

Note that the purpose of this decision-making model, referred to here as the PRECARE model, is not to tell you what particular action to perform in a particular situation, but rather to give you a way to approach difficult ethical cases in a considered and structured manner.

The PRECARE decision-making model

It is one thing to understand the major ethical theories; it is quite another to be able to apply them in practice. This can be especially challenging in the pre-hospital environment. Paramedics often have to make decisions under difficult conditions, such as when under severe time pressure, in dealing with highly emotional people, being unable to consult with clinicians or relatives, and managing patients who may be physiologically and/or psychologically compromised. These challenges are best met by having a decision-making model to hand that can act as a guide in the field. The more practised you are at using a model, the more prepared you are likely to be.

The model we will present here is an adaptation of a model developed by Kerridge, Lowe and McPhee,[1] which in turn incorporates many of the features of the models proposed by Jonsen, Siegler and Winslade,[2] Pellegrino and Thomasma,[3] and Koehn.[4] This model has also been adopted by Staunton and Chiarella.[5]

For ease of memory we shall refer to the model as PRECARE—as in PRE-hospital CARE. The components of this acronym are as follows:

Problem—Identify the ethical problem.

Reconnaissance—Get the facts.

Ethics—Consider the four principles of bioethics.

Code—Consider your professional code of conduct.

Alternative—Consider an argument for an alternative course of action.

Regulations—Consider the relevant legal regulations.

Evaluate—Evaluate the various considerations and make your final decision.

We shall introduce each of these seven steps in turn by applying them to the ethical case outlined in 'An introductory case: Speaking up', at the beginning of this chapter.

Let us begin with the first step of the PRECARE model, which builds on the notion that difficult cases often involve an ethical problem.

Problem

In many cases decision-making can be difficult because one or more ethical problems need to be addressed before you can act in an informed manner, and it is in such cases that an ethical decision-making model can be helpful.

The identification of the ethical problem involved in a case is the first step in the PRECARE model.

P is for problem: identify the ethical problem.

Broadly speaking, an ethical problem is something about a case that needs to be overcome before you can determine the most ethical course of action. In this chapter, we shall focus on ethical problems that involve an ethical dilemma, which is a situation where you are faced with making a choice between equally unfavourable options.

To illustrate this, consider the 'Speaking up' case. This entails a dilemma, as it seems that the paramedic is forced to choose between disclosing confidential information about the alleged assailant to the patient (in order to inform him of the possibility of having contracted hepatitis C) or not disclosing this information (and risking having a possible infection go undiagnosed).

Often these ethical problems are best highlighted by questions, which for the 'Speaking up' case might be:
- Should the alleged assailant's medical information be kept confidential? or, conversely,
- Should the patient be made aware of fact that he has possibly contracted hepatitis C?

Often, the question can be worded in multiple ways. However, what is important is that by identifying this question you have taken the first step to address the problem. Further, by properly phrasing the problem, a response is demanded, in a way that prescribes what actions would logically follow.

Now that the notion of an ethical problem has been introduced, let us turn to the next step in the PRECARE model—reconnaissance.

Reconnaissance

Reconnaissance is a term used to describe the process of going out into the field to gather as many salient facts as possible in order to gain some advantage; in our case, being better informed. The term is commonly associated with a type of military operation, describing situations in which troops venture into enemy territory in order to gather tactical information. However, it also captures well the second step in the PRECARE model.

R is for reconnaissance: get the facts.

In order to assist in addressing the ethical problem identified in the previous step, it will often help to gather various salient facts about the case in question. This means that paramedics, especially if under time pressure, need to take control of a scene and discover what is most likely to be objectively true and of importance, and use these facts to help them to consider possible answers to the ethical question.

For example, in the 'Speaking up' case it was suggested that the central problem could be captured by the question: Should the alleged assailant's medical information be kept confidential? What fact or facts could the paramedic attempt to collect in this case that might help answer this question? The fact that hepatitis C is a significantly debilitating and potentially life-threatening illness will inform any deliberations, and the fact that there is a chance of cross-infection will also play a role. These facts, in the case of a well-known disease such as hepatitis C, should be known to the paramedic, so there may be no need to search for these answers. However, one could imagine a variation of this case where the illness is far less well known, and a paramedic might be required to consult with a clinician or others, either on-scene or not, to determine the facts.

The fact that the assailant has freely disclosed his hepatitis C status is important, since this might indicate a willingness to freely inform the victim or allow him to be informed. Another fact to determine would be whether the alleged assailant might give his permission to disclose his medical condition to the victim. If he agrees, then you may have successfully avoided the dilemma, which is a positive outcome. A dilemma is avoided when you manage to find a way out of the situation without taking either of the hard options, which in this case would mean neither breaking confidentiality nor failing to inform the victim of his possible condition. If you are able to successfully avoid the dilemma, the case no longer involves an ethical problem, in which case the PRECARE model need not be considered further.

Avoiding the dilemma is not always achievable, however, in which case you will have to attempt to resolve the dilemma. Paramedics resolve a dilemma when they consider the ethical problems and legal issues involved in the case and, after due consideration, choose one of the hard options. If you are going to attempt to resolve a dilemma, it is important to first determine the available options open to you as the paramedic.

Any ethical dilemma, once identified, creates at least two or more alternative choices, and there may be more creative options available than initially thought. The production of alternatives is a precursor to marshalling supporting arguments—ethical justification is about supporting one particular decision or behaviour above/over a number of competing alternatives. The rational paramedic should consider all of the relevant realistic alternatives.

Let us assume that the paramedic has identified the following two possible actions in this case:

- Action 1: not disclosing the information to the victim and letting him go home.
- Action 2: disclosing the information to the victim and transporting him to hospital.

Gathering salient facts, including the facts about the possible actions to take, will often help to address the ethical problem and make an informed decision. However, facts alone tell us nothing unless their ethical significance is understood. This is why the next step in the PRECARE model involves an ethical analysis of the situation.

Ethics

Identifying the ethical problem at the heart of a difficult case, and gathering facts pertinent to addressing the problem, are the first two steps of the PRECARE model. The third step involves considering the ethical dimensions of the case.

E is for ethics: consider the four principles of bioethics.

In Chapter 2 we introduced the *four principles of bioethics*. It is at this step of the PRECARE model that we apply these principles. In brief, the four principles of bioethics are four ethical principles which, when applied together to an ethical case, should help you to determine the best course of action.

The four ethical principles are:

1 **Autonomy** You should ensure that your patient is as able as possible to make free and informed decisions about their treatment, and you should respect such decisions.

2 **Non-maleficence** You should not harm a patient, either through action or inaction.

3 **Beneficence** You should help your patient and always act in their best interests.

4 **Justice** You should treat your patient fairly.

In order to illustrate this step, let us work through each of the two alternatives—action 1 (not disclosing) and action 2 (disclosing)—and apply each of the four principles in turn, summarised in Table 3.1.

Our aim is to determine which of the two actions best conforms to the four principles overall.

It is difficult to see which action best satisfies the principle of autonomy. Action 1 seems to fail the principle of autonomy because the patient is unable to make an informed

Table 3.1 Analysis of possible actions in terms of the four principles of bioethics

Principle	Action 1 (Do not disclose the information)	Action 2 (Disclose the information)
Autonomy	As the patient is unaware of all the salient facts, he cannot make an informed decision	The alleged assailant's confidential information has been disclosed and so there is a loss of autonomy
Beneficence	This would not help the patient	This could potentially help the patient
Non-maleficence	This could potentially harm the patient if he has contracted hepatitis C	This would not harm the patient. Nor would it obviously harm the assailant.
Justice	No issues regarding the distribution of resources	No issues regarding the distribution of resources

decision about his treatment as he is unaware of the possibility of contracting hepatitis C. While the risk of infection might be small, should it happen, the effect on the person's welfare could be great. Allowing the patient to make an informed decision affirms his autonomy, as it increases the options open to him, and better allows him to control the direction of his life. However, action 2 also seems to fail this principle in a different kind of way, as autonomy also underpins our right to privacy and confidentiality. Informational privacy is an extension of autonomy, the control of information about one's self. By disclosing this information to the patient, the paramedic is breaking the alleged assailant's right to confidentiality. The attempt to increase the informed decision-making of the patient and allow the assailant a right to confidentiality are both attempts to affirm autonomy. But it seems the autonomy of both people cannot be completely affirmed by either action 1 or action 2.

With respect to the principle of beneficence, only action 2 would help the patient, for only this action results in the patient being informed of his possible condition and, thereby, quickly receiving the appropriate assistance with all of its consequences.

With respect to the principle of non-maleficence, it again seems that action 2 comes out on top. This is because action 1 allows the patient to leave without knowing about his potential infection, which could then lead to further complications. Letting the patient leave constitutes knowingly failing to prevent further harm. And it is difficult to see how disclosing would cause any predictably comparable harm to the assailant.

Lastly, with respect to the principle of justice, no issues seem to arise in this case. You may be tempted to say that action 2 is unfair because the alleged assailant's confidential information has been disclosed. And, because this is unfair, the principle of justice has not been upheld. However, as Freegard states, 'Justice, in an ethical sense, refers to the fair and equitable distribution of benefits, burdens, and duties among and between members of society.'[6] That is, justice here refers to the notion of distributive justice, not to a broader sense of fairness. In this case, there is no issue concerning the distribution of resources. In addition, the issue of confidentiality was considered under the principle of autonomy. So, actions 1 and 2 seem equal in respect to the principle of justice.

Given that action 2 comes out as best with respect to beneficence and non-maleficence, and neither action 1 nor action 2 clearly comes out best with respect to autonomy and justice, it would seem that action 2 better conforms to the four principles of bioethics overall, with two in favour and none against. As such, there is an argument for action 2 being the most ethical course of action. In other words, the paramedic should break confidentiality and inform the patient of the possible risk of hepatitis C infection.

Although the four principles of bioethics are commonly used in the healthcare profession, they should not be followed blindly. Rather, you should also look to your professional code of conduct for further guidance. This is the next step in the PRECARE model.

Code

The four principles of bioethics are a good guide to making ethical decisions in the healthcare profession. However, there are also codes of conduct specific to paramedics that you are professionally bound to consider and act in accordance with. This is the fourth step of the PRECARE model.

C is for code: consider your professional code of conduct.

A code of conduct can be roughly defined as the published basis for the guidance of ethical and professional behaviour. Now that paramedics are registered, you will be required to rely on the Paramedicine Code of Conduct released by the Paramedicine Board of Australia (PBA). The core elements of the code require staff to, in essence, put their patient's interests above their own.

The PBA Code of Conduct at section 3.4 refers to the practitioners' ethical and legal obligations to protect patient confidentiality and privacy. The code almost makes specific reference to public health. Section 5.4(b) reminds practitioners that they have a responsibility to be aware of obligations to report notifiable diseases. The 'Speaking up' case therefore highlights what seems like a tension in this code between protecting patient confidentiality and reporting a notifiable public health condition. So, how exactly has this code helped us?

Help may come from the second sentence on confidentiality in section 3.4, which states that paramedics will hold patient information in confidence 'unless release of information is required by law or public interest considerations'. This 'unless' caveat allows for the possibility that a paramedic may break confidentiality, if there is a legal or professional reason to do so. Thus, the code of conduct might line up with the four principles of bioethics and suggest we may break confidentiality. We shall examine the legal rationale for possibly breaking confidentiality later in this chapter, and in Chapter 6 we explore questions of negligence.

Although we have determined that both the four principles of bioethics and a professional code of conduct may provide arguments for performing action 2 and disclosing the alleged assailant's medical information to the patient, you should remain critically minded and take into consideration the best possible argument for an alternative course of action. This is the next step of the PRECARE model.

seems consistent with the principles outlined in the ACT *Public Health Act 1997* (see Appendix 3.1).

If the alleged assailant does not agree to allow the information to be disclosed to the patient, sections 105 and 108 of the *Public Health Act 1997* might offer more help. These sections apply to instances where a 'responsible person' requests a person with a transmissible notifiable condition to inform a contact of the person at risk from exposure to the notifiable condition; or to give permission to the responsible person to do so. But when those requests are refused, as in the case here, the Chief Health Officer should be informed, and is authorised to trace contacts and notify them of possible infection risks.

Section 108(5) also says that a responsible person may notify the person at risk:

> If a responsible person is authorised under this section to notify the chief health officer or a contact about the contact's potential exposure to a transmissible notifiable condition, that authority operates notwithstanding any duty of confidentiality the responsible person may owe to the person with the condition.

A 'responsible person' is defined as a doctor, an authorised nurse practitioner, a counsellor who has counselled the person in relation to the condition, or a person who is responsible for the care, support or education of the person at risk.

Section 105(2) says that:

> A person who is responsible for the **care, support or education** of someone else must notify the chief health officer of the person if the first person believes, on reasonable grounds, that the other person has, or may have, a notifiable condition.

There is no case law that establishes whether or not a paramedic would fall into this latter category. It would be a matter for the practitioner to make this decision.

So, in short, an examination of the law offers no black-and-white answer to this dilemma. However, given that the *Public Health Act 1997* allows a 'responsible person' who is 'responsible for the care' of the person to break confidentiality with good reason, and that the principles that underpin the Act state that a person who has, or may have, a notifiable condition is accorded the right to receive all reasonably available information about the medical and social consequence of the condition and any proposed treatment, and the right to privacy provided this does not infringe unduly on the wellbeing of others, there does appear to be some legal support for action 2—disclosure.

Therefore, after considering the legal and/or regulatory factors at play, we are now in a position to evaluate our options and decide about the correct course of action. This is the final step of the PRECARE model.

Evaluate

At this point in the process you should have gathered the information you need to make a considered decision. The task now is to evaluate this information: that is, weigh up the competing issues and determine the right course of action. As Staunton and Chiarella state:

> Whatever decision you finally make will be determined by the facts you discover in your decision-making process and the value you place on the differing pieces of information.[10]

Although there is no single straightforward method for evaluating the information you have gathered, what is crucial is a commitment to rationality, which involves both the consideration of all of the possibilities and the ability to give an account of why a decision is made and what thought processes have led to that conclusion. In the same way a particular clinical pathway is taken for good reason, so too is an ethical decision made for good reason. Generally, a good reason has a number of features: it is known or easily explained to the listener, and thus facilitates persuasion; it is relevant to the issue as defined; it is important to all interested parties; it is connected to and provides a support or foundation to the course of action defended. This is the last step of the PRECARE model.

E is for evaluate: evaluate the various considerations and make your final decision.

To demonstrate the evaluation step, let us consider again our case. So far we have considered four different arguments as to how you should act. They were based on:

1   the four principles of bioethics (ethics)
2   your professional code of conduct (codes)
3   an argument for an alternative course of action (alternative)
4   the legal regulations (regulations).

Now it is time to evaluate these considerations—that is, determine how much you value each of these considerations in relation to each other and to our dilemma. What is presented next is a rather crude way of doing this. However, if nothing else, it demonstrates how you need to weigh up each of these considerations and reach a decision.

First, determine how important or influential you think each of the considerations are in comparison to the others. To illustrate this step, consider a simple 1 to 10 scale—with 10 being extremely important and 1 being of little importance. Let us now look at how a particular paramedic, named Paul, ranks these considerations:

Ethics	7
Code	6
Alternative	2
Regulations	8

Paul felt that the legal/regulatory considerations were the most important, rating them as 8. Second in importance were the four principles of bioethics, which Paul rated as 7. Third in importance was the professional code of ethics, rated as 6. Last was the alternative argument, rated here as 2 (perhaps demonstrating that Paul did not find the argument on the basis of deontological ethics persuasive).

Paul might be tempted to stop there. Since he thinks the legal/regulatory considerations are the most important, why not simply follow their recommended course of action in all cases? However, as stated in the previous chapter, as professionals, paramedics are obliged to develop their legal, ethical and professional compasses and apply them together to the situations they encounter. In other words, we are looking for a more holistic

Consideration	Action 1 (Do not disclose the information)	Action 2 (Disclose the information)
Ethics	−7	+7
Code	−6	+6
Alternative	+2	−2
Regulations	−8	+8
Evaluation total	−19	+19

Table 3.2 Applying the PRECARE model to the 'Speaking up' case

decision-making process, rather than one simply informed by a single consideration (such as the law).

This type of cumulative evaluation is illustrated in Table 3.2.

Here we can see that the scores Paul attributed to each consideration have been weighed against one another, alongside the actions in question. If the action is suggested by a particular consideration, it is given a positive number. If the action is discouraged by a consideration, it is given a negative number. For example, Paul rated the alternative viewpoint (suggested by deontological ethics) as only a 2. Thus, you can see a +2 and a −2 in the alternative rows in Table 3.2. The +2 under action 1 denotes that this action was encouraged by this alternative viewpoint. The −2 under action 2 denotes that this action was discouraged by this consideration.[11] The totals at the bottom represent the cumulative evaluation of each possible action. Action 2 clearly outweighs action 1 according to Paul's evaluation. In other words, according to Paul, the answer to the ethical problem captured by the question 'Should the alleged assailant's medical information be kept confidential?' is 'no'.

We should make it clear that this is only a crude illustration of the evaluation process. The complex manner by which these values should be weighed against one another cannot be accurately captured in such a straightforward manner. However, what is being illustrated here is that paramedics should weigh up each of the considerations offered and reach a decision based on the whole picture. Also, note that we are not suggesting that the course of action decided by Paul is necessarily the right one for a paramedic in this situation to take—only that this method of arriving at a decision clearly demonstrates a considered approach.

Once this process has revealed a particular course of action, it is often helpful to imagine how comfortable you would be performing it. You might ask yourself questions such as:

- Would I be comfortable for my actions to be public (that is, known to all)?
- Am I willing to take responsibility for my actions and give account of my reasoning?
- Is my conscience likely to be clear after performing these actions?

Hopefully (especially after carefully working through the PRECARE model) you will be able to answer 'yes' to each of these questions. But if not, this might indicate that you should review your thinking before acting.

The last stage of the evaluation step occurs after you have made your decision, performed the recommended action, and noted the consequences of your actions (as far as is reasonably possible to do so). It is a reflective stage. As Staunton and Chiarella state:

> Evaluation of the process as well as the outcome is essential, otherwise you will have learned little from the process. The opportunity to reflect on our most difficult dilemmas and the choices we made about them is to be welcomed. However, it is important to recognise that the real reflection, as opposed to post-hoc justification, can sometimes be painful. We may honestly feel on reflection that we could have managed the situation better or made better decisions. But clinical–ethical decision making is often made 'on the run' and, with the best will in the world, we will not always get it right. It is important to welcome the evaluation as a learning opportunity and to recognise the potential for improvement.[12]

The final part of the evaluation step, therefore, is to consider your decision in hindsight and determine what you can learn from the experience so that in the future you can approach a comparable problem armed with that knowledge.

Conclusion

The aim of this chapter was to introduce an ethical decision-making model to paramedic practice. This model was designed not to reduce the amount of thought that goes into making such decisions, but rather to provide a structure for such thinking.

The model introduced was the PRECARE model (as in PRE-hospital CARE), which is an adaptation of a model developed by Kerridge, Lowe and McPhee.[13] The components of this acronym are as follows:

Problem—Identify the ethical problem.

Reconnaissance—Get the facts.

Ethics – Consider the four principles of bioethics.

Code—Consider your professional code of conduct.

Alternative—Consider an argument for an alternative course of action.

Regulations—Consider the relevant legal regulations.

Evaluate—Evaluate the various considerations and make your final decision.

It is hoped that by applying this model to the case provided (and also applying the model to further cases presented in this book), your ability to recognise and deal with ethical problems encountered in the field will be strengthened.

Review Questions

1 What is the value of utilising a model like PRECARE to assist with ethical decision-making?

2 What is reconnaissance, and how does it apply to ethical decision-making?

3 What is the difference between avoiding and resolving a dilemma?

4 Which consideration do you value most when attempting to resolve a dilemma: the four principles of bioethics, legal regulations, professional codes of conduct, or some other alternative?

5 Can you identify the normative intersections of the law, the four ethical principles of bioethics and your code of conduct? In other words, can you identify the areas where the same values are repeated?

Appendix 3.1 *Public Health Act 1997* (ACT), s 99

Principles—notifiable conditions

This part shall be construed and administered in accordance with the following principles:

(a) the investigation of notifiable conditions, and any actions taken as a consequence, must be carried out in order to minimise the adverse public health effects of such conditions;

(b) a person who engages in activities that are known to carry a potential risk of exposure to a transmissible notifiable condition, and any person responsible for the care, support or education of such a person, has the following responsibilities:

(i) to take all reasonable precautions to avoid the contracting of the condition by the person who engages in such activities;

(ii) if there are reasonable grounds for believing that the person who engages in such activities has been exposed to the condition—to ascertain whether the condition has been contracted, and what precautions should reasonably be taken to avoid exposing others to the condition;

(iii) if there are reasonable grounds for believing that the person who engages in such activities has contracted, or is likely to have contracted the condition—to comply with preventative measures or treatment that will minimise the risk to others of exposure to the condition;

(iv) if there are reasonable grounds for believing that the person who engages in such activities has contracted, or is likely to have contracted the condition—to take reasonable measures to ensure that others are not unknowingly placed at risk through any action or inaction of the person or any person responsible for the care, support or education of the person;

(c) a person who has, or may have, a notifiable condition, or who engages in activities that are known to carry a potential risk of exposure to a notifiable condition, must be accorded the following rights, to the extent that their exercise does not conflict with the requirements of this part and does not infringe unduly on the wellbeing of others:

(i) the right to privacy;

(ii) the right to receive all reasonably available information about the medical and social consequences of the condition and any proposed treatment.

Endnotes

1   Kerridge, I., Lowe, M. and McPhee, J. (2005) *Ethics and Law for the Health Professions.* Annandale: The Federation Press, ch. 8.

2   Jonsen, A.R., Siegler, M. and Winslade, W.J. (2002) *Clinical Ethics: A Practical Approach to Ethical Decisions in Clinical Medicine.* New York: McGraw-Hill Professional.

3   Pellegrino, E.D. and Thomasma, D.C. (1993) *The Virtues in Medical Practice.* New York: Oxford University Press.

4   Koehn, D. (1994) *The Ground of Professional Ethics.* London: Routledge.

5   Staunton, P. and Chiarella, M. (2008) *Nursing and the Law*, 6th ed. Marrickville: Elsevier, at p. 30.

6   Freegard, H. (2007) Making ethical decisions. In: H. Freegard (ed.), *Ethical Practice for Health Professionals* (pp. 29–46). Melbourne: Thomson, at p. 39.

7   Kerridge, Lowe and McPhee, *Ethics and Law for the Health Professions*, at p. 90.

8   *Public Health Act 1997* (ACT). Available: https://www.legislation.act.gov.au/a/1997-69/ (accessed 27 November 2018).

9   *Privacy Act 1988* (Cth), Sch. 3 (private), s 14 (public).

10   Staunton and Chiarella, *Nursing and the Law*, at p. 32.

11   If you were unsure whether a consideration encourages or discourages an action, you would place a '?' next to the number and not include it in your evaluation total.

12   Staunton and Chiarella, *Nursing and the Law*, at pp. 32–33.

13   Kerridge, Lowe and McPhee, *Ethics and Law for the Health Professions*, ch. 8.

Chapter 4

An introduction to the legal system and paramedic professionalism

Ruth Townsend

Learning objectives

After reading this chapter, you should be able to:

• know where our laws come from
• describe briefly how the law operates
• identify the structure of the legal system
• analyse the law and its relationship to paramedic practice.

Definitions[1]

Act of Parliament See 'Legislation'.

Actus reus Latin for 'guilty act'.

Assault A general term to include both a threat of, and the actual infliction of, personal violence.

Beyond reasonable doubt The standard of proof required to find a person guilty of a criminal offence.

Case law The principles of law arising from the judicial decisions of legal cases.

Common law The law developed by courts over the ages, and applied in similar cases to provide consistency and certainty in law-making, which forms the doctrine of precedent.

Criminal law The body of rules and legislation that prohibits certain conduct and imposes a penalty or punishment on those who are found to have committed such conduct.

Duty of care The obligation owed to anyone who could be injured by a person's lack of care. It must be 'reasonably foreseeable' that an injury could result from the lack of care.

Illegal Describes behaviour that is contrary to criminal law.

Judiciary Those people who adjudicate legal disputes in courts of law.

Jurisdiction The scope or area the law's authority covers.

Legislation A law or body of laws made and enacted by the Parliament (known as a statute or an Act of Parliament).

Mens rea Latin for 'guilty mind'.

Natural justice The notion that proceedings are conducted impartially, fairly and without prejudice.

On the balance of probabilities The standard of proof required to establish liability in a civil matter.

Precedent A decision that interprets law and acts as a guide for future cases. It is an important doctrine that ensures there is a stable legal framework on which to consider each new legal case.

Statute See 'Legislation'.

Unlawful An action that is in breach of civil law (can also be used in reference to breach of criminal law).

An introductory case

Paramedic assault?

Paramedics are called to attend an 18-year-old male with head injuries following an assault outside a pub on a Saturday night. On arrival, the paramedics hear from the crowd that the patient was intoxicated, and verbally provoked another male who subsequently hit him. He fell to the ground, hitting his head. The paramedics approach the patient with a bright light to help them see. They hear the patient say, 'Stay away', 'Don't come near me.' A friend of the patient says, 'Just give him a minute, he is not really with it.' The paramedics continue to approach the patient, and once close enough reach out to commence an assessment. The patient pushes the paramedics away and shouts, 'No, get off me—don't touch me!' The paramedics restrain the patient, holding him down and saying, 'Don't touch us. How do you like this, then?' The paramedics report the patient to the police for assaulting them. Bystanders and the police witness the event.

This chapter will introduce you to some of the methods paramedics can use to determine what the law is, where laws come from, and how the law operates. It will also provide a broad introduction to the machinery of the legal system and how it applies to paramedics.

Introduction

Paramedics have been slowly moving towards professionalism for a number of decades. There are a number of characteristics that define a profession, including altruism, trustworthiness, specialist skills, a body of knowledge, competence and professional autonomy. A professional paramedic would reflect these characteristics, not only with a minimum standard of clinical education and competence, but also with an understanding of the ethical standards regarding conduct and character, and a knowledge of the law and its application to paramedic practice.[2]

The law is essentially a set of rules that establishes community expectations of behaviour, and so establishes the norm of appropriate behaviour in our society. This chapter will introduce you to the legal system, and will outline where paramedics and paramedic services fit into the legal system. The chapter will provide a basic outline of the Australian legal system, its structure and function, and how it applies to paramedics.

What is the law?

Our legal system developed from the British legal system upon colonisation. We have since adapted our laws to meet the needs of our own communities, but the elements of the law that we debate today originated in Britain. The *law* is a system of rules and regulations that are designed to ensure that individual human rights—such as our rights to life, liberty, justice and equality—are upheld. A law is a rule that comes from a legitimate authority (e.g. a democratically elected parliament) and applies to everyone equally. Laws are created to make sure that everyone in a society understands what is expected of them as a member of that society (their *obligations* or *duties*), and what they can expect of others, including their government (their *rights*).

In addition to setting out the *rules* by which we live, another function of the legal system is to *resolve disputes*. The nature of our legal system is largely adversarial. This means that, following the development of a dispute between competing parties, the parties request a hearing by the court to resolve the dispute. The parties bring the evidence that supports their case to the court, and present the material. The court acts as an independent decision-maker, considering the established facts of the case and the law that applies, and deciding who has, in civil cases, on the balance of probabilities, the stronger claim. In criminal cases, the matter is heard and determined by either a judge alone or a judge and a jury. They are required to decide whether the case brought against a person, on behalf of the state, is able to be proved, by the state, beyond reasonable doubt.

There are other instances when the court takes an inquisitorial role, such as coroners' cases, where the purpose of the court is to investigate and determine what has led to the unexpected death of a person. Administrative courts or tribunals are convened to resolve other types of disputes, including, for example, issues of guardianship for patients who may be incompetent to make decisions regarding their healthcare. The differences between these jurisdictions will be discussed later in this chapter.

Legal theory

Our legal system has a core set of principles that includes considerations such as *procedural fairness*, *judicial precedent* and the *separation of powers*. These principles are encapsulated in the concept of *natural justice*, which is the foundation of the system, and its application ensures that legal rights and interests are able to be protected and promoted. Other principles include:

Fairness That it is fair that people know the rules that apply to them and that they must comply with.

Transparency That the legal system is open and transparent, and that decisions are open to review and appeal.

Equality before the law That people have access to the legal system regardless of their ability to pay, and that the system is applied equally, and not more favourably to those who are, for example, richer or hold a higher position in society.

Freedom from bias That decision-makers must excuse themselves from hearing and determining a case if they have an interest in the case.

The right to be heard That each side has a right to put its side of the story to the court for consideration.[3]

The principles of law, and the agreement by citizens to abide by the law, are part of what is known as the *social contract*. The notion that the people have the right to legislate and that all laws must be written and ratified by the people was first proposed by Jean-Jacques Rousseau in 1762, in his treatise titled *Du contrat social ou Principes du droit politique*. (This built on earlier theories developed by Thomas Hobbes and John Locke.) Social contract theory effectively states that some social organisation is preferred over anarchy, and that a government is a way of gathering citizens together to provide that organisation. That group is given authority by members of society to make laws for the benefit of the community. In order to work effectively as a society governed by laws, each individual within the society agrees to relinquish some individual freedom and independence in return for organisation, protection and security. If, however, the government does not provide benefits to the community and attempts to abuse this power, either through bad laws or bad governance, then the community has a legitimate right to rise up and challenge the legitimacy of those laws and, indeed, that government.

Case 4.1 gives an example of how it is necessary to apply the rule of law consistently in order to promote confidence in the system and ensure fairness. It also highlights how the rules of law apply equally to the judiciary as they do to others accessing the legal system. This case highlights the need for all of those within the legal system to act in accordance with the key principles of procedural fairness and due process. If the law is unable to be appropriately applied, even by the members of the judiciary, there is a risk that the public will lose confidence in the rule of law and, therefore, be less likely to comply with it, which could have a negative impact on the safe and effective functioning of our society.

How is the law made?

The highest law in the country is the Constitution, which allows for the Commonwealth Parliament and the High Court to be established. This law was made at the turn of

Case 4.1 Filthy pig (extended)

In August 2011 a young male paramedic, CM, and his female partner, KJ, were called to a patient, W, who had been assaulted. The paramedics assessed the patient, who requested transport to hospital. En route to hospital, the patient became aggressive and spat on the floor of the ambulance. The treating paramedic said, 'Don't f%&*ing do that! This is an ambulance, you filthy pig.'

The situation escalated and the ambulance was pulled over so that the patient could be removed from the vehicle. The patient then threw an icepack at CM's head, shouted and swore at him, and then punched CM in the side of the head. KJ was a witness to these events. As it happened, an off-duty police officer driving past also witnessed these events. In court, the magistrate, Pat O'Shane, heard evidence from the male paramedic, who was the victim of the alleged assault, but failed to take any evidence from the two witnesses. Magistrate O'Shane then dismissed the matter on the basis that it was CM who had initiated the physical interaction, and therefore the actions of W were taken in self-defence.[4]

The dismissal of this case led to a call for an appeal to be lodged and a complaint made to the Judicial Commission, on the basis that Magistrate O'Shane did not apply the foundational principles of law when hearing the matter, which included the right of the prosecutor to bring evidence of the matter before the court so that the judicial officer presiding over the matter relied on all of the evidence to establish the facts of the case.

This was not the first time that Magistrate O'Shane had been accused of failing to properly apply the law. On at least three other occasions she had been criticised for refusing to allow a prosecutor to call further witnesses, and effectively acting as counsel for the defendant rather than as an impartial judicial umpire. As a result of this judicial impropriety, the Supreme Court has criticised her for clear failures to apply procedural fairness.[5]

the 20th century, when the colonies came together and agreed to become a federated nation operating under one Constitution. The Constitution outlines how the federal government is to operate with respect to areas like taxation and trade, its relationship to the states, and defence. The full title of Australia's Constitution is the *Commonwealth of Australia Constitution Act 1900*. The Constitution can be found in libraries or on the internet.[6]

You may have heard of 'constitutional challenges' to pieces of law written by the Parliament that may not be permitted under the Constitution. The High Court of Australia determines whether a law is permissible under the Constitution.

The Constitution does not give any power to the federal government to make laws related to emergency services or, more particularly, paramedic services. These laws are written at a state or territory level, and this is why each is slightly different.

The Australian legal system relies on two sources of law. The first is *legislation* enacted by Parliament, and commonly referred to as an Act or a statute. The second is known as the *common law*, which is a body of law made by judges as a result of decisions from individual legal cases. This is also referred to as *precedent* or *case law*.

An Act of Parliament

Laws made through Parliament by elected representatives are known as *statutes*, *legislation* or *Acts of Parliament*.

A statute is made in a variety of stages. First, an issue is identified either by a parliamentarian via their electorate or raised by a lobby group, or in response to other events. For example, the ACT *Medical Treatment (Health Directions) Act* was introduced to give greater assurances to people who wanted to make choices about their end-of-life care. Other legislation, like the *Public Health Act*, was originally written in response to an outbreak of epidemics,[7] and in an acknowledgment that regulations about sewage, pollution, water cleanliness and the transmission of disease were needed to ensure that those standards were applied by industry, thus allowing for healthier environments and workers, and improved productivity.

Once the issue to be regulated has been identified, a government department is tasked with gathering data on the issue and putting together a document with recommendations about how to best address the issue via laws and other methods. If a law is to be drafted, this is undertaken by the appropriate government ministry, and then tabled as a Bill to the Parliament for debate, amendment and approval. The Bill can be defeated by a vote of the Parliament at any stage of its journey through the process of development (see Table 4.1). A Bill is an Act prior to it being approved and enacted by the Governor (state or territory) or Governor-General (federal).

The difference between an Act and a Regulation

An *Act* of Parliament is the primary instrument in setting out the rules regarding particular matters. A *Regulation* is a document that is subordinate to the Act, but is nonetheless important because it often delegates who has certain powers to do what under the Act, and prescriptively sets out other details required for the implementation of the Act.

For example, the Queensland *Ambulance Service Act 1991* authorises the establishment of an ambulance service. The Queensland *Ambulance Service Regulation 2015* sets out the fee that can be charged for emergency ambulance transport.[8] Regulations are often referred to as *delegated legislation*, because the Act delegates power to the regulation-maker (e.g. a minister of the government, the director-general or chief executive of an organisation) to make the Regulation that holds the details that assist the purpose of the Act to be achieved. For instance, in New South Wales the *Health Services Amendment (Ambulance Service) Regulation 2011* authorises the Chief Executive of the Ambulance Service to take disciplinary action against a member of staff.[9]

Step	Action
Table 4.1 The process of development of a parliamentary Bill	
1	The Bill is introduced to the Parliament.
2	There is a first reading speech, followed by initial debate.
3	The Bill goes to a Select Committee, which hears public submissions on the proposed law. The Select Committee then reports recommended amendments to the Bill to the House, with an explanation of the recommendations.
4	The Bill is read a second time, and there is a significant debate around the principles of the Bill, its purpose, objectives and stated outcomes, and the recommendations that have been forwarded from the Select Committee.
5	The Bill is considered by a full committee from members of the Lower House, where each clause and part is carefully considered and further amendments made. Upon passing as an Act, a Bill's clauses are thereafter referred to as 'sections'.
6	This process occurs again in the Upper House (or in reverse).
7	The Bill is assented to become an Act of Parliament.
8	The Bill is read a third and final time, and any final debate is had at this point prior to the Bill going to the Governor or Governor-General for assent into law.

Precedent

Laws are also developed from cases that come to court. Law that is made in this way is based on the particular circumstances of a case, and how that case relates to legal principles and existing legislation. Interpretation of the meaning of particular pieces of legislation can be determined via individual cases. This is called *case law* or *common law*, and is based on the legal *doctrine of precedent*.

> **Doctrine of precedent** This is the doctrine under which the law is bound to follow previous decisions unless they are inconsistent with a higher court's decision or are wrong at law. This doctrine was developed to promote certainty about what the 'rules' are, and consistency and equity in the way the law is applied.

Common law is different from a statute or an Act, and does not rely on a piece of parliamentary-made law to underpin it. Precedent means that where a similar case has come before a higher court and a decision has been made based on similar facts and circumstances and legislation, a lower court is bound by the decision of the higher court to essentially follow that court's interpretation of the legislation and the way in which it applies to the facts. If the case comes from a different jurisdiction (i.e. not from a higher court within the state where the original decision was made), it is considered to be a *persuasive case*. This ensures a level of consistency and transparency in the system. This also means that, when researching legal cases, you must be aware of the jurisdiction in which the decision was made. For example, some cases from the United States may be interesting, but they have no legal weight here because those decisions are not based on our laws or precedents. Common law is written down in a number of court judgments, and as such it can be difficult to be aware of these laws.

Different types of law

In this section, we shall examine different types of law. These are:

- criminal law
- civil law
- administrative law
- customary law
- human rights law
- international law.

Criminal law

Criminal law essentially reflects the rules and behaviour expected of citizens within our society. It is often punitive (punishing) in nature, meaning that if someone is found guilty of a criminal offence they are often punished by limitations on their freedom (gaol sentence) or something similar (e.g. community service). Criminal laws often mirror society's moral position about an action or an omission to act (i.e. what is considered to be right and what is wrong). For example, murder is a crime, and we would generally argue that to murder another person—that is, to unjustifiably and intentionally take the life of another (as opposed to killing them in self-defence, for example)—is not only legally wrong but also morally wrong.

Each state and territory has its own piece of criminal law like the *Crimes Act*, but essentially the laws in each state and territory regarding criminal acts are the same. Even so, there are some significant differences that relate to health law, including, for example, that abortion is lawful in Victoria and the ACT, but is still a criminal act in New South Wales.

Criminal law forms some of our oldest pieces of law, and from time to time these laws have been amended to bring them up-to-date with modern society. For example, the South Australian *Criminal Law Act* was written around 1913. It was later amended, and in 1972 South Australia became the first state in Australia to decriminalise homosexuality. The members of Parliament who are responsible for writing the laws are also representatives of their communities, and therefore would be expected to reflect the views of their constituents in these laws. There are other pieces of legislation apart from the *Crimes Act* that contain offences punishable by imprisonment or, at the least, financial penalties (fines). For example, the *Road Transport Act* may include laws on drink driving, speeding and running red lights.

Criminal cases are brought to court by the police acting on behalf of the citizens of the state. For a crime to have been committed, it must have two essential elements:

1. that the action is considered an offence (*actus reus*)
2. that there was an intention to carry out the act, or that there was a high degree of reckless indifference as to the outcome of the action (*mens rea*).

So note, in general *criminal law* the following applies:

- It is punitive in nature.
- Actions are brought by police.
- Punishment is often a loss of liberty.
- The act must meet the elements of a crime (including recklessness, intent, statutory offence, etc.).
- The person charged with the offence is known as the *accused*.
- Persons charged with a criminal offence have a right to not incriminate themselves.
- The standard of proof to be found guilty of a criminal offence is *beyond reasonable doubt*.

Civil law

Civil law has nothing to do with the police. Civil law was developed as a way for people to resolve disputes. These disputes often involve issues of property, negligence, workers' compensation, contracts and the like. They usually arise when one party is seeking monetary compensation from another for an alleged breach of contract or agreement. The standard of proof in determining who will be successful in the action is that *on the balance of probabilities* one side's case is stronger than the other's. This standard is lower than that in a criminal case, where the standard of proof is 'beyond reasonable doubt'. This is because in a civil matter a person's liberty is not at stake should they lose their case, and we generally deem that a person's liberty is worth more than any dollar value.

For example, consider Case 4.2. This case demonstrates the complexity of the law and how it applies in clinical practice. If the paramedic were to give the patient the blood despite the patient's refusal of consent for treatment with blood, the paramedic might commit a civil wrong of trespass and battery of the person, for which the patient might later claim compensation. If the patient was not actually competent at the time of the

Case 4.2 Jehovah's Witness car crash

An intensive care paramedic arrives on the scene of a car crash to find a patient conscious but severely haemorrhaging. After slowing the bleeding and providing the patient with a saline solution, the patient's blood pressure continues to drop, and she becomes unconscious. The paramedic is worried that the patient may die before reaching the hospital.

One promising course of action open to the paramedic is to administer packed red blood cells, which should help stabilise the patient.

However, before falling unconscious the patient had informed the paramedic that she is a Jehovah's Witness and did not want to be given a blood transfusion.

refusal and the paramedic had made an error in assessing this, and thus acted accordingly (i.e. did not give the blood), the paramedic may face an allegation of negligence for failing to meet the duty of care to the patient even though there was no intention to harm the patient. If the paramedic were to intentionally refuse to administer the blood knowing that it would cause the patient's death and the patient had not refused to accept it, then it may be that the paramedic's actions go beyond civil negligence and cross into criminal negligence. The issues raised in this case will be discussed in more detail in subsequent chapters, but it is given here as a way of illustrating the difference between a civil act and a criminal act.

In short, in *civil law* the following apply:
- It has nothing to do with the police.
- An action can be brought by one person against another.
- Compensation is usually made in the form of money or goods.
- The person bringing the action is called the *plaintiff*, and the other party is known as the *defendant*.
- The standard of proof for a case is *on the balance of probabilities*.

Torts

Torts are civil wrongs that serve to protect a person's interest in their body, property, finances or reputation. One of the most common torts of particular relevance to paramedics is the tort of negligence, where one party owes a duty of care to another, breaches that duty, harms the person and enables that person to bring an action for compensation to be paid to the injured party. Examples of other torts include trespass (touching a patient without consent) and defamation (making a claim that publicly lowers the reputation of a person).

Administrative law

Administrative law refers to the branch of law that considers matters of government power and authority. For example, the NSW Civil and Administrative Tribunal will consider the most serious disciplinary matters for paramedics—professional misconduct. The Guardianship Tribunal might consider the application of powers of the public guardian. Decisions of the Civil and Administrative Tribunal can be reviewed by the Supreme Court.

Customary law

Although a substantial proportion of the Australian population considers the arrival of the First Fleet in 1788 to be an invasion rather than a settlement, there was no formal declaration of war on the Indigenous Australians, and therefore, under international law, Australia was considered to be peaceably settled.[10] As a result, the laws of the colonising power applied—British laws. There was no legal recognition of the property rights of Indigenous Australians until 1992, when the High Court recognised Indigenous land rights (*Mabo v The State of Queensland (No. 2)*).[11] However, this decision did not result in Indigenous Australians being able to apply their own legal systems, although in some circumstances magistrates have attempted to apply the common law in a way that recognises customary law.

Human rights law

Human rights are the rights all humans have regardless of whether any law exists to support them. These rights include the right to life and the right to non-discrimination on the basis of, for example, race or gender. Federally, at the national level, there is no Bill of Rights in Australia. However, it is important to note that human rights protections exist in other laws. For example, the anti-discrimination laws protect individuals against discrimination on the grounds of gender, race, religion and sexual preference. When interpreting statutes (parliamentary-made law), the courts have recognised rights such as the right to silence (not to incriminate oneself), the right to natural justice, the right of access to the courts, and the protection of property rights. The ACT introduced the first *Human Rights Act* in 2004. This Act protects 20 basic human rights, and has the power to shape the way all legislation in the ACT is interpreted to ensure that it is interpreted in accordance with human rights. Victoria also has the *Charter of Human Rights and Responsibilities Act (2006)*.

Rights have also long been protected by the common law; for example, confidentiality (which is discussed in Chapter 10). It has been suggested that all health practitioners should be aware of human rights for the following reasons:

- Health policy, programs, practices and research may inadvertently violate human rights.
- Violations of human rights may have important adverse health effects on individuals and groups.
- Promoting human rights is now understood as an essential part of efforts to promote and protect public health.[12]

There are different types of human rights, which may be broken down into various sub-categories, including political and civil rights. Civil rights include the right *not to be* subjected to the action of another that would limit your rights. For example, the right to life limits the rights of others to take your life away. Government has a duty to protect these rights. The rights that should be protected include: recognition of the right to life, liberty and security of person; freedom of movement; freedom from torture or cruel, inhumane or degrading treatment or punishment; and freedom from arbitrary arrest and detention.

There are also economic, social and cultural rights that impose a more positive duty on government—that is, the government should provide something, such as work, social security and the highest attainable standard of health, and adequate food, clothing, housing and education.

Australia also has a Human Rights Commission. Its purpose is to promote and protect human rights and equal opportunity, investigate alleged breaches of human rights, and alert government to issues relating to the jurisdiction. The jurisdiction the commission covers includes areas of discrimination on the basis of race, sex, age and disability.

International law

International law is law that has developed between nations to allow for the establishment of rules regarding international relationships. Examples of international law include international treaties and conventions, like the *International Covenant on Civil and Political Rights (ICCPR)*.

International law is relevant for emergency workers such as paramedics, who may, as a requirement of their practice, be sent to work in foreign countries. Without the boundaries and protections of international law, working in these countries could pose many problems.

The structure of the court system

As Fig. 4.1 illustrates, the court system is a hierarchical system.

The jurisdiction of a matter—that is, the court in which a matter will be heard—depends on the nature of the matter. For example, Local Courts (or Magistrates' Courts) deal with minor criminal and civil matters that are heard by a judge alone, whereas the High Court of Australia deals with matters relating to Australia's Constitution and other questions of law that have been unresolved in the lower courts. The court system in Australia is composed of the following eight courts.

Coroners' Courts The primary function of a Coroners' Court is to inquire into the nature and cause of unexpected, violent, unnatural deaths, or deaths that occurred in hospital (e.g. following an anaesthetic), or a death that occurs in prison. The coroner

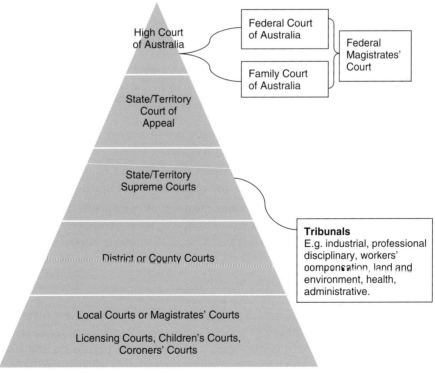

Figure 4.1 The structure of the court system

acts as the judge in this jurisdiction. The coroner's role is not to attribute blame to a particular individual for the death of another person, although if this is reasonably adduced at a coronial inquiry the matter may be referred by the coroner to the police for action; rather, it is to find the cause of death so as to make recommendations about how future deaths from the same cause can be avoided. Many new laws have been developed as a result of coronial inquiries, with the intention of keeping people safe; for example, the mandatory fencing of swimming pools.

Local or Magistrates' Courts The Local Court deals with minor criminal matters and low-claim civil matters; for example, parking fines and speeding charges. The Local Court also has jurisdiction to hold committal hearings to determine whether a serious criminal case is strong enough to go before a jury.

District or County Courts District Courts sit above Local Courts (or Magistrates' Courts) and below Supreme Courts in the hierarchical legal system, with the District Court largely hearing serious criminal matters or large-claim civil matters. The matters can be heard by a judge alone or by a judge and a jury. The judiciary (judges) are those who are appointed (not elected) to impartially adjudicate legal disputes in court. In making decisions regarding disputes, judges are required to not only consider precedent law and statute (Acts of Parliament), but also follow certain legal principles to interpret how those laws apply in a particular situation. A decision of the court is often called a *judgement*, *determination* or *finding*.

Supreme Courts The highest courts in the states or territories, these courts deal with civil claims for damages that may be unlimited in amount. The criminal jurisdiction of these courts deals with the most serious crimes (murder and child sexual assaults).

Court of Appeal A Court of Appeal is the Supreme Court's appellate jurisdiction. That is, the Court of Appeal will hear matters from specified courts and tribunals when there is a matter of law in dispute.

Federal Court The Federal Court has jurisdiction in a range of matters arising under federal law (as opposed to state and territory law).

Family Court This court deals with family disputes, and is able to pursue matters across state and territory lines because the court has federal jurisdiction.

High Court The High Court is Australia's most senior court, with jurisdiction over the Constitution, but it also has the discretion to hear matters on appeal from federal, state or territory Supreme Courts, and is thus Australia's ultimate appeal court. The High Court consists of a Chief Justice and six Justices appointed by the Governor-General.

Tribunals

Each state and territory has its own system of tribunals, which are less formal types of courts. They usually have a number of people sitting on a panel listening to the material presented to them. Often there is only one legally qualified person on the panel. The panel is otherwise made up of appropriately qualified professionals who are able to understand the material that is being presented to them. For example, on a mental health review tribunal, the tribunal is often made up of a lawyer, a psychiatrist and one other person, who may be a layperson with an interest in mental health, or who may be a mental health worker of some sort. Appeals from tribunals will be heard in a higher court.

The tribunals that paramedics are most likely to come into contact with include those related to mental health, workers' compensation, the Guardianship Tribunal, and the Civil and Administrative Tribunal if they are charged with a serious disciplinary offence that may see them struck off the register, like professional misconduct.

How to read law

Law can be confusing to research because it uses a specialised language. However, given that the law governs everyone every day, it is important to be able to find, read and understand it.

When looking up a case of Australian law, the best place to start is with a legal database. The Australian Legal Information Institute (AustLII) is a free public-access database.[13] It has all of the Acts and Regulations for each state and territory, and all of the cases from each state and territory's Supreme Court. Austlii also has material from New Zealand. Some states and territories have access to particular law journals that can be used for research. The Victorian law journal site[14] provides access to decisions made by the Mental Health Review Tribunal. The New South Wales site provides access to decisions made by the Guardianship Tribunal and the Nurses and Midwives Professional Standards Committee.[15] Hopefully this site will also provide access to decisions made by the Paramedic Professional Standards Committee. Having access to the cases and decisions made by each of these tribunals allows health practitioners to gain a better understanding of legal terms such as 'unsatisfactory professional conduct' and 'professional misconduct'. Being found to have engaged in misconduct may result in the loss of employment, so being aware of the terms and what the behaviour encompasses can assist in keeping paramedics and the public safe.

Legal case citations are often given in the following format: *Rogers v Whitaker* (1992) 175 CLR 479. Fig. 4.2 provides an overview of what each part of this citation is referring to. So, in this case, the 'Rogers' in '*Rogers v Whitaker*' refers to Dr Rogers, who was appealing a decision made by the Supreme Court of New South Wales, who had found him to have been negligent in his care of Mrs Whitaker, his patient. Dr Rogers is referred to, therefore, as the 'appellant' and Mrs Whitaker as the 'respondent', because she was responding to his appeal to the High Court of Australia. Mrs Whitaker originally sued Dr Rogers in the Supreme Court of New South Wales for damage she sustained as a result of Dr Rogers' failure to inform her of all of the risks involved in the ophthalmic surgery she underwent. As a result of the surgery, Mrs Whitaker lost the sight in one of her eyes. The Supreme Court agreed that Dr Rogers had been negligent in failing to inform Mrs Whitaker of the risks, and subsequently Dr Rogers appealed the decision to the Supreme Court of Appeal, who dismissed the appeal. That earlier case is recorded as *Rogers v Whitaker* (1991) 23 New South Wales Law Reports 600—or the abbreviated form: *Rogers v Whitaker* (1991) 23 NSWLR 600. Dr Rogers applied and was granted special leave to have the matter heard by the High Court of Australia, and that decision is recorded in the *Commonwealth Law Reports* (CLR).

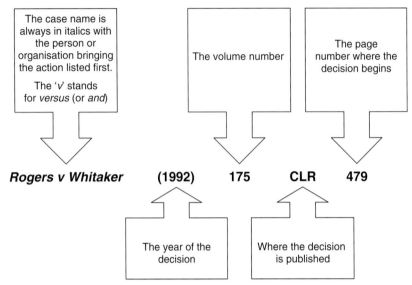

Figure 4.2 Legal case citations

Paramedics, professional regulation and professionalisation

In 2008, the Council of Australian Governments (COAG) established an intergovernmental agreement about health workforce regulation.[16] The aim of this arrangement was to improve health workforce portability across the Australian states and territories, while also providing for improved national governance of health professional regulation.[17] The new system established a single national registration and accreditation system for 10 health professions: chiropractors; dentists (including dental hygienists, dental prosthetists and dental therapists); medical practitioners; nurses and midwives; optometrists; osteopaths; pharmacists; physiotherapists; podiatrists; and psychologists. In June 2012, the Australian Health Ministers' Advisory Council (AHMAC) announced that four further health occupations—Chinese medicine practitioners, medical radiation practitioners, occupational therapists, and Aboriginal and Torres Strait Islander health practitioners—would join the National Registration and Accreditation Scheme.[18] Paramedicine joined the national scheme as the 15th registered health profession, in late 2018.

Objectives of national regulation of health practitioners

The objects of the national scheme are set out in section 3 of the *Health Practitioner National Law Act 2009* (Qld), and are as follows:

(1) The object of this Law is to establish a national registration and accreditation scheme for—
   (a) the regulation of health practitioners; and
   (b) the registration of students undertaking—
      (i) programs of study that provide a qualification for registration in a health profession; or
      (ii) clinical training in a health profession.

(2) The objectives of the national registration and accreditation scheme are—
  (a) to provide for the protection of the public by ensuring that only health practitioners who are suitably trained and qualified to practise in a competent and ethical manner are registered; and
  (b) to facilitate workforce mobility across Australia by reducing the administrative burden for health practitioners wishing to move between participating jurisdictions or to practise in more than one participating jurisdiction; and
  (c) to facilitate the provision of high quality education and training of health practitioners; and
  (d) to facilitate the rigorous and responsive assessment of overseas-trained health practitioners; and
  (e) to facilitate access to services provided by health practitioners in accordance with the public interest; and
  (f) to enable the continuous development of a flexible, responsive and sustainable Australian health workforce and to enable innovation in the education of, and service delivery by, health practitioners.

(3) The guiding principles of the national registration and accreditation scheme are as follows—
  (a) the scheme is to operate in a transparent, accountable, efficient, effective and fair way;
  (b) fees required to be paid under the scheme are to be reasonable having regard to the efficient and effective operation of the scheme;
  (c) restrictions on the practice of a health profession are to be imposed under the scheme only if it is necessary to ensure health services are provided safely and are of an appropriate quality.

These elements will be discussed in more detail throughout this chapter.

Reasons for regulation

The *Health Practitioner National Law Act 2009* (Qld) ('the National Law') is the primary piece of registration on which the National Registration and Accreditation Scheme is based. Regulation under this Act will allow paramedics to regulate themselves, rather than be regulated by their employers, thereby facilitating the professionalisation (self-regulation) of paramedicine in Australia.[19]

Because Australia is a federalised system and health is managed by each state or territory, in order to make the law uniform nationally, each state and territory has used the Queensland version of the legislation as a basis for their own respective state legislation, with some amendments to accommodate the particular state or territory's needs. For example, the NSW version of the legislation—the *Health Practitioner National Law Act 2009* (NSW)— makes reference to the Health Care Complaints Commission, which is a particular body set up for dealing with complaints against all healthcare practitioners (registered and non-registered) in New South Wales. Regulation under the National Law allows paramedics to regulate themselves, rather than be regulated by their employers (as had been the norm). Self-regulation is a big step towards professionalisation for paramedicine in Australia.[20]

Proposed amendments to the Act to include paramedics under the scheme (contained in the *Health Practitioner Regulation National Law Amendment Bill 2017*) were tabled and passed through the Queensland Parliament in September 2017. The amendment was adopted in all states and territories, thus authorising the national regulation of paramedics. The regulatory process commenced with calls for members of the inaugural Paramedicine Board of Australia (PBA). On 19 October 2017, members of the inaugural board were appointed for 3 years by the COAG Health Council. The National Law states that at least half, but not more than two-thirds, of the members of the national board *must* be practitioner members.[21] This demonstrates the element of self-regulation—the profession governed by members of the profession.

Self-regulation takes the form of the PBA having the power to set registration standards particular to paramedicine, as well as education and accreditation standards, which reflect the unique purpose, specialist knowledge and skills and role of paramedics. The appointment of paramedics to the board, along with the powers granted to the board to determine registration and education standards, exemplify the way in which the law allows paramedics to regulate themselves for the first time.

Regulation of paramedics will enable many actions to occur, including the tracking of sanctioned health practitioners across jurisdictions. Before registration, if a practitioner was found to have breached professional standards in one state they could travel to another state and work there. National registration will mean that individual practitioners can move more freely between employers because they have been assessed by the Paramedicine Board of Australia as being fit for registration, which means that practitioners will not have to be reassessed every time they move states.

The national register will also list publicly those practitioners who have restrictions on their practising certificates or who have failed to be assessed as fit for registration by the board. National registration also facilitates the rigorous and standardised assessment of overseas-trained health practitioners, which previously has not occurred. Both of these measures contribute to the establishment and maintenance of a flexible, responsive and sustainable health workforce, which is part of the objective of the national regulatory scheme for health professionals. The idea behind the scheme was to break down the silos between professions that have limited flexibility in healthcare delivery.[22]

National regulation also allows for the accreditation and the setting of national standards of all paramedic programs of education across the country by the PBA, which represents all paramedics in Australia, not just the ambulance authorities as had previously been the case.

National regulation will allow for the establishment of disciplinary bodies particular to paramedicine—such as the Paramedicine Council of New South Wales—to oversee the professional behaviour of paramedics by paramedics, and to act against members who do not meet the required professional standards and thus place patients at risk.

National regulation also allows for regulation of non-state-based ambulance service employees. Before the introduction of the national scheme, paramedics in the private sector were not regulated in the same way as those employed in public ambulance services. The national regulation of paramedics will ensure that those providing private emergency paramedic health services (not just transport services) will have to meet the same conditions for registration, education and practice standards as those employed in public health services.

These benefits of national regulation are discussed in more detail below.

Purpose of the PBA

The primary role of the national board, the Paramedicine Board of Australia (PBA), is to make decisions regarding the regulation of the profession in the public interest. The board does this by: as noted above, making decisions about the profession, including education and practice standards that reflect the unique purpose and specialised knowledge and skills common to paramedics; setting and enforcing disciplinary standards that reflect the conduct expected of a paramedic; and the power to determine who enters, and to some extent exits, the profession. As Eburn and Bendall note, regulation under the National Law means that only registered 'paramedics' who are subject to all of the safety mechanisms accompanying that title (including appropriate clinical and professional education and training, and a level of professional accountability associated with registration) are legally allowed to use that title.[23] This is designed to ensure that patients can make safe and informed choices as to who they allow to treat them, rather than trusting in good faith that those using the title 'paramedic' have the requisite knowledge and skill to do so safely, competently and professionally.

Professional standards

The functions of the Paramedicine Board are set out in section 35 of the National Act (discussed above),[24] but in short give paramedicine the opportunity to determine who will be deemed suitably qualified and competent to enter the profession. With the assistance of the Australian Health Practitioner Regulation Agency (AHPRA), the board will maintain a publicly accessible register of registered paramedic practitioners. It will be authorised to: impose conditions on registration; decide the requirements for registration and registration standards for approval by the Ministerial Council; develop or approve standards, codes and guidelines for the profession, including approval of accreditation standards; accredit programs of study to provide suitable qualification for registration in the profession; assess the knowledge and skills of overseas applicants for registration; receive notifications about persons who are registered with the profession (including students) and who are subject to conduct hearings on health, performance and professional standards; establish panels to deal with conduct and performance issues, and to refer matters to respective tribunals for hearing (with the exception that complaints handling and disciplinary functions in Queensland and New South Wales will be undertaken by their respective co-regulatory mechanisms); manage registered practitioners who have conditions or undertakings on their registration; provide financial or other support for health programs for registered practitioners and students; make recommendations to the Ministerial Council about specialist recognition; and give advice to the Ministerial Council about issues related to national registration and accreditation. These are all elements of being an autonomous profession able to regulate itself by setting its own standards—which paramedics, until they had commenced under the national regulatory scheme, were unable to do.

Registration standard

With regard to the registration standards (s 38), the national board must develop and recommend to the Ministerial Council registration standards; that is, what is required for a practitioner to be registered with the profession. The registration standards include the requirement that the registrant:

- hold professional indemnity insurance;[25]
- meet the criminal history requirements of the board;[26]
- meet continuing professional development requirements;[27]
- meet the minimum English language skill requirements;[28] and
- meet the requirements for the 'nature, extent, period and recency of any previous practice of the profession by applicants for registration'.[29]

In other words, registrants must demonstrate that they have been paramedics and continue to practise as paramedics. This is discussed in more detail below.

What is continuing professional development (CPD)?

The PBA has established that registered paramedics must complete 30 hours of CPD training every year to ensure that they keep their skills and knowledge up-to-date. The standard applies to all registered paramedics. It does not apply to students or those with non-practising registration. You must maintain your CPD portfolio for 5 years. Fortunately, both the Australian and New Zealand College of Paramedicine and Paramedics Australasia professional associations have online CPD folders available for members to record and store their CPD data.

What is 'recency of practice'?

'Recency of practice' is defined by AHPRA as the health practitioner having 'maintained an adequate connection with, and recent practice in the profession since qualifying for, or obtaining registration'.[30] The recency of practice provision developed by the Paramedicine Board may be important in determining who can be registered as a paramedic. There may be paramedics who hold the required qualification, but who have not practised as paramedics for a lengthy period of time. The board will have the power to determine the requisite amount of time that is, for example, required to show 'recency' of practice. This will help determine who can enter the profession, and be listed on the register. Determining entry to the profession is a core self-regulatory element common to all professions.

What is it to 'practise as a paramedic'?

Practising as a paramedic under the National Law does not just mean working on the road as a paramedic, or working in a clinical role. It can also mean, for example, working off-road in an administrative or management role, or as an educator. The PBA says:

> Practice for the purposes of the standard is any role, whether remunerated or not, in which an individual uses their skills and knowledge as a health practitioner in their profession. It is not restricted to the provision of direct clinical care. It also includes using professional knowledge in a direct non-clinical relationship with clients, working in management, administration, education, research, advisory, regulatory or policy development roles, and any other roles that impact on [the] safe, effective delivery of services in the profession.[31]

In other words, for the purpose of maintaining registration, it is possible to demonstrate recency of practice as a paramedic even if the registrant has not been working in a clinical capacity.

Why do a criminal record check?

The PBA will consider whether an applicant for registration is a 'fit and proper person' to join the profession and undertake the paramedic role.[32] Failure to meet this criterion can result in an applicant being denied registration, or a current registrant being removed from the register under section 5(c) of the professional misconduct criteria. This particular registration standard is not something that is applied to unregistered health practitioners.

The way in which a determination is made as to whether someone is a 'fit and proper person' to seek registration as a health practitioner is largely subjective. Although the terms themselves have no precise meaning, in essence the board will consider whether a registrant has a criminal record and, as a result, poses a risk to the public. The legal case in which disgraced former medical practitioner Geoffrey Edelsten attempted to be re-registered, after being struck-off for, among other things, being of poor character, illustrates the way the standard is considered by the courts. The court said:

> [B]y contemplating that a person's character may be a basis for refusal of registration … [the legislation] suggests … that protection of the public, and thus the public interest, extends to ensuring both the reality and the perception that the … profession is comprised of persons who are honest and trustworthy, and in whom the public … [including other professionals] may therefore have confidence.[33]

A criminal record can result from driving offences (e.g. driving while intoxicated), drug offences, domestic violence or other assaults. So those seeking registration, or who are currently registered, should protect their registration, which for many is their livelihood, by avoiding engaging in criminal behaviour.

Complaints handling and disciplinary action

To protect the public from harmful practitioners, the National Law applies a nationally consistent arrangement for the receipt of complaints and the management of health, performance and conduct matters related to all registered practitioners in Australia.[34] The National Law allows for disciplinary action to be taken against practitioners who do, or may, pose a risk to the public. For example, if a paramedic, in the practice of their profession, were to demonstrate knowledge or skill or exercise care that fell below the standard reasonably expected of a paramedic, then that paramedic may be found to have engaged in *unsatisfactory professional performance* and be sanctioned accordingly, with, for example, the requirement to attend extra training to help correct the gap in the practitioner's skill set that led to the complaint against them being upheld.

The board not only is responsible for overseeing various regulatory processes, including registration, but is also responsible for the 'receipt, assessment and investigation of complaint and other notifications' about the practitioners they regulate. The National Law provides for a national board to establish state, territory and regional boards to exercise its functions in the jurisdiction in a way that provides an effective and timely local response to health practitioners and other persons in the jurisdiction. Such a board for paramedicine has been constituted in New South Wales, for example. The national board delegates the necessary powers to the state, territory and/or regional boards,[35] and works with the Health Care Complaints Commission in each state and territory to ensure community concerns are being appropriately dealt with. AHPRA provides material to the respective boards to be dealt with by a professional standards panel or a tribunal, depending on the type and seriousness of the allegation made against the practitioner. The complaint will be investigated and, if deemed to have substance, will be sent to either a performance and professional standards panel to hear, respectively, allegations of 'unsatisfactory professional performance' or 'unprofessional conduct'; or to a tribunal for allegations of 'professional misconduct', the most serious allegation.[36]

Issues of poor professional conduct

The PBA may act against a registered paramedic if the board forms a reasonable belief that the paramedic has engaged in unsatisfactory professional performance, unprofessional conduct or professional misconduct. The terms refer to varying degrees of poor conduct, ranging from the least serious (unsatisfactory professional performance) to the most serious (professional misconduct). If a practitioner is found to have engaged in either unsatisfactory professional performance or unprofessional conduct, the penalties may include being required to attend further education, work under supervision, have another type of condition placed on their practice (e.g. not work with schedule 8 drugs); or report to a panel.[37]

Unsatisfactory professional performance is defined under section 3 of the National Law as:

> **Unsatisfactory professional performance**, of a registered health practitioner, means the knowledge, skill or judgment possessed, or care exercised by, the practitioner in the practice of the health profession in which the practitioner is registered is below the standard reasonably expected of a health practitioner of an equivalent level of training or experience.

Unprofessional conduct is defined in section 3 as:

> **unprofessional conduct**, of a registered health practitioner, means professional conduct that is of a lesser standard than that which might reasonably be expected of the health practitioner by the public or the practitioner's professional peers, and includes—
>
> (a) a contravention by the practitioner of this Law, whether or not the practitioner has been prosecuted for, or convicted of, an offence in relation to the contravention; and
>
> (b) a contravention by the practitioner of—
> (i) a condition to which the practitioner's registration was subject; or
> (ii) an undertaking given by the practitioner to the National Board that registers the practitioner; and
>
> (c) the conviction of the practitioner for an offence under another Act, the nature of which may affect the practitioner's suitability to continue to practise the profession; and
>
> (d) providing a person with health services of a kind that are excessive, unnecessary or otherwise not reasonably required for the person's well-being; and
>
> (e) influencing, or attempting to influence, the conduct of another registered health practitioner in a way that may compromise patient care; and

(f) accepting a benefit as inducement, consideration or reward for referring another person to a health service provider or recommending another person use or consult with a health service provider; and

(g) offering or giving a person a benefit, consideration or reward in return for the person referring another person to the practitioner or recommending to another person that the person use a health service provided by the practitioner; and

(h) referring a person to, or recommending that a person use or consult, another health service provider, health service or health product if the practitioner has a pecuniary interest in giving that referral or recommendation, unless the practitioner discloses the nature of that interest to the person before or at the time of giving the referral or recommendation.

Note that in New South Wales the elements of both unsatisfactory and unprofessional conduct are listed together as unsatisfactory professional conduct (*Health Practitioner Regulation National Law Act 2009* (NSW), s 139B).

Professional misconduct is defined in section 3 as:

(a) **unprofessional** conduct by the practitioner that amounts to conduct that is substantially below the standard reasonably expected of a registered health practitioner of an equivalent level of training or experience; **and**

(b) more than one instance of **unprofessional** conduct that, when considered together, amounts to conduct that is substantially below the standard reasonably expected of a registered health practitioner of an equivalent level of training or experience; **and**

(c) conduct of the practitioner, **whether occurring in connection with the practice of the health practitioner's profession or not,** that is inconsistent with the practitioner being a fit and proper person to hold registration in the profession. (Emphasis added)

Paramedics should note that the board has the power to consider the actions of a practitioner 'whether occurring in connection with the practice of the health practitioner's profession or not', which means that it may consider the conduct of a practitioner out of work hours that may be unrelated to paramedicine. This would include, for example, drink-driving out of work hours, or committing any other type of serious criminal offence as discussed above. The charge of misconduct is so serious, and the penalty so severe (i.e. potentially the loss of a practitioner's form of living if they are struck off the register), that the matters are heard by a tribunal which is headed by a lawyer. The penalties that may be imposed are outlined in section 196(2), and include:

(a) caution or reprimand the practitioner;

(b) impose a condition on the practitioner's registration, including, for example—
   (i) a condition requiring the practitioner to complete specified further education or training, or to undergo counselling, within a specified period; or
   (ii) a condition requiring the practitioner to undertake a specified period of supervised practice; or
   (iii) a condition requiring the practitioner to do, or refrain from doing, something in connection with the practitioner's practice; or
   (iv) a condition requiring the practitioner to manage the practitioner's practice in a specified way; or

    (v) a condition requiring the practitioner to report to a specified person at specified times about the practitioner's practice; or

    (vi) a condition requiring the practitioner not to employ, engage or recommend a specified person, or class of persons,

(c) require the practitioner to pay a fine of not more than $30,000 to the National Board that registers the practitioner;

(d) suspend the practitioner's registration for a specified period;

(e) cancel the practitioner's registration.

The type of offences that usually result in this type of serious penalty include when a practitioner has become impaired through drug or alcohol consumption or a health impairment, or has been involved in some sort of criminal activity that places the public at risk of harm if the practitioner were to remain on the register.

There is as yet no national data on the conduct and competence of paramedics. But behaviour that has been deemed to be unprofessional conduct and/or professional misconduct by doctors and nurses includes: inadequate or inappropriate testing, investigations or treatment; inadequate, inaccurate or misleading documentation/health records; missed, incorrect or delayed diagnosis or referral; communication in a disrespectful manner; inappropriate prescribing; inaccurate prescribing; failure to cooperate with the investigation; breach of undertaking; inappropriate sexual comments and inappropriate sexual conduct; unacceptable breach of confidentiality; inappropriate collection, use or disclosure of patient information; failure to provide adequate or accurate information; failure to assess the patient's capacity to consent; inappropriate sexual or aggressive behaviour; assault; failure to disclose or properly manage a conflict of interest; and having a health impairment that put the public at risk.[38] Because the work that nurses and doctors do is so similar in nature to the work of paramedics, it is likely that paramedics will also be found to have engaged in some of these poor behaviours once there is a national mechanism that will allow such information to be collated and analysed.

The most useful point of analysing the behaviours that commonly result in the sanctioning of doctors and nurses is that it can provide some clue as to what type of behaviours paramedics should avoid engaging in. An analysis of the behaviours listed above shows that these behaviours have one element in common, and that is that they have all resulted from a failure of the health practitioners to put their patient's interests first. Putting the patient's interests first is at the heart of healthcare professionalism. It will be necessary for the Paramedicine Board to ensure that professionalism and patient-centred care are incorporated throughout the paramedic curriculum through its powers to establish education and accreditation standards, so that a culture and ethos of professionalism in paramedicine can be developed, thereby protecting both the public and paramedics from legal action.[39]

An understanding of law and ethics will complement the paramedic's clinical skills and assist the paramedic to conduct themselves in a professional way, thus avoiding any potential charge against their character or conduct. If a paramedic practises competently, compassionately and safely—not so as to avoid a charge of negligence or professional disciplinary inquiry, but because it is in the best interests of their patients to do so—this gives the best evidence of the altruistic nature of their character, and is likely to keep both patients and practitioners safe.

Can paramedics be called to court to justify their actions?

If paramedics fail to treat a patient to the requisite standard, there is a possibility that they will be called to legally account for their actions (or omission to act) in a number of other ways, including civilly (negligence), criminally (manslaughter), or via coronial inquiry (reportable death), parliamentary inquiry or royal commission (service-wide governance). The legal standard of care, and associated legal requirements of paramedic practice, will be discussed in more detail in the following chapters.

In short, paramedics most often present to the Coroners' Court to provide evidence of what they found or what they did with regard to a patient who has died in a way that has required an investigation by the coroner. There are relatively few cases of paramedics being called to court on a charge of negligence, and therefore there is little in the way of evidence to suggest that paramedics should practise 'defensive medicine' in an attempt to minimise their chance of being sued for medical negligence. This is discussed in more detail in Chapter 6.

Policies and guidelines

The Paramedicine Board has powers under the National Law Act to develop policies and guidelines in order to establish a clear and transparent standard of practice for paramedics, and to set public expectations about the paramedic profession's values, culture and ethos. There are four main documents that are important for paramedics to be familiar with: the code of conduct for paramedics (discussed earlier in this book), the mandatory notification guideline, the social media policy, and the professional indemnity insurance policy.

Mandatory notification guideline

The Paramedicine Board has developed a registration standard with regard to the physical and mental health requirements for registration of practitioners,[40] and the suitability of individuals to competently and safely practise.[41] This is an important element of professionalism that paramedics have not, until now, had to consider. The National Law sets out mandatory notification requirements for health practitioners suffering from an impairment or a lack of knowledge, skill or judgement that may cause the practitioner to practise 'below the standard reasonably expected'.[42] This notification may be voluntary,[43] it may be made by an employer,[44] or by another health practitioner[45] or by an education provider.[46] There have been several issues raised by other health practitioners about the way in which the mandatory notification provisions should operate, because it raises concerns about the way in which practitioners who become patients should be managed.

Paramedics are specialist emergency service workers who are routinely exposed to high-risk and high-stakes situations in uncontrolled and unobserved environments. This places them at high risk of developing mental health conditions.[47] Under the National Law, the Paramedicine Board has established mandatory reporting guidelines that help individual paramedics decide whether or not they need to make a mandatory notification to the board.[48]

A range of studies have discussed the mental health risks and mandatory reporting requirements embedded in the National Law,[49] because the requirements raise the potential for professional conflicts to arise between competing duties. For example, practitioners have an obligation to maintain patient confidentiality, but also a duty to report practitioners they believe may place patients at risk because of their own impairment. This potentially creates a tension between treating practitioners' duty to their patient and their duty to the safety of the public, and it is regarding this point that a number of health practitioners and their representative bodies have raised concerns.[50] It has also been suggested that some mandatory reports of mental illness to the respective health practitioners' boards have been made vexatiously or unnecessarily, serving only to increase problems such as anxiety that had not reached the level of endangering public safety, and this has resulted in lobbying to have the law changed.[51]

However, at this time the law remains that a notification to the National Board should be made *only* when a reasonable belief is formed[52] that the practitioner-patient has behaved in a way that constitutes notifiable conduct;[53] that is, when the practitioner-patient's impairment 'affects or is *likely to detrimentally affect* ... the person's capacity to practise the profession'.[54] Monitoring of a paramedic's own or a colleague's mental health has not previously been a mandatory requirement for paramedics, but it will become a matter of professionalism that they will need to become familiar with now they are regulated by the National Law.

Social media policy

The professionalisation of paramedicine has occurred in large part because of advances in technology. The types of technological advances likely to disrupt the role of paramedics and the way in which they perform that role now and in the near future include the use of telemetry, drones, the automated driving of vehicles, and the use of electronic medical records/tablet,[55] medical apps[56] and social media.[57] Technology is likely to continue to disrupt paramedic norms of work, and this poses a challenge for present and future paramedics with regard to safely managing the increasing complexity of their practice and the duty to their patients. Addressing these complexities will require a commitment to not only the maintenance of clinical competencies, but also to the teaching and practice of professionalism, which is particularly important in times of technological and cultural change.[58]

This issue of managing advances in technology in the workplace has particular implications for paramedics because of the particular nature of the work they do. Unlike other health professionals, paramedics work in public places and with public crises, like terrorist attacks,[59] that attract public interest. There is an appropriate way in which paramedics can utilise this technology to protect the public interest while at the same time protecting individual patient privacy. However, there have been many examples, particularly in the United Kingdom, where paramedics have been encouraged by their employers to use technology like social media as a tool that serves to benefit the organisation rather than the public interest. This has resulted in both the public and the profession being placed at risk of harm. This has been discussed more extensively in other forums.[60]

The use of patient information for a marketing benefit is strictly limited under the National Law.[61] There are other laws that limit the use of patient information by public agencies in Australia, including the *Privacy Act 1988* (Cth),[62] (see further details in Chapter 10). The law is relatively weak in this area, and so there has been debate within the paramedic community about not only the legal issues involved in the use of social media by paramedics, but also the ethical issues involved with its use.[63] This is because, although there may be some benefits to using social media for educative purposes, the risks of compromising patient safety, confidence, and trust in the profession to maintain patient privacy—a fundamental element to the practitioner–patient relationship—are necessary to manage, and so the Paramedicine Board has adopted a social media policy that applies to not only paramedics, but all other registered health practitioners in Australia.

The key elements of the policy are that paramedics must comply 'with confidentiality and privacy obligations such as not discussing patients or posting pictures of procedures, case studies, patients, or sensitive material which may enable a patient to be identified without having obtained consent in appropriate situations'.[64] This reiterates the requirements to protect patient confidentiality and privacy, as stressed in the code of conduct.

Requirement to have insurance[65]

The *Registration standard: Professional indemnity insurance arrangements* issued by the Paramedicine Board of Australia says: 'When you practise as a paramedic, you must be covered by your own or third-party PII [Professional Indemnity Insurance] arrangements …'[66] Most paramedics will be practising as employees, and many as employees of state ambulance services. Those services will carry insurance, often under state or territory self-insurance schemes. By virtue of the doctrine of vicarious liability, those employers will be liable for any negligent practice by employed paramedics. Likewise, where a paramedic is working only as an employee, the employer will be vicariously liable for any negligent acts or omissions, and their cover should be sufficient.

However, things get a little more complicated when paramedics are no longer at work and respond to a case while they are off-duty. The unique nature of paramedic work is that, unlike nursing or medicine, it often happens out of the hospital, and so a paramedic who comes across an emergency on the way home from work and stops to assist could be said to be working as a paramedic, whereas a nurse or a doctor might be considered to be acting as anyone else would—essentially as good Samaritans. If paramedics are said to be working as paramedics in a situation like this, then they are required by the board to have professional indemnity insurance in order to comply with their registration requirements, because the registration requirement states that a paramedic can only practise as a paramedic if they have indemnity insurance. So while a paramedic acting in such a situation would likely be covered by the good Samaritan provisions with regards to any claims of negligent action under the various civil liability laws around the country—*Civil Laws (Wrongs) Act 2002* (ACT); *Civil Liability Act 2002* (NSW); *Personal Injuries (Liabilities and Damages) Act* (NT); *Law Reform Act 1995* (Qld) and *Civil Liability Act 2003* (Qld); *Civil Liability Act 1936* (SA); *Civil Liability Act 2002* (Tas); *Wrongs Act 1958* (Vic); *Civil Liability Act 2002* (WA) and *Volunteers and Food and Other Donors (Protection from Liability) Act 2002* (WA)—and so cannot be sued for stopping and offering assistance even when not on duty, they could still be disciplined by the board because they do not have insurance whilst practising as a paramedic, and therefore are in breach of a registration standard. It has been argued[67] that paramedics are *not* practising their profession in a situation like this, and so therefore should not need indemnity insurance, but the matter has not been tested in court, and the board is advising all registered paramedics to get professional indemnity insurance. A paramedic working for themselves should have professional indemnity insurance. Additionally, if a paramedic is called before a disciplinary panel on a liability issue, the legal costs involved will likely be covered by professional indemnity insurance. Nonetheless, it is wise to check exactly what the insurance covers before purchasing it, as this cost may otherwise have to be borne by the paramedics themselves.

Conclusion

The development of policies, guidelines and a code of conduct by the Paramedicine Board of Australia establishes regulatory standards and norms that will influence and shape the paramedic profession's values and identity. This will benefit not just the profession, but also the public the profession serves. It is critical that paramedics develop a basic understanding of the laws that govern their practice and the reasons for them. The objective of the laws that regulate paramedics is to protect the public and ensure that the patient's interests are put before those of the paramedic. If paramedics can apply this principle in their everyday practice, then both patients and paramedics are likely to be safe from harm.

Review Questions

1 List three main features of criminal law, and three different features of civil law.
2 List the two main ways in which laws are made in Australia.
3 What is the benefit of case law over statutory law?
4 How are human rights recognised in law in Australia? Give some examples.
5 Why is an understanding of the legal system important for paramedics?

Endnotes

1 Butt, P. and Hamer, D. (eds). (2011) *Concise Australian Legal Dictionary*, 4th edn. Chatswood, NSW: Lexis Nexis.

2 Townsend, R. (2017) The role of the law in the professionalisation of paramedicine in Australia. (PhD thesis, Canberra, Australian National University.)

3 Townsend, R. and Luck, M. (2013) *Applied Paramedic Law and Ethics* Sydney: Elsevier, p. 70.

4 *R v Kasian Wililo*, unrep, NSW Local Court, 20 January 2012.

5 See further details in Eburn, M. and Townsend, R. (2012, 8 February) Resignation now could help O'Shane preserve a proud legacy. *The Sydney Morning Herald*.

6 Parliament of Australia website. Online. Available: http://www.aph.gov.au/About_Parliament/Senate/Powers_practice_n_procedures/Constitution (accessed 27 November 2018).

7 Baum, F. (2008) *The New Public Health*, 3rd ed. Sydney: Oxford University Press.

8 *Ambulance Service Regulation 2003*, s 5(1)(a).

9 *Health Services Amendment (Ambulance Service) Regulation 2011* (NSW), s 11F.

10 Stewart, C., Kerridge, I. and Parker, M. (2008) *The Australian Medico–Legal Handbook.* Sydney: Elsevier.

11 *Mabo v The State of Queensland (No. 2)* (1992) 175 CLR 1.

12 British Medical Association. (2001) *The Medical Profession and Human Rights: Handbook for a Changing Agenda.* London: Zed Books, at p. 21.

13 Australian Legal Information Institute website. Online. Available: http://www.austlii.edu.au (accessed 11 June 2012).

14 AustLII Victorian Resources. *Victorian Case Law.* Online. Available: http://www.austlii.edu.au/au/vic/ (accessed 19 February 2019).

15 AustLII New South Wales Resources. *New South Wales Case Law.* Online. Available: https://www.austlii .edu.au/au/nsw/ (accessed 19 February 2019).

16 The author would like to thank Dr Ramon Shaban for his contribution to this section of the chapter.

17 Council of Australian Governments. (2008) *Intergovernmental Agreement for a National Registration and Accreditation Scheme for the Health Professions.* Canberra: Commonwealth Government.

18 Australian Health Ministers' Advisory Council. (2011) *National Registration and Accreditation Scheme for the Health Professions—Project for the 2012 Health Professions.* Online. Available: http://www.nras2012 .ahpra.gov.au/ (accessed 19 March 2011).

19 *Health Practitioner Regulation National Law Act 2009* (Qld), Sch, Pt 5.

20 For further discussion, see Eburn, M. and Bendall, J. (2010) The provision of ambulance services in Australia: a legal argument for the national registration of paramedics. *Journal of Emergency Primary Health Care* 8(4). Online. Available: https://www.aph.gov.au/DocumentStore.ashx?id=0e7356a8-1061-48c8-b352-e9773b8c7b4f&subId=408148 (accessed 28 November 2018).

21 *Health Practitioner Regulation National Law Act 2009* (Qld), Sch, Pt 5, s 33(4).

22 Read more about this in Townsend, The role of the law in the professionalisation of paramedicine in Australia.

23 Eburn and Bendall, The provision of ambulance services in Australia.

24 *Health Practitioner Regulation National Law Act 2009* (Qld), Sch, Pt 5, s 35.

25 Ibid., s 38(1)(a).

26 Ibid., s 38(1)(b).

27 Ibid., s 38(1)(c).

28 Ibid., s 38(1)(d).

29 Ibid., s 38(1)(e).

30 The Australian Health Practitioner Regulation Agency (AHPRA) defines 'recency of practice' in its regulation standards. Online. Available: http://www.ahpra.gov.au/Registration/Registration-Standards/Recency-of-practice.aspx.

31 Australian Health Practitioner Regulation Agency (AHPRA). Practice. *Glossary.* Online. Available: https:// www.ahpra.gov.au/Support/Glossary.aspx (accessed 14 February 2019).

32 *Health Practitioner Regulation National Law Act 2009* (Qld), Sch, Pt 7, s 55.

33 *Edelsten v Medical Practitioners Board (Vic)* [2000] VSC 565, at [36].

34 *Health Practitioner Regulation National Law Bill 2009* (Qld), Explanatory notes, p. 5.

35 Ibid.

36 *Health Practitioner Regulation National Law Act 2009* (Qld), Sch, Pt 1, s 6.

37 Ibid., Sch, Pt 8, s 190.

38 Australian Health Practitioner Regulation Agency (AHPRA) AHPRA Panel Decisions 2012–2013. Online. Available: http://www.ahpra.gov.au/Publications/Panel-Decisions.aspx.

39 Townsend, R. and Luck, M. (2013) *Applied Paramedic Law and Ethics*, 2nd ed. Sydney: Elsevier.

40 *Health Practitioner Regulation National Law Act 2009* (Qld), Sch, Pt 5, s 38(2)(a).

41 Ibid., s 38(2)(c).

42 Ibid., Sch, Pt 8, s 144(1)(b).

43 Ibid., s 144.

44 Ibid., s 142.

45 Ibid., s 141.

46 Ibid., s 143.

47 Paramedics Australia Mental Health and Wellbeing Special Interest Group. Online. Available: https://www.paramedics.org/mental-health-wellbeing/.

48 Australian Health Practitioners Regulation Agency (2014, March) *National Board Guidelines for Registered Health Practitioners: guidelines for mandatory notifications*. Online. Available: http://www.nursingmidwiferyboard.gov.au/Codes-Guidelines-Statements/Codes-Guidelines/Guidelines-for-mandatory-notifications.aspx.

49 Worthington, E. and MacKenzie, P. (2017) Doctor suicides prompt calls for overhaul of mandatory reporting laws, *The 7.30 Report* [ABC television]. Available: http://www.abc.net.au/news/2017-04-13/doctor-suicides-prompt-calls-for-overhaul/8443842; Goiran, N., Kay, M., Nash, L. and Haysom, G. (2014) Mandatory reporting of health professionals: the case for a Western Australian style exemption for all Australian practitioners. *Journal of Law and Medicine* 22, 209–220; Bismark, M.M., Spittal, M.J., Morris, J.M. and Studdert, D.M. (2016) Reporting of health practitioners by their treating practitioner under Australia's national mandatory reporting law. *Medical Journal of Australia* 204(1), 24; Avant Advocacy (2015) *Mandatory Reporting Position Paper*. Online. Available: https://www. avant.org.au/mandatory-reporting; Beyondblue are currently conducting a nation-wide study on the wellbeing of police and emergency service users, see https://www.headsup.org.au/news/2017/04/26/measuring-police-and-emergency-services-workers-wellbeing-at-work; Wolf, G. (2017) Compelling safety: reforming Australian treating doctors' mandatory reporting obligations. *Sydney Law Review* 39(2), 199–232.

50 Townsend, The role of the law in the professionalisation of paramedicine in Australia.

51 Ibid.

52 '[T]he assent of belief is given on more slender evidence than proof. Belief is an inclination of the mind towards assenting to, rather than rejecting, a proposition': *George v Rockett* (1990) 170 CLR 104, at [14].

53 *Health Practitioner Regulation National Law Act 2009* (Qld), Sch, Pt 8, s 140.

54 Ibid., Pt 8, s 5 ('impairment').

55 Davison, K. and Forbes, M.P. (2015) Pre-hospital medicine: a glimpse of the future. *Australasian Journal of Paramedicine* 12(5). Available: https://ajp.paramedics.org/index.php/ajp/article/view/242.

56 Hayes, C. and Graham, Y.N.H. (2017) Future of digital technology in paramedic practice: blue light of discernment in responsive care for patients? *Journal of Paramedic Practice*. Online. Available: https://doi.org/10.12968/jpar.2017.9.6.240.

57 Baron, A and Townsend, R. (2017) Live tweeting by ambulance services: a growing concern. *Journal of Paramedic Practice* 9(7), 282–286.

58 Wilson, I., Cowin, L.S., Johnson, M. and Young, H. (2013) Professional identity in medical students: pedagogical challenges to medical education. *Teaching and Learning in Medicine* 25(4), 369–373.

59 Sibson, L. (2012) Paramedics: ready for terrorism? *Journal of Paramedic Practice* 4(8), 439.

60 Baron and Townsend, Live tweeting by ambulance services.

61 *Health Practitioner Regulation National Law Act 2009* (Qld), Sch, Pt 7, s 133.

62 Privacy law in Australia does not provide for the comprehensive publication of health data through social media or other mechanisms, with National Privacy Principle 2, for example, providing a clear prohibition

on the disclosure of personal information other than in exceptional circumstances or as authorised by the person whom the information is about: *Information Privacy Act 2009* (Qld), sch 4.

63   Baron and Townsend, Live tweeting by ambulance services.

64   Paramedicine Board of Australia. (2018) Social media policy (interim). Available: https://www.paramedicineboard.gov.au/professional-standards/codes-guidelines-and-policies/social-media-policy.aspx (accessed 10 January 2019).

65   This discussion is based on and drawn from Eburn, M. and Townsend, R. (2018) Professional insurance for paramedics. *Response* 45, 20–21.

66   Paramedicine Board of Australia. (2018) *Registration standard: Professional indemnity insurance arrangements.*

67   *R v Kasian Wililo*, unrep, NSW Local Court, 20 January 2012.

Chapter 5
Consent and refusal of treatment

Bronwyn Betts

Learning objectives

After reading this chapter, you should be able to:

- identify the elements of a valid consent
- explain the circumstances in which consent to treatment is not required
- discuss the law relating to the refusal of treatment
- identify situations whereby a substitute decision-maker may provide consent or refuse healthcare for another
- discuss the law relating to consent and children.

Definitions

Adult A person who has reached full legal capacity—18 years of age in Australia, and 20 years in New Zealand.

Assault Unlawful touching of a person without consent, giving rise to criminal charges and prosecution.

Attorney A person who has been appointed by another to make decisions for them, and on their behalf, at a time when they are no longer capable of making decisions.

Capacity The ability to understand the nature, purpose and consequences of a decision.

Child A child or minor (see below) is a person who has not yet reached the age of majority; however, the definition of a 'child' for the purposes of providing consent for medical treatment may vary between jurisdictions.

Competence Used interchangeably with 'capacity'. A person who is deemed to have the capacity to make decisions about a matter is deemed to be competent.

Guardian A person appointed, usually by a court or tribunal, to make decisions on behalf of another who has impaired decision-making capacity.

In loco parentis In place of a parent.

Minor A person who has not yet reached the age of majority—18 years in Australia, and 20 years in New Zealand.

Parens patriae The jurisdiction of the court to intervene and make decisions to ensure the welfare of those who are vulnerable and unable to care for themselves.

Substitute decision-maker A person appointed to make decisions for, and on behalf of, another with impaired decision-making capacity.

Trespass Tort of trespass. Touching a person without their consent, or a threat or conduct that creates an apprehension that the said conduct will occur.

An introductory case

The embarrassed paramedic

A paramedic arrives on the scene to find a 50-year-old male patient experiencing severe chest pain. The paramedic determines that a glyceryl trinitrate (GTN) spray should be used to lower the patient's blood pressure and reduce the strain on the heart.

However, before administering the drug, the paramedic realises that she should ask the patient whether he has taken any erectile dysfunction drugs (such as Viagra) in the previous 24 hours; if he has, the GTN spray may drop the patient's blood pressure to a dangerously low level.

The paramedic decides not to enquire, as she is embarrassed to ask. She is also embarrassed to inform the patient that the administration of GTN can, in these circumstances, pose a significant risk because of the sudden drop in blood pressure.

The patient agrees to the administration of the GTN spray.

Has the paramedic obtained a valid consent for the administration of GTN spray?

This chapter will provide you with the means to determine the legal responsibilities of the paramedic in cases such as this one.

Introduction

Patients have a right to make decisions about medical treatment, whether to accept what is recommended by their health provider, to reject it or to choose one of a number of treatment options that may be available.[1] This right of choice is founded on the ethical principle of autonomy, and has been recognised by the common law in numerous cases before courts and tribunals,[2] and is enshrined in several statutes.[3]

In New Zealand, the right to choose is strengthened by the *Code of Health and Disability Services Consumers' Rights*,[4] which provides:

> Services may be provided to a consumer only if that consumer makes an informed choice and gives informed consent, except where any enactment, or the common law, or any other provision of this Code provides otherwise.

The right to make decisions about medical treatment would logically extend to include decisions about ambulance treatment and ambulance transportation to a hospital or health facility. It is therefore essential that paramedics appreciate the need to obtain consent before ambulance treatment is delivered, are aware of the various means by which consent can be provided, are knowledgeable of the elements of a valid or lawful consent, and are conversant with the circumstances in which the law provides an exception to the requirement that consent be obtained before treatment is administered.

This chapter will discuss the law relating to consent to ambulance treatment and transportation, including the potential consequences for you as a paramedic if treatment is provided without consent. Topics that will also be discussed include:

- consent and children
- consent from a substitute decision-maker
- refusal of treatment and transport.

Consent

To consent is to agree.[5] It is essential that the patient agrees to the treatment, and does so *before* treatment is provided. Consent can be provided in a number of different ways. It can be in writing, provided verbally or be implied by way of conduct or actions. Irrespective of the form the consent takes, or the manner in which it is provided, it is essential that the consent is valid; that is, it meets the legal requirements.

Paramedics, by the very nature of the work that they do, and the circumstances in which paramedic services are required, will often encounter patients who are not capable, due to their underlying physical or psychological condition, of providing a valid consent to treatment and ambulance transportation.

The law recognises that these circumstances exist, and provides, under a legislative scheme in each jurisdiction, a means whereby another person, a substitute decision-maker, may be authorised to provide consent to treatment and transport on behalf of the patient. In the event that there is no other person authorised to provide consent on behalf of the patient, the law provides an exception to the requirement of consent in circumstances where urgent and necessary treatment is required to avoid a serious risk to the patient's life, health or wellbeing.

Obtaining consent before treatment is administered is essential for two reasons. First, it respects the patient's right to make their own decisions regarding healthcare, and, secondly, it protects the paramedic from a potential civil claim (trespass to person) and/or criminal prosecution (assault).

Forms of consent

Consent can be provided in a number of ways. It can be provided orally, in writing, or be implied by conduct or actions.

Implied consent

Implied consent is probably the most common form of consent provided for a range of minor or routine investigations and treatments. The patient indicates, via an act or some form of conduct, that they have no objection to the treatment or procedure that has been proposed. For example, following a discussion about the need to check a patient's blood pressure, the patient may roll up their sleeve and hold out their arm, indicating they have no objection to the paramedic conducting this assessment. This would amount to implied consent.

Implied consent is only intended to apply in circumstances where the procedure is minor and where general knowledge of the procedure is commonplace. In circumstances where the patient is not familiar with the procedure, or has not undergone it previously, the paramedic is encouraged to obtain verbal consent.

The fact that the patient may have requested that the ambulance attend cannot be taken to amount to implied consent to conduct an assessment or implement treatment.[6]

Verbal consent

Verbal consent is probably the most common form of consent that paramedics seek and obtain. Following a conversation with the patient during which the paramedic provides information about the assessment's findings and the recommended treatment, the patient verbally agrees to what the paramedic recommends.

Written consent

Many healthcare agencies have standard consent forms in place that are used for the purpose of obtaining a patient's written consent for a specific procedure. Written consent is usually sought and obtained in circumstances where the proposed procedure is invasive in nature, or where the treatment carries considerable risk. As a general statement, and probably for practical reasons, obtaining a patient's written consent for treatment is not something that ambulance service providers require of paramedics. There may, however, be some exceptions to this statement.[7]

Elements of a valid consent

There are four elements of consent, and each of the elements must be satisfied for the consent to be deemed valid or lawful. The elements are:

1 The consent is voluntary.
2 The patient has been provided with sufficient information.
3 The consent covers the treatment that is to be provided.
4 The patient has the capacity to make the decision about the treatment.

Voluntary decision

When making decisions regarding treatment options, it is not uncommon for a patient to look for advice and support from others, most commonly family members and health providers. It is appropriate that this advice and support are provided; however, the decision that the patient ultimately makes regarding treatment must be their own, and not one that is made merely to appease another person.[8]

The decision regarding treatment options must also be based on accurate information, not false or misleading details that may ultimately influence the patient's decision.[9]

If the paramedic is suspicious that a patient has not made a voluntary choice about treatment options, and that they may have been unduly influenced by another person, the paramedic should evaluate the situation and, when doing so, consider (1) the strength of will of the patient, and (2) the nature of the relationship that the patient shares with the person whom the paramedic suspects may be influencing the patient to make a decision that may not be their own.[10]

The strength of will of a patient can be affected by factors such as pain, fatigue, fear and grief. A patient exposed to these factors could easily be placed in a position in which they are vulnerable, and in which it is possible that their wishes could be overborne by those of another. Paramedics should be alert to this possibility.

The relationship that the patient shares with the other person is relevant insofar as it may be one in which influence is a common feature. This is particularly pertinent in circumstances where there is a relationship that involves an element of dominance between the person and the patient. In view of the limited time that a paramedic will spend with a patient, it is unlikely that the paramedic will be able to ascertain whether dominance is a factor in the relationships the patient shares with others. However, it is important to be mindful of this factor, particularly when information is shared that indicates that strong religious and cultural beliefs may exist.

Case 5.1—*Re T (Adult: Refusal of Medical Treatment)*—highlights these factors.[11]

Informed consent

A valid consent requires that the patient is provided with details regarding their condition, the proposed treatment, the risks associated with the proposed treatment, and alternative treatment options where they are available. (Consider Case 5.2.)

Under the common law, a patient must be 'informed in broad terms of the nature of the procedure which is intended'.[12]

In New Zealand, the *Code of Health and Disability Services Consumers' Rights* provides that a 'consumer' has a 'right to the information that a reasonable consumer, in that consumer's circumstances, needs to make an informed choice or give informed consent'.[13]

Consent covers the treatment

The requirement that the consent must 'cover the act' or 'treatment' essentially means that the consent will only extend to, or relate to, the specific treatment that has been discussed, and to which the patient has agreed. Some authors describe this as 'specificity'.[14]

In some cases, the paramedic may consider that the patient's changing condition necessitates the administration of additional treatment or procedures that were not previously anticipated and so were not discussed with the patient. The scope of the original consent will not extend to include these additional treatments unless it can be demonstrated that they were provided out of necessity in order to protect the life and health of the person, and it was not possible or practical to discuss the additional procedures with the patient, and obtain their consent, before the procedures were performed.[15] See the discussion below in the section 'Emergencies', regarding the principle of necessity.

Case 5.1 *Re T (Adult: Refusal of Medical Treatment)*

Ms T was admitted to hospital with right-shoulder pain, chest pain and shortness of breath. She was 20 years of age at the time, and 34 weeks' pregnant. Four days prior to the hospital admission, Ms T had been involved in a road traffic crash after which she had been medically assessed. Hospital admission was not considered to be necessary at that time.

Ms T was diagnosed as suffering from pneumonia, and treatment was commenced. Her condition deteriorated rapidly. She was in severe pain, for which she was receiving a narcotic analgesic, her breathing was laboured and she was intermittently confused. Some hours later, Ms T went into labour. A decision was made to deliver the baby by caesarean section. Ms T informed the midwife and, shortly after, the doctor, that she did not wish to receive a blood transfusion should one be considered necessary, but that the doctors could administer blood substitutes. The doctor reassured Ms T that she would be unlikely to require a blood transfusion following a caesarean section.

Ms T's condition deteriorated further and a blood transfusion was considered essential; however, it was withheld due to Ms T's express refusal to consent to the transfusion. Ms T's partner and father sought assistance from the court and a direction that the blood transfusion be administered on the basis that her decision was not valid due to the undue influence of Ms T's mother.

Ms T's parents had separated when Ms T was 3 years old. Ms T's mother was a devout Jehovah's Witness and her father was not. Ms T had spent most of her childhood living with her mother; however, a custody order expressly forbade Ms T being raised as a Jehovah's Witness. When Ms T was 17 years old, she moved to live with her paternal grandmother, and then, at the age of 19 years, with her partner.

Ms T's mother had spent time alone with Ms T during the hospital admission, and it was immediately following these visitations that Ms T informed the hospital staff of her wish regarding not receiving a blood transfusion.

The court took these factors into account, along with other factors, such as: Ms T's vulnerable state evidenced by her severe pain, fluctuations in her state of orientation and the effect of the narcotic analgesia; the relationship that Ms T shared with her mother and her mother's strong opposition to blood transfusions. After reviewing each of these factors, the court concluded that the combined effect had resulted in Ms T reaching a decision that was not entirely her own.

Case 5.2 The embarrassed paramedic

A paramedic arrives on scene to find a 50-year-old male patient experiencing severe chest pain. The paramedic determines that they should use a glyceryl trinitrate (GTN) spray to lower the patient's blood pressure and reduce the strain on the heart.

However, before administering this drug the paramedic realises that she should ask the patient whether he has taken any erectile dysfunction drugs (such as Viagra) in the previous 24 hours, as, if he had, the GTN spray might drop the patient's blood pressure to a dangerously low level.

The paramedic decides not to enquire as she is embarrassed to ask. She is also embarrassed to inform the patient that the administration of GTN can in these circumstances pose a significant risk because of the sudden drop in blood pressure.

The patient agrees to the administration of the GTN spray. Has the paramedic obtained a valid consent for the administration of GTN spray?

Capacity

A valid consent requires that the patient has the capacity to make the decision at the time that the decision is made. Capacity is about understanding. A patient is said to have the capacity to make a decision, and is legally competent, if they have the ability to understand the nature and effect of the decision.

The terms 'capacity' and 'competence' are often used interchangeably.[16] A patient is said to lack the capacity to decide whether to consent or refuse treatment if: the patient is unable to comprehend and retain information that is material to the decision; and the person is unable to process that information and arrive at a clear choice.[17] See the section 'Capacity', below, for a more detailed discussion of the capacity to make decisions.

Circumstances where consent is not required

In very limited circumstances, a paramedic would be justified in providing treatment to a patient without consent. These circumstances would include:
- an emergency situation
- a non-emergency where a patient lacks decision-making capacity and requires treatment of some kind
- a situation where the law authorises prescribed treatment in very specific circumstances.

While the circumstances may be limited, the frequency with which paramedics may encounter a situation involving any one of these circumstances is high.

Emergencies

Paramedics are often required to attend a patient who is unable to provide consent and whose condition is such that urgent and necessary treatment is required. In these circumstances, the common law provides an exception to the need for consent. McHugh, in *Marion's case*, stated the exception in the following terms:

> Consent is not necessary … where a surgical procedure or medical treatment must be performed in an emergency and the patient does not have the capacity to consent and no legally authorised representative is available to give consent on his or her behalf.[18]

This common law exception is referred to as either the *principle of necessity* or the *emergency principle*,[19] and would apply in the following circumstances:

- It is not practical to obtain consent (e.g. the patient is unconscious, confused or unable to communicate with the paramedic).
- There is no authorised person available to provide consent on behalf of the patient.[20]
- Treatment is considered to be necessary to avoid a risk to the life, health or wellbeing of the patient.
- The treatment provided is reasonable having regard for all the circumstances.[21]

Most Australian jurisdictions have legislated to give effect to the common law principle of necessity. This has been achieved through the various guardianship regimes. The provisions in each jurisdiction differ slightly; however, for the most part, they achieve the same objective—that is, to authorise the administration of urgent treatment that is considered necessary to:

- save the patient's life, or
- prevent serious damage to their health, or
- prevent significant pain or distress.

There is some variation as to which health providers are authorised under these various legislative provisions. In some jurisdictions, it is a medical or dental practitioner or a person working under their supervision. In other jurisdictions, terms such as 'health provider' or 'health professional' are used. Table 5.1 sets out the legislation that operates in each jurisdiction, the circumstances in which urgent treatment can be administered, and the health provider authorised under the relevant legislation to administer urgent treatment.

Non-emergencies

Other than in the context of an emergency, there are very limited circumstances in which treatment or ambulance transport can be provided without consent. Authorisation in these limited circumstances is provided under various statutory provisions.

For example, the paramedic may be authorised under mental health or public health legislation to detain a patient and, thereafter, transport the patient to a health facility for assessment. This authority, and the circumstances in which it would apply, are discussed further in Chapter 9, 'Mental illness and the law in the pre-hospital emergency care setting'.

The guardianship legislation in each jurisdiction may also include provisions for the administration of treatment, other than emergency treatment, to a person with impaired

Table 5.1 Emergency provisions				
Jurisdiction	**Act**	**Section**	**Treatment**	**Provider**
Australian Capital Territory	*Guardianship and Management of Property Act 1991* (ACT)	s 32N	**Adults** Common law 'right' to provide urgent medical treatment without consent is preserved	**Health professional** defined as 'doctor or dentist'
New South Wales	*Guardianship Act 1987* (NSW)	s 37	**Adults** 'Medical or dental treatment' to save life, prevent serious damage to health, or prevent pain or distress Medical treatment includes a medical or surgical procedure, an operation or an examination normally carried out by or under the supervision of a medical practitioner, including prophylactic, palliative or rehabilitation care	**Medical practitioner Dentist** Person supervised by a medical practitioner or a dentist
	Children and Young Persons (Care and Protection) Act 1998 (NSW)	s 174(1)(2)	**Child or young person** Medical or dental treatment to save life or prevent serious damage to health	**Medical practitioner Dentist**
Northern Territory	*Emergency Medical Operations Act* (NT)	s 3(1)	**Adults and children** Surgical operation, anaesthetic or blood transfusion to prevent death or permanent disability	**Medical practitioner**
Queensland	*Guardianship and Administration Act 2000* (Qld)	s 63	**Adults** 'Health care' to meet imminent risk to an adult's life or health, or prevent significant pain or distress **'Health care'** defined as care, treatment, services to diagnose physical or mental condition carried out by or *under supervision* of a 'health provider'	**Health care provider** defined as a person who provides healthcare in the practice of a profession or in the ordinary course of business

Table 5.1 Emergency provisions continued				
Jurisdiction	**Act**	**Section**	**Treatment**	**Provider**
South Australia	*Consent to Medical Treatment and Palliative Care Act 1995* (SA)	s 13(1)	**Patient over 16 years** Treatment to meet an imminent risk to life or health	**Medical practitioner**
Tasmania	*Guardianship and Administration Act 1995* (Tas)	s 40	**Adults and children** 'Medical or dental treatment' to save life, prevent serious damage to health, or prevent pain or distress Medical treatment includes a medical or surgical procedure, an operation or an examination normally carried out by or under the supervision of a medical practitioner, including prophylactic, palliative or rehabilitation care	**Medical practitioner Dentist** Person supervised by a medical practitioner a or dentist
Victoria	*Guardianship and Administration Act 1986* (Vic)	s 43A	**Adults** 'Medical or dental treatment' to save life, prevent serious damage to health, or prevent pain or distress Medical treatment includes a medical or surgical procedure, an operation or an examination normally carried out by or under the supervision of a medical practitioner, including prophylactic, palliative or rehabilitation care	**Medical practitioner Dentist** Person supervised by a medical practitioner a or dentist
Western Australia	*Guardianship and Administration Act 1990* (WA)	s 110ZI	**Adults** 'Urgent treatment' to save life, prevent serious damage to health, or prevent pain or distress Treatment includes a medical or surgical procedure and treatment, palliative care and other healthcare	**Health professional** defined as 'a registered practitioner or any other person who practises a discipline or profession in the health area that involves the application of a body of learning'

decision-making capacity. The authority provided in these circumstances is restricted to the administration of treatment that is minor, uncontroversial and necessary to promote the patient's health and wellbeing.[22]

Refusal of treatment

Every adult person has the right to make choices about treatment, including the right to reject the treatment that is recommended by that person's health provider, even if that decision may result in otherwise avoidable death.[23] This right of choice is not limited to decisions that others, such as a family member or the attending paramedic, may regard as sensible or even rational.[24]

Patient-initiated refusal of ambulance treatment and/or transport to hospital is a situation that paramedics encounter on a regular basis.[25] The critical issue that the paramedic must resolve is whether or not the patient's decision to refuse treatment and/or transport is valid. This necessarily requires the paramedic to consider the requirements of a valid decision to refuse, and to conduct the necessary assessment that is directed towards these legal requirements.[26]

If the patient has provided a valid refusal, the paramedic must respect the patient's wishes, but if the decision to refuse treatment and transport is not valid, the paramedic must consider the patient's immediate health and safety needs and implement a course of action to ensure that the patient's life, health and wellbeing are not compromised.[27]

Provided that the patient has sufficient decision-making capacity at the time the decision to refuse treatment is made, the only other requirements of a valid decision to refuse treatment are that the decision is made voluntarily and that it relates to the situation that has arisen.[28] Decision-making capacity will therefore be the central issue in cases involving a patient-initiated refusal of treatment, and will be the focus of the paramedic's assessment.

In addition to the three requirements of a valid refusal, the paramedic is also required to provide the patient with information that will assist them in their decision-making.[29]

Informed choice

A decision by a patient in a hospital or health agency to refuse medical treatment is usually made within the context of a medical condition that the patient knows to exist, or is made with a conscious objection to a particular form of treatment that may be contrary to the patient's religious or cultural beliefs.

However, a decision to refuse ambulance treatment is often made in circumstances in which the patient has no prior knowledge, awareness or insight into the existence of an illness or injury, and no understanding of their immediate health needs and the potential consequences if those health needs are not addressed and treatment is not provided.[30]

If the patient is to make a choice regarding whether or not to accept treatment, and whether to accept the recommendation that paramedics transport them to hospital for further assessment, it is only logical that the patient be provided with information so they can make this choice.[31]

In the case of *Brightwater Care Group (Inc) v Rossiter,*[32] Martin J expressed the view that 'full information as to the consequences of any decision should be provided in circumstances where it is "perfectly feasible" to do so'.[33]

This requirement is reinforced in New Zealand by the *Code of Health and Disability Services Consumers' Rights,* which relevantly provides that a consumer has a 'right to the information that a reasonable consumer, in that consumer's circumstances, needs to make an informed choice …'.[34]

The information that a paramedic should provide to a patient, where it is practical to do so, should include: details of the clinical assessment and likely diagnosis; the treatment that the paramedic recommends; transportation to hospital for further assessment, if indicated; and the possible risks associated with the condition if the recommended treatment is not provided or medical supervision at a hospital or health agency is not accessed.

Voluntary decision

See the discussion in the section 'Voluntary decision', above.

Specific to the situation

The refusal must be clear and unambiguous, and must relate to the current circumstances. A refusal that is ambiguous is one in which the patient may make a broad statement regarding treatment, but fail to stipulate exactly what they are willing to accept and what they are refusing. For example, if you were discussing resuscitation with the patient and the patient said 'Do what you think is best, but nothing heroic', this would leave the paramedic in some doubt as to the extent of the intervention refused by the patient.[35]

The paramedic should clarify with the patient the precise treatment they are choosing to reject, for it is possible that the patient may choose to consent to some procedures but not to others. Or they may choose to consent to treatment, but not consent to transportation to a health facility, or vice versa.

Once it has been ascertained exactly what the patient is refusing, the paramedic should confirm with the patient whether or not they intend that their decision (to refuse treatment) is to apply in changed circumstances; that is, if the patient's condition were to rapidly deteriorate. As an example, see Case 5.3.[36]

However, if the patient's condition does rapidly deteriorate and no clarification as to consent or refusal to treat has been determined, the paramedic may act under the doctrine of necessity.

It is possible that the patient may have completed an advance health directive in which they have specified exactly what treatment or procedures they do not wish to receive. For a more detailed discussion regarding advance health directives, and the operation of these documents in these circumstances, see Chapter 7, 'End-of-life care'.

Capacity

The question of decision-making capacity becomes a central issue in circumstances where a patient is suffering from a condition that has the potential to cause some degree of cognitive impairment and refuses ambulance treatment.

While the test to determine decision-making capacity is a legal test, the assessment of capacity is one that is frequently, and necessarily, carried out by paramedics and other health providers in their respective practice settings.[37]

Case 5.3 Jehovah's Witness car crash

An intensive-care paramedic arrives on the scene of a car crash to find a patient conscious but severely haemorrhaging. After slowing the bleeding and providing the patient with a saline solution, the patient's blood pressure continues to drop, and she becomes unconscious. The paramedic is worried that the patient may die before reaching the hospital.

One promising course of action open to the paramedic is to administer packed red blood cells, which should help stabilise the patient. However, the patient informed the paramedic before falling unconscious that she is a Jehovah's Witness and does not want to be given a blood transfusion.

Did the paramedic determine the scope of the patient's refusal and whether or not she intended her decision (to refuse a blood transfusion) to apply in these changed circumstances?

Presumption of capacity

The starting point when considering issues of capacity is the presumption, at law, that every adult has the capacity to make decisions, unless it can be shown that this presumption is rebutted; that is, the patient is not capable of understanding matters relating to the decision at hand.[38]

Factors that can reduce capacity

The next step is to identify whether the patient is suffering from a condition that has the potential to reduce decision-making capacity. A patient may be permanently deprived of capacity as a consequence of a chronic and debilitating illness, a severe intellectual disability or as a result of a serious brain injury. Capacity may also be deprived on a temporary basis by such factors as: alcohol intoxication; the effects of drugs and other substances; hypoxia; confusion; fatigue; severe pain; or other manifestations of an acute illness or traumatic injury.[39] It is important that the paramedic is aware of the conditions and circumstances that could reduce capacity; however, the mere presence of one or more of these conditions does not, of itself, mean that the patient lacks capacity. The paramedic must assess whether the patient has the ability to understand the nature and effect of their decision.

Assessment of capacity

The common law test to assess capacity was formulated in the English case of *Re C* (Case 5.4).[40]

The original test involved three steps:

1 The patient is able to take in, retain and comprehend the treatment information.

2 The patient believes the information.

Case 5.4 *Re C (Adult: Refusal of Medical Treatment)*

Mr C was 68 years of age and suffered from paranoid schizophrenia. He was also delusional and thought that he was a doctor. The diagnosis of schizophrenia was made at a time when Mr C was serving a prison term for attempted murder. He was subsequently transferred to a secure psychiatric facility, where he remained for several years.

While an inpatient in the secure facility, Mr C developed a gangrenous leg ulcer on his right lower leg. He was advised that the only effective treatment would be a below-knee amputation, without which he would most certainly die. Mr C refused to give consent for a below-knee amputation, but consented to other forms of conservative treatment, including antibiotics and surgical debridement of the wound.

It was evident that Mr C's general capacity was impaired by his chronic mental illness; however, the issue the court was required to resolve was whether Mr C's schizophrenia and delusional state had rendered him incapable of making a decision regarding treatment for his gangrenous leg. That is, did Mr C understand the nature, purpose and effect of the treatment (below-knee amputation), and the consequences of refusing that treatment?

The court applied the three-stage test (referred to above) to analyse Mr C's decision-making process, and found:

1 that Mr C did understand and retain the treatment information
2 that he believed it
3 that he had weighed up the risks and benefits and arrived at a clear choice with respect to the treatment he wished to receive, and that which he did not.[41]

---

3 The patient is able to weigh up the risks and benefits of the treatment and arrive at a clear choice.[42]

Assessing a patient's ability to *retain and understand* treatment information could possibly be achieved by asking the patient to repeat, using their own words, what they understand the treatment information to mean. If the patient is cooperative and willing to provide an answer, this will make it easier for the paramedic to assess this first step.

Assessing to determine whether a patient *believes* the treatment information could be achieved by asking the patient to express, using their own words, what they think could be wrong (with their health) and how they think it should be addressed.[43]

Assessing a patient's ability to *weigh up* the risks and benefits in order to arrive at a clear choice may be achieved by exploring with the patient the factors they considered when making their decision, and what may have influenced them to arrive at the decision they did. However, it must be stated that the reason a patient makes a decision is relevant only insofar as it may demonstrate that the patient was able to weigh up information and arrive at a choice. The fact that the paramedic may not agree with that choice, or considers the patient's choice and reasons for making the choice to be illogical or irrational, is not relevant.[44]

Sufficient understanding

Capacity is assessed in the context of the decision that is to be made. It is possible for a patient to have capacity to make some decisions, yet lack decision-making capacity in respect of another decision.[45] The seriousness of the decision, and the gravity of the risk involved, dictate the level of understanding that is required.

> … the [health provider] should consider whether at the time [the patient] had a capacity which was commensurate with the gravity of the decision which he purported to make. The more serious the decision, the greater the capacity required.[46]

This issue has been the subject of considerable debate.[47] Some commentators have suggested that capacity is a yes/no proposition, and have interpreted this statement to mean that a greater degree of scrutiny is required by the health provider to determine whether the patient has capacity when the decision is a serious one.[48] The alternative and accepted view is that capacity is measured along a sliding scale, and, in circumstances where the decision is serious and carries a greater degree of risk, the patient requires a greater level of understanding of the nature and effect of their decision.[49]

In circumstances where the patient is making a decision that may have grave consequences, the paramedic should take great care to assess the patient's decision-making capacity, and seek advice if they are concerned that the patient may not understand the nature and effect of the decision that is being made.[50]

Outcome of the assessment

Option 1: Valid decision Where the paramedic has provided the patient with information relevant to their condition, and about the proposed treatment and risks, and thereafter considers that the patient's decision to refuse treatment and/or transport is valid, that is:

- the patient has made a voluntary decision
- the patient's decision relates to what is recommended, and is intended to apply in the current circumstances
- the patient has decision-making capacity that is commensurate with the decision being made.

The paramedic must respect the patient's decision, irrespective of whether or not they agree with it. This requirement was articulated by the then Queensland State Coroner in the following statement:

> In this case I consider the officers reasonably concluded that [the patient] had the capacity to understand the nature of her condition and their advice to her; she was therefore entitled to make an informed decision to refuse further treatment.

> Even though the ambulance officers did not agree with her, in the circumstances I consider they had no authority to compel [the patient] to accompany them to hospital.[51]

Case 5.5 Possible fall from a second-level balcony

Paramedics are called to attend a 27-year-old man who was found lying unconscious in a pool of blood on the concrete path under the balcony of his second-floor home unit. The caller also resided in the unit block, and was well known to the man. Before the paramedics arrived at the scene, the man regained consciousness and staggered to his unit. With the assistance of the caller, the paramedics located the man's unit and were able to gain entry. They found the patient lying on a bed and, when they announced their presence and inquired whether he was injured, the man demanded, in a very angry tone, that they leave his unit immediately. The paramedics persisted, and the man told them that he did not call an ambulance and that he did not want or need an ambulance, and that they should leave.

Option 2: Invalid decision Where the paramedic considers that the patient's decision to refuse treatment and/or transport is not valid, the paramedic should seek immediate advice and explore options to ensure that the patient's life, health or safety is not compromised.

Tip: Take care to document The paramedic should ensure that the ambulance record is completed and that it reflects everything that took place. Details should include:
- the assessment findings (both clinical findings and those conducted to determine the validity of the decision to refuse)
- the paramedic's interpretation of the assessment findings
- the information provided to the patient regarding the condition, treatment and possible risks (if treatment is not provided)
- the assessment of the patient's decision-making capacity.

Case 5.5 illustrates these concepts.

Substitute decision-making

In circumstances where a patient lacks the capacity to make decisions regarding their healthcare, a substitute decision-maker may be appointed, or authorised to make decisions on behalf of the patient. The appointment and authorisation of a substitute decision-maker is achieved by way of legislation that has been enacted in New Zealand and in each Australian state and territory.[52]

The legislative scheme in each jurisdiction—often referred to as the *guardianship regime*—creates a framework in which decisions for those with impaired decision-making capacity can be made, by the person appointed for this purpose, a health provider responsible for the care and treatment of the patient (in limited circumstances), or through a direction issued by the patient at an earlier time when their decision-making capacity was intact.

There is some uniformity between the guardianship regimes that operate in each jurisdiction; however, there is a lack of consistency between jurisdictions with respect to the terminology that is used when referring to various aspects of each scheme, including the names that are used when referring to a substitute decision-maker.

Paramedics will undoubtedly attend patients with impaired decision-making capacity and in circumstances where a substitute decision-maker has been appointed to make decisions regarding healthcare for, and on behalf of, the patient. The paramedic should therefore be aware of the following information as it relates to the jurisdiction in which they practise:

- How a substitute decision-maker may be appointed to make decisions for a person with impaired decision-making capacity, and the name of the document used for this purpose.
- The terms used to refer to a substitute decision-maker.
- When the substitute decision-maker's authority to make decisions is activated.
- What decisions the substitute decision-maker is authorised to make on behalf of the patient.

How is a substitute decision-maker appointed?

There are three possible mechanisms by which a person may be appointed to make healthcare decisions on behalf of another:

1 The appointment is made in advance, by the individual, at a time when their decision-making capacity is intact.

2 The appointment is made by a court or tribunal.

3 A decision-maker is authorised, under the relevant legislation, by default.

A person who has decision-making capacity can appoint in advance[53] an individual or a number of individuals, of their choosing, to make decisions regarding their healthcare should they lose, at some future time, the capacity to make their own decisions.[54]

In three Australian jurisdictions (Queensland, Victoria and South Australia), 'health care specific' appointments can be made by an individual; that is, the substitute decision-maker is appointed specifically to make decisions about healthcare, and not decisions relating to other matters.[55] In all other Australian jurisdictions (with the exception of the Northern Territory) and in New Zealand, 'general' appointments can be made by an individual; that is, the substitute decision-maker is appointed to make decisions about a range of matters, including decisions about healthcare for the individual. General appointments can also be made in Queensland, Victoria and South Australia.

In circumstances where a substitute decision-maker has not been appointed in advance, the legislation may identify a default decision-maker.[56] The default decision-maker is selected from a list of possible substitute decision-makers, set out in order of priority, who could be authorised to make health decisions for, and on behalf of, a person with impaired decision-making capacity. The list includes, for example, family members and those who share a close relationship with the person and have an interest in their welfare.

In circumstances where a substitute decision-maker has not been appointed or authorised by one of the two mechanisms referred to above, an application can be made to the relevant court or tribunal in each jurisdiction, seeking the appointment of a person as a substitute decision-maker.[57]

It is likely that paramedics will encounter, in the pre-hospital setting, both substitute decision-makers who have been appointed by the individual in advance, and have been authorised to make healthcare decisions on that person's behalf at a time when they are not capable of making decisions for themselves, and default substitute decision-makers.

Terms to describe a substitute decision-maker

The term used to describe a substitute decision-maker varies between jurisdictions, and in some jurisdictions different terms may be used to describe substitute decision-makers appointed by different mechanisms. Terms used include: *attorney, statutory health attorney, enduring attorney, guardian, agent, medical agent, responsible person* and *appropriate person.*

When can a substitute decision-maker make decisions for a patient?

The authority to make decisions about healthcare for, and on behalf of, another person is not activated unless and until the person suffers from impaired decision-making capacity. It is not uncommon for capacity to fluctuate, and it is the very nature of the patient's condition that may result in these fluctuations. In these circumstances, the authority of the substitute decision-maker to make decisions for, and on behalf of, the patient will depend on the patient's decision-making capacity *at the relevant time.*

What decisions can a substitute decision-maker make?

In most jurisdictions, a substitute decision-maker is able to make decisions to consent to and refuse healthcare for the patient. However, there are a number of limitations with respect to decisions to refuse treatment, and these limitations vary between jurisdictions. Table 5.2 sets out the various guardianship regimes in each jurisdiction, the terms used to refer to a substitute decision-maker in that jurisdiction, and the decisions that a substitute decision-maker is authorised to make.[58]

Case 5.6 provides an example of a scenario you may encounter.

Consent and children

As with an adult patient, a paramedic is required to obtain consent before treatment is administered to a child. An exception to this requirement would involve an emergency situation in which it was not possible, or reasonably practical, to obtain consent from either the child or a person authorised to provide consent on behalf of the child. See the discussion in the section 'Emergencies' regarding the emergency exception.

Questions that commonly arise when considering the topic of consent and children include:
- What age is a person considered to be a child?
- Who is authorised to provide consent on behalf of a child?
- What if the child's parent is not present at the time the paramedic attends?
- Can a child provide consent for their own treatment?

Table 5.2 Substitute decision-makers

Jurisdiction	Act	Substitute decision-maker (health-specific)	Substitute decision-maker (general)	Substitute decision-maker (default)	Authorisation (health-specific and general substitute decision-makers)
New Zealand	*Protection of Personal and Property Rights Act 1988*	–	Enduring attorney	–	Decisions relating to personal care and welfare
Queensland	*Powers of Attorney Act 1988* (Qld)	'Attorney' under an advance health directive			Consent and refusal of 'healthcare'[a] Cannot consent for 'special health care'[b]
New South Wales	*Guardianship Act 1987* (NSW)	–	Enduring attorney	Statutory health attorney	Personal matters and health matters Cannot consent for special healthcare
			Enduring guardian	Person responsible	Consent for medical and dental treatment
Victoria	*Medical Treatment Act 1988* (Vic)	'Agent' under an enduring power of attorney (medical treatment) s 5A	–	–	Consent and refusal of 'medical treatment'[c] Cannot consent to 'special health care'[d] Strict requirements regarding refusal *Refusal of Treatment Certificate* must be completed
	Guardianship and Administration Act 1986 (Vic)		Enduring guardian	Personal representative	
Tasmania	*Guardianship and Administration Act 1995* (Tas)		Enduring guardian	Person responsible	Consent and refuse medical and dental treatment Cannot consent for 'special treatment'[e]

Jurisdiction	Legislation	'Medical agent' under a medical power of attorney		Consent and refusal of 'medical treatment'[f]; Cannot consent for 'prescribed treatment'[g]; Limits on refusal
South Australia	Consent to Medical Treatment and Palliative Care Act 1995 (SA)	'Medical agent' under a medical power of attorney	–	Consent and refusal of 'medical treatment'[f]; Cannot consent for 'prescribed treatment'[g]; Limits on refusal
	Guardianship and Administration Act 1993 (SA)	Enduring guardian	Appropriate authority	Consent and refusal of medical and dental treatment, except where a 'medical agent' is available to act
Western Australia	Guardianship and Administration Act 1990 (WA)	Enduring guardian	Person responsible	Consent and refusal of medical, surgical and dental treatment
Northern Territory	Adult Guardianship Act 2009 (NT)	–	–	'Adult guardian' appointed by court can consent and refuse medical and dental treatment
Australian Capital Territory	Powers of Attorney Act 2006 (ACT)	Enduring attorney	–	Consent for medical treatment
	Guardianship and Management of Property Act 1991 (ACT)	–	Health attorney	

[a] Means the care or treatment of, or a service or procedure to diagnose, maintain or treat carried out by, or under the supervision of a health provider. Does not include first-aid treatment or non-intrusive examination made for diagnostic purposes. *Powers of Attorney Act 1988* (Qld), Sch 2, s 11.

[b] Includes: removal of tissue while alive for purposes of donation; sterilisation; termination of pregnancy; participation in research; electroconvulsive therapy; and psychosurgery. *Powers of Attorney Act 1988* (Qld), Sch 2, s 7.

[c] Means the carrying out of a operation or the administration of drugs or other medical procedure, but does not include palliative care. *Medical Treatment Act 1988* (Vic), s 4.

[d] Includes: sterilisation; termination of pregnancy; and removal of tissue to transplant into another. *Guardianship and Administration Act 1986* (Vic), s 3.

[e] Includes: treatment to render infertile; termination of pregnancy; and removal of non-regenerative tissue for purposes of transplantation into another. *Guardianship and Administration Act 1995* (Tas), s 4.

[f] Includes: treatment or procedure administered or carried out by a medical practitioner in the course of medical or surgical practice, or a dentist, in the course of dental practice, and includes the prescription or supply of drugs. *Consent to Medical Treatment and Palliative Care Act 1995* (SA), s 4.

[g] Includes sterilisation and termination of pregnancy. *Guardianship and Administration Act 1993* (SA), s 61.

Case 5.6 Daughter insists on hospital transport

Paramedics are called to attend an 85-year-old woman following a fall. The woman told the paramedics that she had stumbled when walking on the uneven floor tiles. Following a thorough assessment, the paramedics could not identify any serious injuries. However, they recommended that it would be prudent for her to be assessed by a doctor, and that they transport her to the local hospital for this purpose. The woman declined. The paramedics had no reason to doubt the woman's decision-making capacity. However, the woman's daughter was present and insisted that her mother go to hospital. The daughter informed the paramedics that she had been appointed as her mother's enduring attorney, and that they should comply with her directions and transport her mother immediately.

- Can a child refuse treatment?
- Can a parent refuse treatment for their child?
- How is conflict between a parent and child (regarding treatment options) resolved?

Who is a child?

The age of majority, or the age at which a person reaches full legal capacity, is 18 years in all Australian states and territories, and 20 years in New Zealand. It is at this age that a person is recognised as an adult. A person less than 18 years of age in Australia, and less than 20 years of age in New Zealand, has not yet reached majority. Terms that are used to refer to a person less than 18 and 20 years, respectively, include *child, minor* and *young person*.[59]

Although a person attains full legal capacity at 18 and 20 years, respectively, legislation in each jurisdiction may enable a person who is not yet an adult to make certain decisions,[60] or be deemed responsible for certain actions.[61]

Table 5.3 sets out the legislation that determines the age of majority in each jurisdiction, and the legislation that provides that a person can consent to healthcare from an age other than the age at which the person is deemed to be an adult.

Who is authorised to provide consent on behalf of a child?

As a general statement, the parent of the child is legally authorised to provide consent for treatment to be administered to the child, unless it has been established that the child is sufficiently intelligent and can understand the nature and purpose of the proposed treatment.[62] See the discussion in the section 'What is the test to determine whether a child has capacity to consent to treatment?' regarding a child who is capable of providing consent.

Parental rights and obligations are founded in the common law, and have been enshrined in legislation in both Australia and New Zealand. In Australia, the responsibilities of a

Table 5.3 Legislation—age of majority and capacity to consent

Jurisdiction	Act	Section	Age of majority	Capacity to consent (other than age of majority)	Section	Age	Treatment
New Zealand	*Age of Majority Act 1970*	s 4	20 years	*Care of Children Act 2004*	s 36(1)(2)	16 years	Donation of blood Medical, surgical, dental treatment and procedures
Queensland	*Law Reform Act 1995*	s 17	18 years	–	–	–	–
New South Wales	*Minors (Property and Contracts) Act 1970*	s 9	18 years	*Minors (Property and Contracts) Act 1970*	s 49(2)	14 years	Medical and dental treatment provided by, or pursuant to directions from, a medical or dental practitioner
Victoria	*Age of Majority Act 1993*	s 3	18 years	–	–	–	–
Tasmania	*Age of Majority Act 1993*	s 3	18 years	–	–	–	–
South Australia	*Age of Majority (Reduction) Act 1993*	s 3	18 years	*Consent to Medical Treatment and Palliative Care Act 1975*	s 6 See also: s 3(a)(i) s 4	16 years	Decisions about own medical treatment—provided by doctor or dentist
Western Australia	*Age of Majority Act 1972*	s 5	18 years	–	–	–	–
Australian Capital Territory	*Age of Majority Act 1974*	s 5	18 years	–	–	–	–
Northern Territory	*Age of Majority Act 1981*	s 4	18 years	–	–	–	–

parent with respect to their child are defined in the Commonwealth *Family Law Act 1975*, and include 'all the duties, powers, responsibilities and authority which, by law, parents have in relation to children'.[63] These responsibilities include the authority to make decisions regarding medical treatment.[64]

In New Zealand, the responsibilities of a parent or guardian are defined in the *Care of Children Act 2004*, and include 'all duties, powers, rights and responsibilities that a parent of the child has in relation to the upbringing of the child'.[65] Defining a 'parent' is not as straightforward as it may seem, however. Family structures vary greatly, and a family involving two biological parents and their children is just one of many such structures in which children may be raised. In Australia, the *Family Law Act* does not define 'parent', but refers to a parent as a person who has, by law, parental responsibilities for a child.[66]

For the purposes of providing consent to medical treatment, some jurisdictions have defined 'parent' to include any person who has parental responsibilities for the child or young person.[67] The authority to provide consent to medical treatment includes one or both parents,[68] and, subject to the existence of a court order that may stipulate otherwise, the authority exists irrespective of whether the parents are married to each other, separated or divorced.[69]

Can someone other than the parents provide consent?

In the vast majority of cases in which a paramedic will attend a child, a parent will be present and will be able to make decisions regarding treatment for their child. However, in some cases a paramedic may be required to attend a child who is not, at the time of the attendance, in the care of their parent, and it is not possible or reasonably practical to establish contact with the parent. Examples of possible circumstances in which this may occur include the following:

- The child is alone or in the company of other children, and no parent or adult is present. For example, the child may be playing in a suburban park or riding a push-bike along a bike path or road.
- The child is in the short-term and temporary care of another, such as a casual sitter/carer, family friend or older sibling.
- The child is in the regular daily care of another, such as a childcare worker, boarding-school supervisor or school principal.
- The child is in the long-term and permanent care of another person, such as a grandparent or other family member, and the child's parent has little or no involvement in the provision of the care or direction regarding how care will be provided.
- The child does not live at home, is emancipated from their parents, and may even be homeless.

If the situation involves an emergency, consent is not required for the administration of urgent and necessary treatment.[70]

If the situation does not involve an emergency, and the parent is not present and cannot be contacted, and there is no other person available who can authorise treatment for the child, it would be reasonable for the paramedic to provide all necessary first aid, which, in the opinion of the paramedic, is considered to be in the best interests of the child, and thereafter explore available options to ensure that the child's health and safety are not compromised.

If the child is in the short-term or temporary care of someone other than the parent, and the parent cannot be contacted, this person would most likely be able to provide consent for first aid and minor treatment—for example, the application of a dressing to a small abrasion.[71]

If the child is in the care of another person on a regular day-to-day basis, and the care that is provided is subject to directions issued by the parent, the carer would be authorised to act in accordance with those directions, which may also include directions regarding the provision of any medical treatment that may be required.

An example of a situation in which this may occur is where a child is in the care of a school principal at a school the child is attending, or the master of a school boarding house in which the child is residing during the school term. The parent's directions to the school principal or boarding-house supervisor may include directions regarding the healthcare of the child, including a general consent for first aid and previously prescribed medical treatment, in the event that it is required. It is unlikely that this general consent would extend to include treatments or procedures that were not contemplated by the parent at the time the general consent was provided.[72]

In circumstances where the child is in the long-term care of someone other than the parent or legal guardian, and the care is being provided on a permanent basis without involvement from the parent, the carer is said to be *in loco parentis* to the child, or 'in place of the parent'.[73] A person *in loco parentis* may be a family member who has assumed the responsibility for the care and upbringing of a child in circumstances where the parent is not able or willing to do so. In some jurisdictions, a person *in loco parentis* will have the same responsibilities and authority as that of the parent.[74]

Can a parent refuse to provide consent to treatment for their child?

A parent has the authority to provide consent, and to refuse consent, to treatment for their child. This authority is linked to the parental responsibility to care for the child and, as such, the authority to refuse medical and other healthcare is not unconditional. When making decisions regarding treatment for their child, a parent must at all times act in the best interests of the child.[75]

What constitutes 'best interests' is determined on a case-by-case basis. Courts will consider all factors relevant to the child's welfare; however, the dominant consideration will be the child's physical welfare. The best interests of a child in the context of decisions regarding medical treatment and other healthcare would, almost certainly, be that which achieves a state where the child is free from physical distress or discomfort, and where the child's physiological or psychological health is not at risk.[76]

The administration of treatment recommended by a health provider, which could reverse a situation in which the child may suffer irreparable harm or perhaps die, would most likely be deemed to be in the child's best interest.[77] There have been a number of cases in both Australia and New Zealand where the courts have intervened, in their *parens patriae* (welfare) jurisdiction,[78] to override a parent's decision to refuse lifesaving medical treatment for their child.[79]

What if the parent refuses to provide a paramedic with consent to urgent and potentially lifesaving treatment for their child? It is not possible or practical for a paramedic to urgently refer such a case to a court or tribunal to override a parent's decisions that may not be in the child's best interests.

Paramedics are often confronted with these time-critical dilemmas. In New Zealand and in each Australian jurisdiction, child protection legislation has been enacted to safeguard the welfare of children, and may be used in these circumstances, where it is practical to do so.[80] See Chapter 8, 'Protective jurisdiction', for a discussion regarding the child protection schemes and how they operate.

If the situation is one in which the child's condition is grave, and urgent lifesaving treatment is required, the paramedic may need to explore alternative options. In the case of *Gillick v West Norfolk Area Health Authority* (*Gillick's case*), Lord Templeton made the following statement, which may serve as a guide for paramedics and other health providers confronted with these difficult and time critical circumstances:

> Where a doctor and parent disagree, the court can decide and is not slow to act. I accept that if there is not time to obtain a decision from the court, a doctor may safely carry out treatment in an emergency if the doctor believes the treatment to be vital to the survival or health of an infant and notwithstanding the opposition of a parent or the impossibility of alerting the parent before the treatment is carried out. In such a case the doctor must have the courage of his convictions that the treatment is necessary and urgent in the interests of the patient and the court will, if necessary, approve after the event treatment which the court would have authorised in advance, even if the treatment proves to be unsuccessful.[81]

Case 5.7 provides an example of time-critical circumstances.

Can a child provide consent for their own treatment?

There is no set age at which all children are deemed capable of making decisions about healthcare, including the decision to consent to treatment. Legislation in South Australia, New South Wales and New Zealand each sets an age at which a child in those jurisdictions can provide consent to treatment. Table 5.3 sets out the legislation in each jurisdiction, indicating the age at which a child can consent to treatment, and the type of treatment to which a child can consent.

In South Australia, a child is authorised to make decisions about medical and dental treatment provided by either a doctor or a dentist, and can do so from the age of 16.[82] In New South Wales, if a child aged 14 years or above provides consent, that consent will be sufficient to defend a claim of assault or battery in relation to the medical or dental treatment that was provided to the child.[83] In New Zealand, a child from the age of 16 can make decisions regarding medical, surgical and dental treatment or procedures, and can also consent to the donation of blood.[84]

If a child marries, parental responsibility comes to an end, and thereafter the child can consent to treatment irrespective of their age.[85]

Under the common law in Australia and New Zealand,[86] a child or young person may have capacity to consent to treatment if the child is sufficiently intelligent and has the ability to fully understand the nature and purpose of the proposed treatment.[87] This

Case 5.7 Snake bite

Paramedics working in a rural coastal community are called to a local primary school to attend a 10-year-old boy who has been bitten on the leg by a brown snake. The highly venomous brown snake is well known to the area, and there have been several recent sightings of this particular snake in the school grounds.

First-aid treatment is applied immediately. The boy's parents are notified. They provide instructions that the child is not to go to hospital, but to be kept quiet and in a darkened room. They advise that they will collect him from school during the afternoon, and will take him to a herbalist who will be able to administer natural therapies to counteract the snake venom. The paramedic speaks directly with the parent, and informs her that it is possible that the brown snake that bit the boy is one of the highly venomous species, and if this is the case the appropriate antivenene must be administered as a matter of urgency, otherwise the boy will die.

Are the parents of this 10-year-old boy acting in the child's best interests?

What course of action should the paramedics take?

common law position is based on the 1986 decision of the English House of Lords in *Gillick's case* (Case 5.8),[88] which was subsequently adopted by the High Court of Australia in *Secretary, Department of Health and Community Services v JWB and SMB* ('*Marion's case*').[89]

What is the test to determine whether a child has capacity to consent to treatment?

The test to determine whether a young person has the capacity to consent to treatment is the *Gillick test* or the *mature minor test*. A young person is said to be *Gillick competent* if they demonstrate that they fully understand the nature and purpose of that which is proposed.[90] The test focuses on the individual level of maturity and intellect of the young person, and whether they can understand fully the potential seriousness of their condition and the consequences of the treatment options.

The nature of the decision to be made, and the circumstances in which it is made, are relevant factors in determining Gillick competency. It is possible that a young person may be capable of understanding a decision relating to a minor procedure, yet is not capable of fully understanding one in which the clinical issues are complex and the potential consequences are grave.[91]

The *Gillick principle*, and what is required to be assessed in order to determine *Gillick* competency, is clear. The court or the health provider conducting the assessment must be satisfied that the young person:

Case 5.8 *Gillick's case*

The Department of Health and Social Security issued guidelines regarding family planning services to each of the area health authorities in England and Wales. The guidelines addressed a range of matters relating to family planning services, including the provision of services to people under the age of 16.[92]

While the guidelines recommended that people under 16 should be encouraged to involve a parent when availing themselves of the family planning services, it provided that doctors could exercise their clinical judgement in each case, and determine whether contraceptive advice, and a prescription for oral contraception, should be provided without the knowledge or consent of a parent of the young person.

Mrs Gillick, a mother of five young girls, sought an assurance from the area health authority that contraceptive advice and treatment would not be provided to her daughters without her consent. The health authority refused to provide Mrs Gillick with an assurance that this would not occur. Mrs Gillick then commenced legal action, seeking a declaration from the court that the guidelines, and the practice which it supported, were unlawful.

The House of Lords refused to grant the declaration that was sought, and held that the guidelines were lawful, because a child under the age of 16 is capable of providing consent to medical treatment, 'if the child has sufficient understanding and intelligence to enable him or her to understand fully what is proposed'.[93]

- is mature
- is intelligent
- fully understands the proposed treatment and consequences, and
- has a level of understanding commensurate with the seriousness of decision.

What is less clear is the means by which this test is applied in the various clinical settings in which young people are provided with healthcare.[94] Factors that may be helpful and should be considered include:[95]

- the age of the young person
- the young person's level of maturity and intellect
- the nature of the young person's condition and the seriousness of the decision to be made
- the young person's ability to take in, retain and comprehend fully the treatment that is proposed
- the young person's ability to understand the health and broader consequences of the decision

- the young person's psychological state at the time, and
- any medical or other health assessments that may be relevant.

Can a child refuse treatment?

The legislative schemes in both South Australia and New Zealand that provide authority for a young person to consent to healthcare before reaching full legal capacity, also provide authority for a young person to refuse treatment. In the remaining jurisdictions, the common law applies.

In South Australia, the *Consent to Medical Treatment and Palliative Care Act 1995* authorises a person over 16 years of age to 'make decisions' about medical and dental treatment,[96] and a child less than 16 years of age to provide consent for medical treatment, if the medical practitioner who is to administer the treatment, and one other medical practitioner who is to examine the patient, are of the opinion that the patient is capable of understanding the nature, consequences and risks of the treatment, and the treatment that is to be administered is in the best interests of the child.[97] In relation to decisions made by a person over 16 years, there is nothing in the Act that indicates a decision would be limited to only those decisions involving a consent to treatment.

In New Zealand, the *Care of Children Act* provides that the 'consent or refusal of consent' of a young person aged 16 or over, or a young person of any age if that person is married or living in a de facto relationship, will have the same effect as if the consent or refusal of consent was provided by a person of full age.[98] In addition to the provisions of the *Care of Children Act*, the *New Zealand Bill of Rights Act*,[99] which applies to both adults and children in New Zealand, expressly states that 'every person has a right to refuse to undergo medical treatment'.[100]

The remaining Australian jurisdictions rely on the common law principles enunciated in *Gillick's case* to determine whether a young person less than 18 years of age has the capacity to make decisions regarding healthcare and medical treatment. The *Gillick* principles would also apply to determine whether a young person in New Zealand, who is less than 16 years of age, had the capacity to decide to refuse treatment.[101]

Gillick's case focused on the capacity of a young person to consent to medical treatment, and did not specifically address the issue of a young person's capacity to make decisions to refuse medical treatment. Subsequent English decisions have concluded that a *Gillick*-competent young person cannot refuse treatment if that refusal is contrary to the wishes of the young person's parent.[102] This approach has not been adopted in Australia.[103]

In Australia, a *Gillick*-competent young person can refuse to consent to treatment, and can do so even if that decision is contrary to the wishes of their parent. However, the young person's decision to refuse must not be contrary to their own best interest. A court, in its *parens patriae* jurisdiction, can intervene and override the young person's decision if it considers that the young person's best interests would be served by the administration of the treatment that is the subject of the refusal.[104]

What if a *Gillick*-competent young person refuses to consent to urgent and potentially lifesaving ambulance treatment and transportation to hospital? It is not possible or practical for a paramedic to urgently refer such a case to a court or a tribunal to review the young person's decision and determine whether it is in their own best interests. Paramedics are

Case 5.9 Fall from a horse

Paramedics are called to attend a 15-year-old girl following a fall from a horse. The young girl had been riding with friends when her horse spooked, throwing her to the ground. She has suffered a compound fracture to her femur, and is losing a significant amount of blood from the open wound. When the paramedics arrive, she is pale, clammy, hypotensive and in severe pain.

Her friends have been trying to contact her parents, but neither of them is answering their mobile phones.

The paramedics decide that the fractured limb needs to be splinted immediately, and that an intravenous infusion and pain relief are necessary. The young girl refuses to allow the paramedics to splint her leg or provide any of the treatments discussed. She asks them if they can take her home.

How would the paramedics determine if this 15-year-old is *Gillick*-competent?

What factors may be relevant when turning their mind to the issue of *Gillick* competence in this 15-year-old patient?

What lawful course of action is available to the paramedics in this case?

often confronted with these time-critical dilemmas. If there is any doubt as to the capacity of the young person to make a decision about treatment, or doubt regarding the decision that has been made (in terms of it being in the person's own best interests), the paramedic should seek immediate advice and transport the young person to a hospital or health facility where these decisions can be made, including the decision to refer the matter urgently to a court or a tribunal. For example, see Case 5.9.[105]

Conclusion

The ethical principle underpinning this area of the law is patient autonomy. A patient has an autonomous right to make decisions that affect their own body, and the laws relating to the consent and refusal of healthcare, and that which facilitates substitute decision-making, protect and preserve this right.

The aim of this chapter was to introduce you to these areas of the law, and to provide guidelines that may assist you as you apply these laws in your everyday practice.

It is not possible to create a checklist that can be readily applied by paramedics in all cases. However, an understanding of the principles that underpin the law of consent and refusal, coupled with the guidelines provided in this chapter, will assist you to make appropriate decisions within a legal framework, and ultimately act in a manner that respects patient autonomy.

Review Questions

1 What are the elements of a valid consent for treatment?

2 A person is presumed to have capacity to make decisions regarding healthcare. How would a paramedic assess whether a patient has decision-making capacity for a matter?

3 When can a substitute decision-maker make healthcare decisions for, and on behalf of, another?

4 Who is authorised by law to provide consent for a child?

5 What is the common law test to determine whether a child is capable of providing consent for treatment? What does the code of conduct say about informed consent?

6 Can a parent refuse to provide consent for treatment?

7 In what circumstances would a court intervene and override a parent's decision to refuse to provide consent for treatment for their child?

Endnotes

1 A person cannot demand that a form of treatment be provided, if the medical practitioner is of the opinion that the treatment is not indicated and will offer no benefit.

2 *Schloendorff v Society of New York Hospital* 105 NE 92 (NY 1914); *Secretary, Department of Health and Community Services (NT) v JWB and SMB (Marion's case)* (1992) 175 CLR 218.

3 The *New Zealand Bill of Rights Act 1990*, the *Code of Health and Disability Services Consumers' Rights*, and the guardianship legislation in each jurisdiction protect the right to make decisions in advance, and preserve the requirement that treatment is provided in accordance with the patient's wishes.

4 *Code of Health and Disability Services Consumers' Rights*, Right 7(1), discussed in Skegg, P. (2006) Consent to treatment: introduction. In: P. Skegg and R. Paterson, R. (eds), *Medical Law in New Zealand* (pp. 145–169). Wellington: Thomson Brookers; Manning, J. (2002) Autonomy and the competent patient's right to refuse life-prolonging medical treatment—again. *Journal of Law and Medicine* 10(2), 239–247.

5 The term 'consent' is derived from the Latin *consensere*, meaning 'to agree'.

6 *Hart v Herron* (1984) Aust Torts Reports ¶80-201, discussed in Forrester, K. and Griffiths, D. (2010) *Essentials of Law for Health Professionals*, 3rd ed. Sydney: Elsevier. The case involved a patient who presented to a psychiatric hospital seeking information about deep sleep and electroconvulsive therapy, which the patient was scheduled to undergo. The patient was in an agitated state and agreed to take medication to 'calm him down'. The deep sleep and electroconvulsive therapy was then provided to him without his knowledge. The hospital argued that his presentation to the facility for the purposes of the treatment was implied consent. The court rejected this proposition.

7 For example, paramedics in Queensland are required to obtain written consent from a patient prior to the administration of thrombolytic therapy. This is also the case for paramedics employed by the Wellington Free Ambulance in New Zealand. Written consent may also be required if the proposed treatment forms part of a clinical trial.

8 *Re T (Adult: Refusal of Medical Treatment)* [1992] 4 All ER 649; *Beausoleil v La Communauté des Soeurs de la Charité de la Providence et al (Sisters of Charity)* (1964) 53 DLR 65.

9 *Appleton v Garrett* (1997) 8 Med LR 75. Right 6(3) of the New Zealand *Code of Health and Disability Services Consumers' Rights* sets out providers' obligations to provide honest and accurate answers to questions relating to services, including a recommendation from the provider: Right 6(3)(b).

10 These factors were considered by the court in *Re T (Adult: Refusal of Medical Treatment)*. See Case 5.1.

11 Ibid.

12 *Chatterton v Gerson* (1981) QB 432, at 443. Cited with approval in *Rogers v Whitaker* (1992) 175 CLR 479, at 490. In addition to the requirement that the patient is informed in broad terms for the purposes of providing consent, a doctor has a duty to inform a patient of any material or significant risk associated with the treatment that is to be provided. A failure to do so may give rise to an action in negligence in circumstances where the patient suffers harm.

13 *Code of Health and Disability Services Consumers' Rights*, Right 6. For a detailed analysis of this right, and what constitutes sufficient information to make an 'informed choice', see Skegg, P. (2006) The duty to inform and legally effective consent. In: P. Skegg and R. Paterson (eds), *Medical Law in New Zealand* (pp. 105–253). Wellington: Thomson Brookers, at pp. 222–227.

14 See, for example, Stewart, C., Kerridge, I. and Parker, M. (2008) *The Australian Medico–Legal Handbook*. Sydney: Elsevier.

15 *Murray v McMurchy* [1949] 2 DLR 442; *Walker v Bradley*, unrep, District Court of New South Wales, No. 1919/89, 22 December 1993.

16 Both terms are used to refer to the legal requirement that a person understands the nature and effect of a particular decision. The case law dealing with matters relating to this requirement in the context of a decision to consent or refuse medical treatment predominately uses the term 'capacity'. The term 'capacity' will be used in this chapter.

17 *Re MB (Medical Treatment)* [1997] 2 FCR 426; *Re B (Adult: Refusal of Medical Treatment)* [2002] 2 All ER 449.

18 *Marion's case*, at 310.

19 Historically, the terms 'necessity' and 'emergency' have referred to different circumstances in which it was appropriate to act without consent. In *Re F (Mental Patient: Sterilisation)* [1990] 2 AC 1, at 75–77, Lord Goff differentiated between the two terms in the following way: *necessity* applied to circumstances involving a patient who lacked decision-making capacity on a permanent or semi-permanent basis, and where treatment or care was necessary for the health and wellbeing of the patient. *Emergency*, however, involved a situational crisis in which treatment was necessary to preserve life. There does not appear to be any distinction drawn between the two terms in Australia, and both are used interchangeably to justify treatment without consent in circumstances where it is necessary to act. See *Hunter and New England Area Health Services v A* (2009) 74 NSWLR 88, at [31]–[33]. See discussion in Richards, B. (2010) General principles of consent to medical treatment. In: B. White, F. McDonald and L. Willmott (eds), *Health Law in Australia* (pp. 93–111). Sydney: Thomson Reuters, at p. 109.

20 For example, a health attorney appointed or authorised under legislation. See the section, 'Substitute decision-making' in this chapter.

21 *Rogers v Whitaker* (1992) 175 CLR 479, at 489; *Hunter and New England Area Health Service v A* (2009) 74 NSWLR 88, at [31].

22 In New South Wales, the *Guardianship Act 1987* (NSW), s 37(2); and Queensland, the *Guardianship and Administration Act 2000* (Qld), s 64.

23 This right has been recognised in each of the major common law jurisdictions, including the United Kingdom, Canada, New Zealand and, most recently, in Australia. See *Re B (Adult: Refusal of Medical Treatment)* [2002] 2 All ER 449; *Re C (Adult: Refusal of Medical Treatment)* [1994] 1 All ER 819; *Re T (Adult: Refusal of Medical Treatment)* [1992] 4 All ER 649; *Malette v Schulman* (1990) 67 DLR (4th) 321; *Re G* [1997] 2 NZLR 201; *Auckland Area Health Board v A-G (NZ)* [1993] 1 NZLR 235; *Hunter and*

New England Area Health Service v A (2009) 74 NSWLR 88; *Brightwater Care Group (Inc) v Rossiter* (2009) 40 WAR 84; *Australian Capital Territory v JT* (2009) 232 FLR 322; *H Ltd v J* (2010) 240 FLR 402. The right has also been strengthened in New Zealand by the *Code of Health and Disability Services Consumers' Rights*, Right 7(7), and the *Bill of Rights Act 1990*, s 11.

24 *Re T (Adult: Refusal of Medical Treatment)*, at 653.

25 There is no publicly accessible data in Australia that identifies the frequency and circumstances in which paramedics are required to manage a situation in which a patient refuses ambulance treatment, although a number of ambulance service providers collate this information. The Queensland State Coroner, in the 2007 inquest into the death of a patient who refused ambulance transport following a road traffic crash, noted that 'refusal of patients to accept treatment is an issue ambulance officers must deal with frequently': *Inquest into the death of Nola Jean Walker*, unrep, Queensland Coroner's Court, State Coroner Barnes SM, 22 November 2007. Online. Available: http://www.courts.qld.gov.au/__data/assets/pdf_file/0003/106347/cif-walker-nj-20071123.pdf (accessed 28 November 2018).

26 The test to determine the validity of a decision to refuse treatment is a test at law; however, it is one that is necessarily carried out by health providers in a variety of clinical settings. This factor was noted by Dame Butler-Sloss in the English case *Re B (Adult: Refusal of Medical Treatment)* [2022] All ER 449. See also, discussion in Queensland Law Reform Commission (QLRC) (2010) *A Review of Queensland's Guardianship Laws*, Report No. 67. Brisbane: QLRC, at p. 300.

27 This is reflected in the New Zealand *Code of Health and Disability Services Consumers' Rights*, Right 7(4), which provides 'where a consumer is not competent to make an informed choice and give informed consent, and no person entitled to consent on behalf of the consumer is available, the provider may provide services where— (a) it is in the best interests of the consumer; and … '.

28 *Re T (Adult: Refusal of Medical Treatment)* [1992] 4 All ER 649.

29 *Brightwater Care Group (Inc) v Rossiter* (2009) 40 WAR 84.

30 Burstein, J. (1999) Refusal of care in the prehospital setting. *Topics in Emergency Medicine, Advanced Emergency Medical Journal* 21(1), 38–42; Shah, M., Brazarian, J., Mattingly, A. et al. (2004) Patients with head injuries refusing emergency medical services transport. *Brain Injury* 18(8), 765–773.

31 Some commentators advocate that the failure to provide information should not vitiate an otherwise valid decision to refuse treatment, for reasons that it would be inconsistent with established legal principles, that being, the right to make a choice irrespective of the reasons. See discussions in: Freckelton, I. (2011) Patients' decisions to die: the emerging Australian jurisprudence. *Journal of Law and Medicine* 18(3), 427–438; Willmott, L., White, B. and Then, S. (2010) Withholding and withdrawing life-sustaining medical treatment. In: White et al (eds), *Health Law in Australia* (pp. 449–490); Willmott, L., White, B. and Mathews, B. (2010) Law, autonomy and advance directives. *Journal of Law and Medicine* 18(2), 366–389.

32 *Brightwater Care Group (Inc) v Rossiter* (2009) 40 WAR 84.

33. Ibid., at [32]–[34]. The view held by Martin J was inconsistent with that expressed by McDougall J in *Hunter and New England Area Health Service v A* (2009) 74 NSWLR 88. The patient in the latter case had provided an earlier advance directive and was no longer competent, whereas the patient in the *Brightwater* case made a contemporaneous decision to reject treatment, and was still competent to make decisions at the time of the hearing. Whether or not these distinguishing factors are relevant will ultimately be determined when judicial clarification of the need for information is provided.

34 *Code of Health and Disability Services Consumers' Rights*, Right 6.

35 *W Healthcare NHS Trust v H* [2005] 1 WLR 843, discussed in: Willmott, White, and Matthews, Law, autonomy and advance directives, at 370.

36 *Werth v Taylor* 475 NW 2d 426 (1991). See also: *Re T (Adult: Refusal of Medical Treatment)* [1992] 4 All ER 649. In this latter case, T was informed by the doctors that there were alternatives to a blood transfusion, and that these alternatives could be administered if her condition was to change and a transfusion was warranted. This information was not accurate. T's condition deteriorated and, in the

opinion of her treating doctors, a blood transfusion was needed. T had not been required to consider whether she would still refuse a blood transfusion in these changed circumstances, for she incorrectly assumed that it would not be necessary.

37 See comments in endnote 25 above. Also, see the discussion in Appelbaum, P. (2007) Assessment of patients' competence to consent to treatment. *New England Journal of Medicine* 357, 1834–1840.

38 *Re MB (Medical Treatment)* [1997] 2 FCR 426. The presumption of capacity is also embodied in the New Zealand *Code of Health and Disability Services Consumers' Rights*, Right 7(2).

39 *Re B (Adult: Refusal of Medical Treatment)* [2002] 2 All ER 449; *Re T (Adult: Refusal of Medical Treatment)* [1992] 4 All ER 649.

40 *Re C (Adult: Refusal of Medical Treatment)* [1994] 1 All ER 819.

41 Ibid., at 822.

42 Ibid.

43 See the discussion in: Stewart et al., *The Australian Medico–Legal Handbook*, at p. 83. It is interesting to note, however, that a number of recent decisions examining issues relevant to a patient's decision-making capacity do not refer to the requirement that the patient believes the information regarding the nature, purpose and effect of the proposed treatment.

44 Lord Donaldson MR in *Re T (Adult: Refusal of Medical Treatment)* [1992] 4 All ER 649, at 653, stated: 'the right of choice is not limited to decisions which others might regard as sensible. It exists notwithstanding that the reasons for making the choice are rational, irrational, unknown or even non-existent.'

45 This is reflected in the New Zealand *Code of Health and Disability Services Consumers' Rights*, Right 7(3), which provides: 'where a consumer has diminished competence, that consumer retains the right to make informed choices and give informed consent, to the extent appropriate to his or her level of competence.'

46 *Re T (Adult: Refusal of Medical Treatment)* [1992] 4 All ER 649, at 641.

47 See Parker, M. (2004) Judging capacity: paternalism and the risk-related standard. *Journal of Law and Medicine* 11(4), 482–491.

48 Devereux, J. and Parker, M. (2007) Competency issues for young persons and older persons. In: I. Freckelton and K. Petersen (eds), *Disputes and Dilemmas in Health Law* (pp. 54–76). Sydney: The Federation Press; Stewart, C. and Biegler, P. (2004) A primer on the law of competence to refuse medical treatment. *Australian Law Journal* 78(5), 325–342; Parker, Judging capacity, at 487.

49 This view is consistent with that expressed by McDougall in the New South Wales Supreme Court decision *Hunter and New England Area Health Services v A* (2009) 74 NSWLR 88, at [24]. See, also, the discussion regarding the interpretation and application of the New Zealand *Code of Health and Disability Services Consumers' Rights* as it relates to Right 7 generally and Right 7(4) specifically, in: Greig, K. (2000) Informed consent in the *Code of Health and Disability Services Consumers' Rights*. Presentation to the 8th Annual Medico–Legal Conference, 8 February 2000.

50 In some jurisdictions, the ambulance service provider has issued procedural guidelines to assist the paramedic to assess decision-making capacity in the pre-hospital setting. See, for example, the guidelines published by the Queensland Ambulance Service. *Clinical Practice Manual.* Online. Available: https://www.ambulance.qld.gov.au/clinical.html (accessed 28 November 2018).

51 *Inquest into the death of Nola Jean Walker*, at 17. This finding also reflects the High Court decision involving police officers in *Stuart v Kirkland-Veenstra* [2009] 15 HCA; 237 CLR 215. Online. Available: http://www.austlii.edu.au/au/cases/cth/HCA/2009/15.html (accessed 28 November 2018).

52 An excellent overview of this area of the law, as it relates to each of the Australian jurisdictions, is provided in: White, B., Willmott, L. and Then, S. (2010) Adults who lack capacity: substitute decision-making. In: White et al. (eds), *Health Law in Australia* (pp. 149–207). And, in New Zealand: Skegg, P. (2006) Capacity to consent to treatment. In: P. Skegg and R. Paterson (eds), *Medical Law in New Zealand* (pp. 171–202). Wellington: Thomson Brookers, at pp. 180–187.

53 The guardianship legislation in New Zealand, and in each Australian jurisdiction, with the exception of the Northern Territory, provides for the advance appointment of a substitute decision-maker.

54 Generally, the individual appointed for this purpose is required to be an adult, and required to have the capacity to make decisions.

55 In Queensland, this appointment is made under an 'advance health directive', *Powers of Attorney Act 1998* (Qld), ss 35(1)(c), 36(3)–(5). In Victoria, the appointment is made under an 'enduring power of attorney (medical treatment)', *Medical Treatment Act 1988* (Vic), ss 5A, 5B. In South Australia, the appointment is made under a 'medical powers of attorney', *Consent to Medical Treatment and Palliative Care Act 1995* (SA), ss 8, 9.

56 The guardianship legislation in each Australian jurisdiction, with the exception of the Northern Territory, provides for the authorisation of a substitute decision-maker by default. The guardianship legislation in New Zealand does not provide for a substitute decision-maker by default.

57 All jurisdictions make provision for the appointment of a substitute decision-maker by a court or a tribunal.

58 See White, Willmott and Then, Adults who lack capacity, at pp. 164–165. The authors have provided a comprehensive table in which key legislative terms for each Australian jurisdiction have been provided.

59 The terms 'child', 'minor' and 'young person' are used to describe a person who has not yet attained the age of majority. See Chapter 8 for more information.

60 For example, the decision to consent to medical and dental treatment.

61 For example, the age at which minors are deemed to be criminally responsible for their actions.

62 *Gillick v West Norfolk and Wisbech Area Health Authority* [1987] AC 112 *(Gillick's case).*

63 *Family Law Act 1975* (Cth), s 61B.

64 *Marion's case.*

65 *Care of Children Act 2004* (NZ), ss15, 17(1).

66 *Family Law Act 1975* (Cth), s 4, Div 2.

67 In South Australia, 'parent' is defined to include a person *in loco parentis* to the child (in place of the parent): *Consent to Medical Treatment and Palliative Care Act 1995* (SA), s 4. In Tasmania, 'parent' includes a 'guardian or a person acting *in loco parentis*': *Guardianship Act 1995* (Tas), s 3. In New Zealand, consent can be provided under the *Guardianship Act 1968*, s 25(3)(b), by a person 'acting in place of the parent', in circumstances where there is no guardian in New Zealand or no guardian that is capable of giving consent. In New South Wales, a 'parent' is defined for the purposes of the *Children and Young Persons (Care and Protection) Act 1998* (NSW) as one who has 'parental responsibility for the child or young person' (s 3).

68 In Australia, *Family Law Act 1975* (Cth), s 61C. In New Zealand, *Care of Children Act 2004*, s 7(1), and *Guardianship Act 1968*, s 6, 'the father and the mother shall *each* be guardians' (emphasis added).

69 *Family Law Act 1975* (Cth), s 61C(2).

70 *Marion's case*, at 310.

71 This has not been the subject of judicial consideration. See the opinion expressed by Skene, L. (2008) *Law and Medical Practice: Rights, Duties, Claims and Defences*, 3rd ed. Sydney: Lexis Nexis. At page 122, the author opines that the basis on which a casual carer would have authority to provide consent in these limited circumstances is by virtue of the principle of necessity (discussed further in the section 'Emergencies') and the need to act in the best interests of the child.

72 See the discussion in: Queensland Law Reform Commission (QLRC) (1996) *Consent to Health Care of Young People*, Report No. 51. Brisbane: QLRC, at p. 93.

73 *In loco parentis* is a Latin term that means 'in place of the parent'.

74 See endnote 67, above.

75 *State of Queensland v B* [2008] 2 Qd R 562; *Minister for Health v AS* (2004) 33 Fam LR 223; *Re Heather* [2003] NSWSC 532; *Re J (an infant): B and B v Director General of Social Welfare* [1996] 2 NXLR 134; *Marion's case*, at 339–340.

76 Manning, J. (2001) Parental refusal of life-prolonging medical treatment for children: a report from New Zealand. *Journal of Law and Medicine* 8, 263–285.

77 *Minister for Health v AS*. See, also, Manning, Parental refusal of life-prolonging medical treatment for children, at pp. 263–285. The author summarises a number of cases in which courts have intervened and reversed a parent's decision to refuse treatment, and those in which the parental decision has been upheld. For an excellent, and recent, summary of this area of the law, see: Matthews, B. (2010) Children and consent to medical treatment. In: White et al. (eds), *Health Law in Australia* (pp. 113–147), at pp. 119–136.

78 *Parens patriae* jurisdiction relates to the authority of the court to intervene and make decisions to ensure the welfare of those who are vulnerable and unable to care for themselves. For example, children and persons with impaired decision-making capacity.

79 *Royal Alexandra Hospital for Children v J* (2005) 33 Fam LR 448; *Re J (an infant)*.

80 There has been no judicial consideration of the use of child welfare legislation in these circumstances. However, the intention of the legislative scheme in each jurisdiction is to protect a child who may be exposed to harm, which would certainly be the case if a parent was refusing, against advice, to consent to the administration of urgent and lifesaving first aid and medical treatment in the pre-hospital setting.

81 *Gillick's case*, at 200. This issue has not been considered by an Australian court.

82 *Consent to Medical Treatment and Palliative Care Act 1995* (SA), s 6. See also ss 3(a)(i), 4, and 12(b)(i) and (ii), the last of which provides that a child less than 16 years of age may also consent to medical treatment if: the medical practitioner who is to administer the treatment is of the opinion that the child is capable of understanding the nature, consequences and risks of the treatment; the treatment is in the best interest of the child; and this opinion is supported by one other medical practitioner who personally examines the child.

83 *Minors (Property and Contracts) Act 1970* (NSW), s 49(2). See discussion in: New South Wales Law Reform Commission (NSWLRC) (2004) *Minors' Consent to Medical Treatment*, Issues Paper No. 24. Sydney: NSWLRC, at pp. 30–36, 88–91. The purpose of the section is to provide protection for medical and dental practitioners (from liability for assault and battery) where the practitioner has acted with reasonable care and with the consent of a person aged 14 years or older. The section does not provide that a person has the capacity to make decisions regarding healthcare from the time the person reaches the age of 14 years.

84 *Care of Children Act 2004*, s 36(1).

85 Section 36(2) of the *Care of Children Act 2004;* this also extends to children living in a de facto relationship. See Bunny, L. (1997) The capacity of competent minors to consent to and refuse medical treatment. *Journal of Law and Medicine* 5, 52–80, at 57–58.

86 See commentary in: Skegg, Capacity to consent to treatment, at p. 195. The author states that it is not entirely clear as to whether the enactment of the *Care of Children Act 2004*, which does not expressly preserve the common law, had the effect of distinguishing the common law capacity to consent to medical treatment of young people who are under 16 years of age. The uncertainty in this regard arises from a number of 'indecisive and conflicting High Court (NZ) decisions'. Notwithstanding, the author opines that the better view is that the New Zealand legislation has not extinguished the common law rights, and that a young person under 16, if deemed to have the requisite capacity, can made decisions regarding healthcare.

87 The common law *Gillick* principle applies in each Australian jurisdiction in relation to decisions made by a young person under the age of 18, and in New Zealand and South Australia to decisions made by a young person under the age of 16. In South Australia, the common law *Gillick* principle has been enshrined in the *Consent to Medical Treatment and Palliative Care Act 1995* (SA), s 12(b)(i) and (ii).

88 *Gillick's case.*

89 *Secretary, Department of Health and Community Services (NT) v JWB and SMB (Marion's case)* (1992) 175 CLR 218.

90 A *Gillick*-competent young person must demonstrate a level of understanding, in relation to the proposed treatment, that is higher than that required of an adult in similar circumstances.

91 *Re Alex* (2004) 31 Fam LR 503, discussed in Matthews, Children and consent to medical treatment, at pp. 128–129.

92 The age at which a young person in England could consent to medical treatment.

93 *Gillick's case*, at 188–189.

94 See the discussion in: New South Wales Law Reform Commission (NSWLRC) (2008) *Young People and Consent to Health Care*, Report No. 119. Sydney: NSWLRC, at pp. 86–89.

95 See the discussion in Matthews, Children and consent to medical treatment, at p. 139.

96 *Consent to Medical Treatment and Palliative Care Act 1995* (SA), s 6.

97 Ibid., s 12(b)(i) and (ii).

98 *Care of Children Act 2004*, s 36(1) and (2).

99 *New Zealand Bill of Rights Act 1990*, s 11.

100 The right to refuse medical treatment is subject to limits that may be prescribed by other laws. See *New Zealand Bill of Rights Act 1990*, ss 4, 5.

101 See comments in endnote 86, above.

102 *Re R (A Minor) (Wardship: Medical Treatment)* [1991] 3 WLR 5; this decision was criticised by McHugh J in *Marion's case*, at 316, where His Honour stated that it was 'inconsistent with *Gillick*'. See also: *Re W (A Minor) (Medical Treatment: Court's Jurisdiction)* [1992] 3 WLR 758. Commentators have criticised these decisions for the reason that they fail to recognise the principle of autonomy that underpinned *Gillick's case*, and effectively preserved the right of a parent to consent to treatment for their child until such time as the child reaches majority. See: Bunny, The capacity of competent minors to consent to and refuse medical treatment, at 70–71; Matthews, Children and consent to medical treatment, at pp. 139–140.

103 See the discussion in New South Wales Law Reform Commission, *Young People and Consent to Health Care*, at pp. 83–89.

104 *Minister for Health v AS.*

105 While there had been no judicial consideration on this point, it is likely that the administration of urgent first-aid treatment and the transportation of a child to a safe place would be authorised under the common law principle of necessity.

Chapter 6
Negligence and vicarious liability

Peter Jurkovsky

Learning outcomes

After reading this chapter, you should be able to:

- understand how the law of negligence applies to a paramedic in a personal and professional capacity
- identify and apply the elements of negligence in a particular situation
- recognise the relevant defences to a claim in negligence
- understand the principles underpinning the doctrine of vicarious liability, and how it applies in a professional capacity
- effectively review key cases in negligence law as they relate to paramedic practice, and recognise their effect on future practice.

Definitions

Common law The law developed by courts over the ages, and applied in similar cases to provide consistency and certainty in law-making, which forms the doctrine of precedent.

Defendant The party who responds to proceedings initiated by another party seeking relief in formal legal proceedings.

Duty of care A requirement that a person act towards others in a manner that a reasonable person in the circumstances would behave to avoid reasonably foreseeable harm.

Legislation A law or body of laws made and enacted by the Parliament (known as a statute or an Act of Parliament).

Negligence The failure to exercise appropriate levels of care, which causes reasonably foreseeable harm.

Non-economic loss Damage suffered that cannot be directly calculated in monetary terms, and may include pain and suffering, disfigurement and loss of enjoyment of life; while noting that any actual compensation under this head of damages will still be provided in monetary terms.

Plaintiff The party who initiates formal legal proceedings seeking relief against another party.

Precedent A decision that interprets law and acts as a guide for future cases. It is an important doctrine that ensures there is a stable and consistent legal framework on which to consider each new legal case.

Strict liability Where liability is not based on any form of culpability or fault, but only on proof that the act in question occurred.

Tort A civil wrong or wrongful act, as distinct from a criminal proceeding.

Vicarious liability The liability imposed on one person or corporation for the wrongful act of another on the basis of the legal relationship between them.

An Introductory case

Negligence

A paramedic has been called to a scene where a man has had a fall and suffered a non-life-threatening head injury that will require hospital treatment for suturing the wound. When the paramedic arrives, the patient behaves aggressively, appears intoxicated and refuses transport despite continued requests. The patient then leaves the scene after the paramedic bandages the head wound. The man is later struck by a car and sustains significant injuries.

He sues the ambulance service for negligence, on the basis that his treatment was below the required standard in two areas: first, that he should have been convinced to go to hospital; and, secondly, that the bandage the paramedic applied was not adequately secured, and slid down over his face, obscuring his vision, which caused him to be struck by the car.

This chapter will provide the reader with the means to determine the responsibilities of a paramedic in cases such as this one.

Introduction

This chapter will explore the law of negligence by describing the key elements that are required to establish negligence generally, reviewing a number of relevant cases, discussing a number of associated aspects of the law in this area, and, finally, reviewing and analysing three specific Australian cases that offer extensive, and extremely contextual, applications of negligence principles.

The law of negligence potentially plays a part in every aspect of an individual's personal and professional lives. Most of us, fortunately, will not be exposed to the law of negligence, in a formal litigious sense, during our lives. Nevertheless, an awareness of the law remains vitally important when acting in a professional or personal capacity, as paramedics practise in a growing and increasingly litigious environment, which, in this electronic age, has a particularly heightened public profile.

What is a tort?

A tort is a civil wrong. It signifies:

- an actionable, wrongful act, other than a breach of contract, which is
- performed intentionally, negligently or in circumstances involving strict liability, and which
- affords a remedy in the form of damages to the person who has sustained an injury as a result.[1]

There is significant overlap between many of the torts and the criminal law. The difference between a crime and a tort is that the former is concerned with the protection of society and punishing the wrongdoer, whereas the latter involves some form of compensation for the harm done.[2] Examples of this overlap include the torts of assault, battery and false imprisonment.

The most widely applied tort is negligence.

What is 'negligence'?

Negligence is based on foreseeability of risk and the reasonableness of a person's conduct in particular circumstances. The tort of negligence recognises that people should take reasonable care and consideration of the foreseeable harm one person may cause another in respect to their relationship to them. For example, it is reasonable for a patient to expect that a paramedic would take reasonable care when treating them in individual circumstances to avoid harming them.

The elements of what might constitute negligence are well defined, as they have been formulated through common law principles over the past century. These principles are now embedded in legislation in all states and territories, which operates in conjunction with the common law.

In order for an action in negligence to succeed, the person bringing the case, the plaintiff, must essentially prove, on the balance of probabilities: that a duty of care was owed by the defendant; that the duty has been breached because it fell below the required standard; that, as a result of this breach of duty, harm was caused that was reasonably foreseeable and was not too remote to allow for the recovery of recognised damages.

To summarise the requirements to uphold a negligence claim, a party must:

- establish a **duty of care** (*duty*)
- prove a **breach of duty of care** (by proving that the care given fell below the *reasonable standard*)
- demonstrate that the breach resulted in physical, emotional or pecuniary **damage** or loss (*damage*)
- establish that the harm **caused** was not too remote from the breach, and that there is a causal link between the act and the injury (*causation*).

These terms will be discussed in more detail below.

Although negligence laws have emanated from hundreds of years of common law evolution, more rapid development ensued during the past century, with the most significant reforms in Australia taking place in the early 2000s when a crisis in the area of professional liability insurance saw the implementation of various reforms to stabilise the law and fundamentally cap the amount of damages available to successful litigants for non-economic loss.

These reforms came about after an extensive review of the laws of negligence through the *Review of the Law of Negligence Report* (The Ipp Report)[3] in 2002. The main reforms as they relate to negligence laws include:

- the imposition of caps on damages for non-economic loss in personal injury claims
- stricter rules around defences
- modification of the tests for the standard of care for professionals
- waivers of liability in relation to recreational activities.

These reforms effectively mean that an action in negligence is more difficult to bring than it was prior to the introduction of these laws. Table 6.1 lists the respective laws in each state and territory.

The various legislative enactments around negligence also operate in conjunction with the common law, where the laws state that, 'except as provided by this Part, this Part is not intended to affect the common law',[4] meaning that express areas in the legislation state the relevant laws, while still allowing the courts to apply precedent from earlier negligence cases where the statutory law is unclear or silent.

What is 'a duty of care'?

A duty of care is owed in circumstances where there is a foreseeable risk of harm to others. The duty of care operates to define the scope and substance of negligence law. It addresses the major questions of what we regard as behaviour for which a plaintiff should be compensated.[5]

The modern requirements to establish a duty of care are founded in the famous case of *Donoghue v Stevenson*,[6] which describes the scenario in which Mrs May Donoghue

Table 6.1 Legislation incorporating negligence in all states and territories	
Australian Capital Territory	*Civil Law (Wrongs) Act 2002*
New South Wales	*Civil Liability Act 2002*
Northern Territory	*Personal Injuries Act 2003*
Queensland	*Civil Liability Act 2003*
South Australia	*Civil Liability Act 1936*
Tasmania	*Civil Liability Act 2002*
Victoria	*Wrongs Act 1958*
Western Australia	*Civil Liability Act 2002*

drank a bottle of ginger beer at the Wellmeadow café in Scotland in 1928. The manufacturer of the drink was Mr Stevenson.

Mrs Donoghue suffered severe gastroenteritis and nervous shock as a result of ingesting a decomposed snail that was concealed in the bottle. As the law stood at the time, she had no *direct relationship*, known as *privity of contract*, with the manufacturer in a legal sense. The direct contractual relationship, which would normally establish the duty of care, was between the manufacturer and the retailer, and would not have included a duty to the consumer, in this case Mrs Donoghue.

The case wound its way through the court system until it finally rested with Lord Atkin's judgment in the English House of Lords in 1932. To establish this crucial missing link in negligence law, Lord Atkin drew on biblical propositions that neighbours have a responsibility to each other. He famously stated:

> Who, then, in law is my neighbour? The answer seems to be—persons who are so closely and directly affected by my act that I ought reasonably to have them in contemplation as being so affected when I am directing my mind to the acts or omission which are called in question.[7]

This statement created the '*neighbour*' *principle* in negligence, which is now the cornerstone of the law when evaluating a duty of care. With this assessment, the vast majority of situations will give rise to a duty of care when considering factors such as the relationship between the persons involved, proximity and the ability to take precautions.

In most cases that come before the courts, whether the defendant owes the plaintiff a duty of care will usually be determined by reference to the precedents established by similar cases,[8] noting that it is acknowledged that the categories of duty remain open to development under the common law and relevantly associated legislation in each jurisdiction.

Assessing the duty of care in new and novel circumstances has been an area that has caused some disquiet and controversy for the courts over the years, with the High Court of Australia developing various approaches in its attempts to provide a clear guide for litigants. The application of these different approaches has arguably created some uncertainty, whereas the codification of these common law factors has now provided the courts with a more structured assessment tool when considering whether a duty of care exists in less defined circumstances.

The various state and territory wrongs and civil liability Acts have codified the core principles around a duty of care and the factors that may give rise to a breach of duty in a general sense, while noting that the particular circumstances of each case are considered when assessing liability.[9] The statutory provisions state that a person is not negligent in failing to take precautions against a risk of harm, unless: the risk was foreseeable; the risk was not insignificant; and, in the circumstances, a reasonable person in the defendant's position would have taken those precautions.[10]

The on-duty paramedic will always owe a duty of care to their patients and others with whom they may come into contact while fulfilling their professional duties. The contentious position of the off-duty paramedic will be discussed later in the chapter.

What are the standards of care and the assessments that identify a breach of duty of care?

As described above, a duty of care can normally be readily identified in most factual situations where one party is in some way responsible for another party's welfare, whereas more complicated scenarios may arise and require a supplementing detailed analysis.

Once a duty of care has been established, the next step in the investigation is to discern whether the party who owes a duty of care has breached that duty, and therefore fallen below the standard required by law.

In determining whether a reasonable person would have taken precautions against a risk of harm, the Acts also affirm that a court is to consider, among other relevant matters: (1) the probability that the harm would occur if care were not taken; (2) the likely seriousness of the harm; (3) the burden of taking precautions to avoid the risk of harm; and (4) the social utility of the activity that creates the risk of harm.[11] These assessments are known as the factors that incorporate the *calculus of negligence*. None of these four factors will of itself be determinative of liability, with the courts balancing them against each other to decide whether the defendant should have taken additional precautions to avoid the risk of injury.[12]

A number of the wrongs and civil liability Acts identify an extended test where the standard of care, and its potential breach, is being assessed for 'professionals'. The definition of a 'professional' is an 'individual practising a profession'.[13] Although this definition does not necessarily assist our analysis to any great degree, the cases that have developed around this aspect of negligence law normally revolve around medical practitioners. Kerridge et al., however, suggest that the term is not limited to the medical profession, and that it would be up to a court to decide whether or not, in the circumstances of a particular case, a person was practising as a professional.[14]

Paramedics are now registered health professionals with the Australian Health Practitioner Regulation Agency (AHPRA) under the *Health Practitioner Regulation National Law Act 2009* (the 'National Law'), and would definitively meet this threshold.

Legislation in Victoria and South Australia[15] also extends the base classification in relation to the standard of care to 'persons holding out as possessing a particular skill',[16] where that person is assessed on the basis of 'what could reasonably be expected of a person possessing that skill and the relevant circumstances as at the date of the alleged negligence and not a later date'. This would also cover paramedics in their role.

This principle also gives rise to the question as to what standard of care a student paramedic will be held to when operating in the field. In most situations, a student paramedic will be unrecognisable to patients and members of the general public as an inexperienced paramedic unless it is made clear to the patient or an insignia is obvious or pointed out to those involved. Therefore, two options arise: first, that a clearly recognisable student paramedic will be held to the standard of care of a reasonable student in the circumstances; second, that an unrecognisable student will be held to the standard of a reasonable paramedic, remembering that the ultimate duty of care lies with the employer, who must ensure that ambulance crews are operating in the field with competence.

While the common law definitions will continue to hold significant weight and the statutory interpretations will develop over time, when considering that the negligence additions to the wrongs and civil liability Acts are less than 20 years old, the primary assessment for the standard of care will always be a fundamental question of whether a person acted with reasonable care in avoiding foreseeable injury to others in the circumstances.

In short, the clinical standard of care required to be given to a patient is determined by the peer group. This is evidenced by protocols, clinical guidelines, codes of conduct, policy documents and evidence from peers as to how they would act if they were in a similar situation. The provision of information to the patient also forms part of the standard of care, and is discussed separately.

The provision of information and the standard of care

Although the basic standard of care required in giving information to a patient will be similar to the standard of care in the treatment of a patient, the requirements when providing information extend the standard in a key area.

The case of *Rogers v Whitaker*[17] is the lead case in this area of negligence law (see Case 6.1).

The important extra element in cases where the provision of information is involved is that, although the standard of care will be assessed in the light of what a reasonable professional should have done in the circumstances, the decision-making process of the receiver of the information (normally the patient in medical cases) will play a role and be analysed to ascertain whether reasonable care was taken in providing that information. As Mendelson describes, 'except in cases of emergency, the choice as to whether to proceed with medical treatment is to be made by the patient on the basis of the information provided by the medical practitioner' (or relevant medical professional).[18]

The key cases in this area have typically involved medical practitioners. The principle can be applied to paramedic practice with a precautionary note when genuine emergency situations arise, while also recognising that a paramedic's diagnostic and treatment armoury is restricted within the framework of their relevant clinical guidelines. The doctrines of emergency and necessity allow medical professionals to undertake treatment without the consent of patients in select circumstances. When a patient has complete capacity and is able to understand all of the information provided to them, despite the acute nature of the circumstances in common ambulance scenarios, they will be entitled to be afforded all of the relevant details of the treatment being proposed, including any inherent material risks associated with the procedure.

For example, when introducing an intravenous pain relief agent, a paramedic should provide the patient with details regarding the broad nature and effect of the treatment and any material risks that the patient has concerns about, or that the treating paramedic thinks the patient would be concerned about, prior to commencing the treatment. If the patient does not have the capacity to understand, believe, weigh and communicate a decision about the treatment, and there is no recognised substitute decision-maker available, the paramedic may be able to instigate the treatment if it will prevent further

Case 6.1 *Rogers v Whitaker* (1992) 175 CLR 479

Mrs Whitaker had been almost totally blind in her right eye for nearly 40 years since suffering a severe injury to the eye at an early age. Despite the injury, she had lived a substantially normal life. Dr Rogers, an ophthalmic surgeon, advised her that an operation on the injured eye would not only improve its appearance, but would potentially restore sight to it.

Following the surgery, which was conducted without any negligence, Mrs Whitaker developed a condition known as 'sympathetic ophthalmia' in her left eye. She subsequently lost all sight in her left eye, and, as there had been no restoration of sight in her right eye, she was left almost totally blind.

She sued Dr Rogers, alleging that his failure to warn her of the risk, albeit remote, of sympathetic ophthalmia was negligent. While she had not specifically asked whether the operation to her right eye could affect her left eye, she had incessantly questioned the appellant as to possible complications. Evidence provided at the trial was that the risk of sympathetic ophthalmia is about 1 in 14,000, and, even then, not all cases lead to blindness in the affected eye.

The majority stated that, in circumstances such as this, doctors are required to inform their patients of any 'material' risks inherent in a procedure. They suggested that a 'material' risk was one where a reasonable person in the patient's position, if warned of the risk, would be likely to attach significance to it, and that it was a matter for the court to determine whether the doctor had provided adequate information and advice as to the material risks.

The court decided that Dr Rogers was negligent in not informing Mrs Whitaker of this inherent material risk in the circumstances, thus denying her of the chance to decline to have the operation.

harm or save the patient's life. See the section on 'Capacity' in Chapter 5 for more details.

Although the law recognises that the circumstances in pre-hospital care are often quite different from the controlled environs of a medical facility, the duty to warn of inherent material risks in the treatment of patients remains a paramount consideration.

In short, if a paramedic fails to give a competent patient (or their recognised substitute decision-maker) the information on the broad nature and effect of treatment proffered and the material risks associated with it, they expose themselves to an allegation of negligence.

What is 'damage'?

A claim of negligence can succeed only if a recognisable form of damage has been sustained. To be compensable, damage must be of a kind, class, character or type that was reasonably foreseeable.[19] The damage cannot be insignificant, and the various states and territories identify 'significant' injury through a variety of criteria, including medical assessment as to the degree of impairment.[20]

The damage can be an economic or a non-economic loss. *Economic loss* includes medical expenses, care services, lost income and anticipated loss of future earnings—anything that can have a monetary value assigned to it—whereas *non-economic loss* can include pain and suffering, disfigurement and loss of enjoyment of life.

What is 'causation', and what is 'remoteness'?

The notion of *causation* is used to establish whether the breach of duty 'caused' or was responsible for the damage or harm suffered by the patient. The legal principles associated with causation have created some challenging questions for courts over the years, particularly in negligence cases.

The plaintiff must prove causation on the 'balance of probabilities', as distinct from the higher level of proof required in criminal cases, being 'beyond reasonable doubt'.

Causation has often been assessed by courts using the 'but for' test, where the court poses the theoretical question 'Would the damage have occurred, *but for* the defendant's negligence?' This test has received some criticism, despite its widespread application as a basic legal tool when assessing whether a defendant should be held liable for the damage caused.

The wrongs and civil liability Acts have now codified the requirements of causation into two distinct inquiries. The first is known as *factual causation*, where the requirements state that 'the negligence was a necessary condition of the occurrence of the harm', whereas the second is known as *legal causation*, or the *scope of liability*, which requires 'that it is appropriate for the scope of the negligent person's liability to extend to the harm so caused' as it relates to *remoteness of damage*.[21]

What is 'vicarious liability'?

Vicarious liability refers to the liability that is automatically transferred from one party to another because of the legally recognised relationship between them. The most common type of vicarious liability covers the employer–employee relationship, whereas other forms are deemed through some agency and partnership associations, and an extended version, known as a *non-delegable duty of care*, applies in some specific cases.

A number of legal and policy-based grounds underpin the principle of vicarious liability. It is appropriate to review the principle as it applies to the employer–employee relationship and discuss its impact on paramedic practice (see Case 6.2).

Applying this to practice, if a paramedic inadvertently delivers an overdose of a drug that is within their scope of practice and clinical guidelines, the employer will be liable for the potential damage unless it can be proven that some deliberateness or criminality was at play in the conduct of the paramedic. If, however, a paramedic were to act outside

Case 6.2 *Deatons Pty Ltd v Flew* (1949) 79 CLR 370

A barmaid who was employed by Deatons Pty Ltd threw a glass of beer into the face of a patron after he had been abusive. He suffered an injury that caused him to lose sight in one eye.

The court found that the barmaid was acting outside the 'scope' of her employment, and therefore her employer was not vicariously liable for the damage caused to the plaintiff. It stated:

> It was an act of passion and resentment done neither in furtherance of the master's interest nor under his express or implied authority nor as an incident to or in consequence of anything the barmaid was employed to do. It was a spontaneous act of retributive justice.

The decision in *Deatons Pty Ltd v Flew* is often criticised as being too harsh. The analysis falls to a decision as to what might constitute a particular employee's 'scope' of employment.

their scope of practice and they harmed the patient as a result, it is possible that they will not be vicariously covered by their employer for that action, and will potentially be personally liable for that harm.

Is there a duty to rescue, and where do the obligations of the off-duty paramedic lie?

There is no general duty to go to the rescue of others in emergency situations.[22] Off-duty paramedics will often come across medical emergencies, and the decision whether to assist is not a legal but a personal one, although it should be noted that some extension to this lack of duty may potentially arise where a paramedic is in uniform. In this situation, a 'community expectation' duty of care may arise, where the public perception is, or is likely to be, that the uniformed paramedic would go to someone's aid in a medical emergency. It should be noted that this is not an area of duty of care that has been legally tested.

The duty of care owed by professionals was reviewed in great detail in the case of *Stuart v Kirkland-Veenstra* [2009] HCA 15; (2009) 237 CLR 215. Here, the High Court was asked to consider whether two police officers owed a duty of care to a potentially suicidal man whom they found sitting in his vehicle with a vacuum hose running from the exhaust pipe in through the window. After talking with the man for some time and making various inquiries, the police officers assessed that he was not at current risk of self-harm. They also formed the opinion that he was rational and coherent and did not appear to be mentally ill. The man committed suicide later that day in his car via carbon monoxide poisoning. The partner of the deceased sued the police officers, alleging that they were

> ## Case 6.3 *Lowns v Woods* (1996) Aust Torts Reports ¶81-376
>
> The case involved a mother who found her 11-year-old son, Patrick Woods, fitting. She sent his brother to summon an ambulance from the branch nearby, and his sister to a local general practitioner to ask the doctor to attend to help her brother. The daughter ran to the surgery of Dr Peter Lowns, which was approximately 300 m away, and advised him that her brother was having an epileptic fit and asked the doctor to attend to provide assistance.

negligent and had breached their duty of care in not apprehending the deceased pursuant to section 10 of the *Mental Health Act 1986* (Vic). The case was peculiar on its facts, and the decision was based on a narrow interpretation of duty of care, with the court ultimately deciding that a duty of care should not be imposed, as the police officers did not have the requisite control over the risk of harm to the deceased.

This lack of duty has long been recognised for all citizens, including paramedics, but doctors have found themselves in a slightly different situation, following a well-known case in the mid-1990s: *Lowns v Woods* (1996) Aust Torts Reports ¶81-376. See Case 6.3.

Although the case was again peculiar on its own facts in some ways, the duty bestowed on doctors has arguably been extended beyond those of other members of the community.

Although there was a factual dispute about whether the request was made, the court found that the doctor had been advised of the boy's situation, had refused to attend the house to provide assistance, and had instead told his sister to bring him to the surgery. The prolonged epileptic fit prevented adequate oxygenation, which resulted in significant brain damage that left the child permanently and totally disabled.

The court found that the doctor did have a duty of care to help the child, and, if the doctor had attended to help, it was likely that the child would not have suffered the serious consequences that eventuated.

The court imposed a duty while recognising that there was no Australian case that had previously imposed liability on a doctor for failing to attend and treat someone despite there being no pre-existing doctor–patient relationship.

The reasons for this are particular to this case, but are nonetheless important to take account of, and include:

- The doctor had a sign holding out that he was a general practitioner and the surgery was open to attending patients.
- A direct request was made for the doctor to attend.
- The patient was very close, so there was a 'physical' proximity.

- The doctor had no other patients more urgent to deal with at the time, and therefore there was nothing to prevent him from attending.

Good Samaritans

The often-cited 'Good Samaritan Act' does not actually exist as a separate piece of legislation. Rather, the good Samaritan provisions can be found in the various wrongs and civil liability Acts throughout Australia.[23] The legislation is aimed at protecting citizens who act in 'good faith' in an 'emergency or accident', where, in most instances, they have no expectation of 'financial reward', therefore creating a barrier against civil liability.

The off-duty paramedic will be protected by this legislation, while also noting that a number of states and territories specifically indemnify 'medically qualified' persons within the definitions where the assistance might extend to the provision of medical 'advice' in an emergency situation.[23] The definition of a 'medically qualified person' in these statutes incorporates paramedics through wording such as 'a person who works or has worked as an ambulance officer or in some other recognised paramedical capacity'.[24]

Intoxicated patients

The vexed questions that accompany the treatment of intoxicated patients create difficulties for paramedics in the field. These complexities often involve a delicate balance between various considerations, and the law of negligence has recognised this aspect of human relationships generally, which can be applied to paramedical practice.

Although the common law treatment and assessment of intoxication remain relevant, some Australian jurisdictions have codified this area of negligence law.[25] New South Wales has addressed this component of the *Civil Liability Act 2002* in definite terms, by expressly excluding recovery for negligence-based injury, potentially by 100%, where the person 'was at the time of the act or omission that caused the death, injury or damage intoxicated to the extent that the person's capacity to exercise reasonable care and skill was impaired'.[26] The Victorian statute applies against a person alleging negligence, and states, 'in determining whether the plaintiff has established a breach of the duty of care owed by the defendant, the court must consider, among other things—(a) whether the plaintiff was intoxicated by alcohol or drugs voluntarily consumed and the level of intoxication'.[27] The patient's intoxication does not relieve the paramedic of the duty to provide the required reasonable standard of care. Indeed, if it were the paramedic who was intoxicated while treating a patient and the paramedic failed to meet the required standard of care as a result, the paramedic could in no way rely on intoxication as a defence. This is codified in civil liability legislation. However, it may be that the intoxication of the patient contributes to, or exacerbates, the harm they experience as a result of the negligence of a paramedic. This is known as the *voluntary assumption of risk*, or *contributory negligence*, which will be discussed in the following section.

Defences to a negligence claim—contributory negligence and the voluntary assumption of risk

The two major defences to a negligence claim are contributory negligence and the voluntary assumption of risk.

The defence of contributory negligence re-examines the elements of a breach of the duty of care and causation from the defendant's perspective, analysing the plaintiff's conduct and its contribution to the injury, whereas the plea of voluntary assumption of risk focuses on the existence and scope of the duty of care.[28] Broadly, contributory negligence is a relatively straightforward concept that requires a more detailed assessment after its acceptance in a particular fact scenario.

Plaintiffs will be found to have contributed to their own injury if they generally fail to take precautions against the risk of harm in a given situation. The person's failure to take precautions is assessed in the same fashion as primary liability at the breach of duty stage in negligence is assessed, being an objective test whereby the plaintiff is judged on what a reasonable person in the given situation would have, or should have, done.

The various wrongs and civil liability Acts identify the coverage of contributory negligence and the standard of care required to found liability,[29] while the provisions now allow a defendant to fully escape liability in negligence where it can be established that the plaintiff was entirely responsible for their injuries when not taking precautions against the risk of harm. Although a 100% reduction is available under the legislation, its application remains rare, and most successful defence cases proving contributory negligence fall into the 20–30% range.

Voluntary assumption of risk—or the Latin term *volenti non fit injuria*—is a defence pleaded where people, being aware of the risk that they face, nevertheless decide to act and accept the risk of injury occurring.[30]

While the defence is again codified through the wrongs and civil liability Acts, the historical common law basis of the defence was predicated on the requirement that a person must 'perceive, understand and appreciate the full extent of both the risk of an injury and the legal consequence of the waiver of the duty of care'.[31] This has been identified as a narrow defence because the defendant has the burden of proving that the plaintiff agreed to take responsibility for the particular risk that had materialised.[32]

The statutory coverage of this defence takes a different approach, with the central enquiry being whether a particular risk was 'obvious'. The statute undertakes a balancing inquiry in which, primarily, 'the person who suffered harm is presumed to have been aware of the risk, unless the person proves on the balance of probabilities that the person was not aware of the risk',[33] while noting that this does not apply 'to the provision of or the failure to provide a professional service or health service',[34] whereby the common law will still apply. The statutes go further in attempting to clarify the meaning of the risks, by stating, among other definitions, that an obvious risk is one that 'would have been obvious to a reasonable person in the position of that person' and would 'include risks that are patent or a matter of common knowledge'.[35]

Voluntary assumption of risk has a wider application beyond negligence when considering human activities such as high-risk recreational sporting pursuits. A provider of these types of services can now eliminate certain normally non-excludable consumer guarantees,[36] whereas in some states the participation in a recognised 'dangerous recreational activity'[37] is excluded for persons who suffer harm as a result of 'obvious risks of dangerous recreational activities'.[38]

Negligence case study 1

The key case of *Ambulance Service of NSW v Worley* [2006] NSWCA 102 (Case 6.4) offers an excellent overview of negligence principles from the perspectives of the treating paramedics and the Ambulance Service itself.

The case provides a typical factual scenario, and analyses the crucial aspects of breach of duty from the employer and employee's positions, while also delivering an excellent overview of the rigour of the Australian court system, which saw a fundamentally flawed decision overturned.

The case review will assess the scenario through the lower court's initial finding and the appeal court's alternative decision, and then discuss the contentious aspects of the findings, finally providing some further commentary in the context of contemporary ambulance practice.

Case 6.4 *Ambulance Service of NSW v Worley* [2006] NSWCA 102

Mr Worley was a 46-year-old postman. While delivering mail on a motorcycle on 7 October 1998, he sustained a bee sting at approximately 11:30 h. He had been stung on four previous occasions over the preceding 6 years, with increasing allergic reactions.

He noted that his neck was starting to redden and he decided to go back to the mail delivery centre. The trip took him approximately 20 minutes.

On arrival at the mail delivery centre, Mr Worley dismounted from his motorcycle and felt that in doing so he had lost control of his bowels. Mr Worley said that he found it 'a bit hard to breathe' on the trip back, but otherwise negotiated the 5.4 km without anything adverse occurring. He agreed that his throat had begun to swell up at that time. He had a severe pain in his chest by the time he reached the mail delivery centre; despite the significance of this symptom, noted by the patient in his evidence, it did not form part of the paramedic's clinical findings and was not therefore at issue.

At 12:01 h, the manager of the mail delivery centre rang for an ambulance. The ambulance arrived at 12:17 h. The Ambulance Service records contain the following entry in relation to the condition of Mr Worley:

Pt c/o feeling itchy/dyspnoeic. Pts face red/swollen. Pt c/o severe pain to neck associated c bite. Audible exp wheeze. Obvious swelling to face. Tongue not swollen. Nil difficulty swallowing. Pt post treatment. Pt c/o severe itching to genitalia.

The patient report also noted that at 12:20 h Mr Worley's pulse rate was 100 and his blood pressure was 78 systolic, with a respiration rate of 28 breaths per minute. At

Continued

Case 6.4 *Ambulance Service of NSW v Worley* [2006] NSWCA 102 continued

12:21 h, Mr Page (the case refers to him as an 'ambulance officer' whom we shall identify as a 'paramedic' when commenting on the case) administered 0.4 mg adrenaline IV in four equal parts at 30-second intervals. The result was indicated as a reduction in dyspnoea and increase in blood pressure. At 12:25 h, he administered haemacell intravenously, with a consequent improvement in perfusion.

By 12:30 h, when the Hartmann's solution was administered intravenously, the pulse rate was down to 80 and the blood pressure up to 90 systolic. The respiratory rate was recorded at 24.

Mr Worley was conscious throughout this treatment, and was sitting on the bed in the first aid room. As Mr Page inserted a cannula in the patient's right hand, Mr Worley made a joke, indicating that he was mentally alert.

The ambulance left with Mr Worley at 12:30 h. Mr Page travelled with him in the back of the ambulance, which Mr Parsell (the second paramedic) drove. Shortly after the trip commenced, Mr Worley complained of a severe pain in his head, which caused him to remove the oxygen mask and say 'My head feels like it's about to explode.'

Mr Worley suffered an intracranial haemorrhage, which left him with a number of permanent disabilities that were mainly physical, although they were accompanied by some change in personality and a mild cognitive disability.

The court found that the intracranial haemorrhage was caused by a sudden spike in blood pressure as a result of the adrenaline treatment, which was also found to be a possible side effect of this type of treatment.

The initial finding by the lower court

Mr Worley was awarded $2,628,032.57 in the NSW Supreme Court, at first instance, on the basis that the treating paramedic was negligent in administering the adrenaline in the circumstances. The Ambulance Service, as his employer, was found to be vicariously liable for the damages payout.

A defence of 'contributory negligence' on the part of Mr Worley for not taking precautions or undertaking desensitisation treatment for his known allergy to bee stings was rejected.

This decision was found to be fundamentally flawed when the NSW Court of Appeal overturned the finding.

The finding by the NSW Court of Appeal

The NSW Court of Appeal focused on two areas. The first was whether the paramedic was negligent in his treatment, and the second was whether the protocol of the Ambulance Service of New South Wales directly relating to this treatment regimen was negligent, in that it was inadequate and/or not in keeping with the currently recognised treatments for anaphylaxis.

Was the paramedic negligent?

The relevant protocols in relation to anaphylaxis involved two parts: diagnosis and treatment.

They stated:

DIAGNOSIS

- May occur in response to drugs especially antibiotics, X-ray contrast media, certain foodstuffs and insect bites especially bee stings.
- May present with:
  Upper airway obstruction due to swollen tongue or laryngeal oedema
  Lower airway obstruction with bronchospasm
  Hypotension
  Bright red skin with sometimes urticaria

TREATMENT

1 Basic protocol 2.

Nasopharyngeal airway may be useful if tongue is swollen.

2 Cannulate and administer Hartmann's.

3 Adrenaline is indicated if any one of the following are present:
  Upper airway obstruction.
  Lower airway obstruction.
  The 'keys signs' of severe shock except skin is often warm and pink.

4 If hypovolaemic shock persists despite adrenaline follow Protocol 42.

5 Salbutamol for mild bronchospasm.

6 URGENT TRANSPORT.

The guide for the administration of adrenaline for this presentation was:

ASTHMA OR ANAPHYLAXIS

- 1ML OF 1:10,000 ADRENALINE IV EVERY 30 SECONDS until the patient is no longer 'in extremis' or a maximum of 5 mL.
- Monitor E.C.G. continuously.
- Can be repeated every 5 minutes.
- Give IM as a bolus if a vein is not available.

The court also noted that 'the indications for use of adrenaline in relation to anaphylaxis in the protocol did not use the term "in extremis", although the indications in relation to asthma did'.[39]

The term 'in extremis' became highly contentious at the initial trial. The findings by the lower-court judge were that the paramedic had not interpreted the protocols correctly, and had given the patient IV adrenaline when he was not, in fact, showing signs of being 'in extremis'. ('In extremis' was found, within the context of this case, to mean 'on the point of death', although it was noted to be a term without precise meaning.)

The NSW Court of Appeal also clarified its thoughts on this issue when it found that:

> Given the findings in relation to the expectations of ambulance officers … and the symptoms of anaphylaxis (as compared with asthma), it seems inherently unlikely that the protocols were intended to impose on ambulance officers an obligation to determine how close a seriously compromised and deteriorating patient was to death.[40]

In relation to the negligence of the paramedic, the first hearing took extensive evidence from numerous medical specialists. Although this evidence was critical at first, the NSW Court of Appeal found that this was not the correct approach in cases such as this. It explained its reasoning this way:

> Ambulance officers are not medical practitioners, let alone specialists in emergency medicine. Their training is by no means insignificant, but it does not equip them with the theoretical knowledge which would permit a fine evaluation of alternative treatments. In a case such as the present, their two functions were to stabilize the condition of a patient, so far as their skills and resources permitted, and to ensure his speedy transfer to an available hospital. There was no complaint in relation to their performance of the transfer function.

Perhaps surprisingly, and not including the treating medical practitioners, each party at trial called five medical specialists, whose evidence was directed mainly to the question as to what was accepted medical and pharmacological practice in relation to the administration of adrenaline in 1998. Without objection, experts in emergency medicine discussed their own practices in well-equipped teaching hospitals, with far less attention being given to the position of ambulance officers and the nature and purpose of the protocols which governed their conduct.[41]

Therefore, after reassessing all of the evidence available, the NSW Court of Appeal overturned the initial finding and held that the paramedic was not negligent in his treatment of Mr Worley.

Conclusion as to the paramedic's negligence

The various elements of negligence were analysed. Although some would have been uncontroversial in the analysis, the key finding was that what the paramedic did was 'reasonable', in that he followed the protocols that were within the range of his training after correctly diagnosing the patient's condition. He could do no more and, although there was an unfortunate adverse outcome, he was not negligent.

The paramedic obviously had a duty of care, but did not breach that duty of care because he did not fall below the standard required of a person, when assessed objectively within the circumstances of the particular case, acting in the role of a paramedic.

After finding that the paramedic was not negligent, it became unnecessary to consider the other elements of negligence, such as causation and damage.

Was the Ambulance Service negligent in relation to the protocols?

The court introduced this contention by stating:

> It was open to the plaintiff to establish that, even if Mr Page followed the protocol, with adverse results, the Ambulance Service would be liable in negligence because it had failed to exercise due care in the preparation of the protocols. To establish that case, the plaintiff sought first to establish that the administration of IV adrenaline was not part of accepted medical practice and, to the extent that the protocol permitted such administration to a patient who was not on the point of death, it was formulated negligently.[42]

The court again took evidence from numerous medicals specialists, while also comparing the protocols for the treatment of anaphylaxis with those from other ambulance jurisdictions, including Victoria, to assess whether the protocol being used in New South Wales was reasonable and appropriate when taking the available information into account.

On this issue, the case of the respondent (Mr Worley, who was the 'plaintiff' in the original case) was founded on the contention that IM adrenaline was the more appropriate treatment regimen because it was less likely to cause catastrophic effects such as those suffered by Mr Worley.

Conclusion as to the negligence of the Ambulance Service

The NSW Court of Appeal again analysed the various elements of negligence, and found that the Ambulance Service was not negligent in its development and administration of the protocols.

The Ambulance Service of New South Wales did have a duty of care to Mr Worley, but did not breach that duty of care, because it met the required standard in the development and administration of protocols for the treatment of patients with anaphylaxis within the scope of the information available to it at the time.

The NSW Court of Appeal concluded by stating:

> It follows that the plaintiff was a most unfortunate victim of misadventure. He is entitled to receive benefits in the nature of workers compensation, for an injury suffered in the course of his employment. He is not, however, entitled to damages for negligence on the part of the Ambulance Service.[43]

Comments on the case

This was clearly a difficult case for all concerned, including the patient, the paramedics and their families. Mr Worley was, as the court stated, an unfortunate victim of misadventure, and he sustained significant injuries in the form of a cerebral haemorrhage as result of the treatment.

The case was also appealed to the High Court in 2007, where special leave to hear the case was declined.

The result was a significant one for a number of reasons. The first is a procedural one, in that the findings will hold significant precedent value in Australian courts when similar cases come to trial because of the high level of the decision, as it was handed down by the NSW Court of Appeal. The more substantive value of the decision for paramedics in practice and ambulance services in Australia is that the case highlights the fact that paramedics obviously have a duty of care to patients when treating, or when omitting to treat, under the principles of negligence, but they will not be found negligent if they correctly diagnose and treat patients, even if the patient suffers an adverse outcome.

The benefit of the judgment from the perspective of the ambulance service is that it reiterates the reality that all services must be fully up-to-date in their design, development and application of treatment protocols. If they are diligent in this way, they, too, will be able to avoid negligence findings, even when a patient suffers a major adverse outcome that may occur within the treatment guidelines.

Negligence case study 2

Masson v State of Queensland [2018] QSC 162 (Case 6.5) is a recent case heard and decided by the Supreme Court of Queensland sitting in Cairns.

Case 6.5 *Masson v State of Queensland* [2018] QSC 162

Ms Masson was a 25-year-old chronic asthmatic. She had previously suffered severe asthma attacks, which, unbeknown to the paramedics (this title is used interchangeably with 'ambulance officers', in line with the case descriptors) had been successfully treated by the administration of adrenaline. On the night of 21 July 2002, Ms Masson drove to the home of her friend, where she collapsed and Queensland Ambulance Service (QAS) was called.

According to the QAS case record, the call was received at 22:52 h and the paramedics were at the scene at 22:58 h. Mr Peters was the senior officer and the determinative decision-maker among the officers. On arrival, he noticed Ms Masson lying supine on the grass while a male performed external compressions on her. The paramedics were given a history of Ms Masson having had a history of severe asthma, suffering an asthma attack, having used her puffer to no effect, asking to be taken to hospital, and collapsing into respiratory arrest, after which a friend performed 'EAR/CPR'.

Mr Peters concluded that Ms Masson was hypoxic and required oxygen immediately. His response to the risk inherent in oxygen deprivation was to ventilate and oxygenate her by the application of a bag valve mask. Mr Peters applied an intravenous cannula into her cubital fossa to administer intravenous drugs. One minute after arrival, at 22:59 h, he commenced administering intravenous salbutamol in aliquots of 250 mcg. In all, eight

Case **6.5** *Masson v State of Queensland* [2018] QSC 162 continued

aliquots, a total of 2 mg, of salbutamol were progressively administered between 22:59 h and 23:20 h. The administration of salbutamol appeared at first to have been effective. The apparent improvement in some of Ms Masson's symptoms continued through to and beyond the point when she was loaded into the ambulance and transportation commenced.

Once transportation from the scene to the hospital was underway, Mr Peters noted an unexpected increase in Ms Masson's heart rate to 136 beats per minute (bpm) as at 23:17 h. The records show that at that time she was again cyanosed and her Glasgow coma scale (GCS) score had descended to three, reflecting the fact that her eyes were no longer opening. By 23:19 h her heart rate had dropped markedly to 40 bpm, her respiratory rate had reduced to 12 retractive breaths per minute and blood pressure was absent. Cardiac arrest was imminent. A minute later, at 23:20 h, Mr Peters administered 300 mcg of adrenaline. Of his reasoning for doing so he testified:

> I then changed my pharmacology. I changed from IV salbutamol to low-dose IV adrenaline … in accordance with the clinical practice manual for adrenaline at that time. … Her vital signs had deteriorated to the point where adrenaline was the most appropriate drug for her clinical presentation … [S]he was now bradycardic. She had a slow heart rate; less than 60. And—although it's not recorded there—she either was or about to be hypotensive.

Mr Peters explained the adrenaline was administered in three 100 mcg aliquots, 60 seconds apart. The initial dose had no effect. Intubation commenced in the meantime. A second dose totalling 2 mg at 23:24 h produced some return of cardiac output, but only for 30 seconds or so.

Mr Peters diagnosed Ms Masson was suffering bilateral tension pneumothoraces (air trapped in the pleural space causing collapsed lung). The ambulance was stopped, not far from the hospital, and Mr Peters conducted an emergency left-side thoracostomy (an incision of the chest wall allowing trapped air to escape). This achieved the decompression of the left lung, accompanied by immediate improvement in heart rate and blood pressure. In light of that improvement and the proximity of the hospital, a right-sided thoracostomy was not attempted, and instead, to avoid further delay, the ambulance proceeded to the hospital.

At the hospital, Ms Masson was noted to be centrally and peripherally mottled and cyanosed. She had no respiratory effort. There was no carotid pulse. She was bagged

Continued

Case 6.5 *Masson v State of Queensland* [2018] QSC 162 continued

with resistance with inspiration. Adrenaline was administered at 23:41 h, 23:43 h and 23:45 h, provoking an immediate response, with a carotid pulse becoming discernible and increasing. Other measures were taken, including the relief of a right-sided pneumothorax, and she was transferred from emergency to intensive care at 00:30 h.

Subsequent to her arrival at the hospital, it became apparent that Ms Masson had suffered severe hypoxic brain damage as a result of oxygen deprivation. It is not in dispute that this was caused as a result of events prior to her arrival at hospital. The plaintiff contends the deprivation of oxygen giving rise to the hypoxic brain injury occurred in the course of her treatment by the ambulance officers, because adrenaline was not administered during the initial phase of her treatment at the scene. On the other hand, the defendant contends that Ms Masson's severe hypoxic brain damage had already irreversibly occurred prior to intervention by the ambulance officers.

The court described the issues for determination as being focused on the paramedic's assessments and decision-making at the scene; specifically, the decision that the pharmacological intervention at the scene should involve salbutamol and not adrenaline.

While the case was concluded in 2018, the events giving rise to the litigation occurred 16 years earlier. Jennifer Masson suffered hypoxic brain damage as a result of a severe asthma attack in 2002. It is alleged that she would have avoided the injury if the paramedics who attended her had promptly administered adrenaline. Their decision not to do so was said to have been contrary to Queensland Ambulance Service (QAS) guidelines, and amounted to a breach of the QAS's duty of patient care. Ms Masson lingered, catastrophically brain-damaged in around-the-clock care, for many years before her death in 2016. The action survived in the hands of her estate, and the amount of fiscal damages was agreed in the amount of $3 million prior to the 9-day trial of her action on the issue of the state's liability in negligence. The relevant QAS *Clinical Practice Manual for Asthma* in use at the time is reproduced below:

Dyspnoea
Asthma

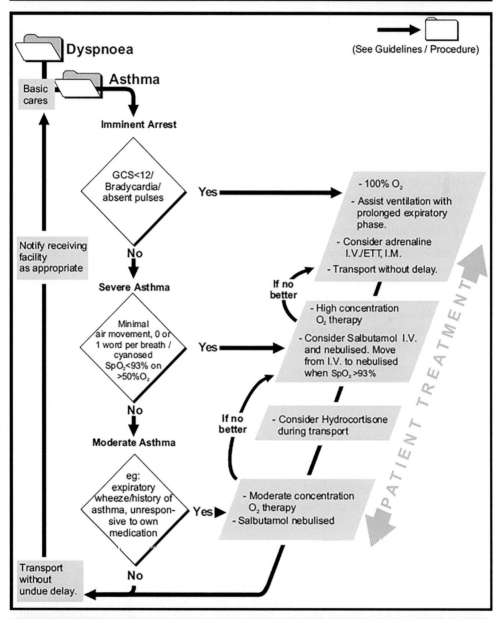

Version 2.1 issued by authority of the Queensland Ambulance Service - revised January 02　　　A2-8

As with all negligence cases, the four elements of the cause of action were at play; namely, duty of care, breach of duty, causation and damage. Interestingly, due to the timeframe of the events (2002), the case was decided solely on common law principles, without the overlay of the more modern statutory provisions under the *Civil Liability Act 2003* (Qld), while also noting that the ultimate result would not have turned on any of these newer provisions.

The elements of negligence are fundamentally four hurdles that must be collectively overcome to successfully prosecute a claim. Here, a duty of care was simple and obvious, where a paramedic acting in a professional capacity has a straightforward duty to a patient in their care. Additionally, the employer (QAS) was vicariously liable for the acts or omissions of the paramedic while acting within their scope of employment, which was clearly the case here.

Progressing to the final element of damage: this was an exceptional case where the quantum amount recoverable if negligence was proven, as described earlier, had preemptively been declared.

The remaining elements of breach of duty and causation were therefore the only contentious issues remaining, where one (causation) can only follow if the other (breach of duty) is proven.

Justice Henry summarised the requirements by stating:

> If the risk was such that the exercise of reasonable care and skill in emergency treatment by ambulance officers called for the administration of adrenaline at the time of the treatment administered at the scene by the ambulance officers ('the time of initial treatment') then the defendant was in breach of its duty of care in not then administering adrenaline. This aspect of the case requires consideration in a general sense of what was warranted by the known circumstances, as well as consideration of the QAS Clinical Practice Manual, particularly the QAS asthma guideline.

> It follows the real issues for determination relevant to breach may be shortly stated as follows:

> (i) In 2002 was adrenaline ordinarily the preferred drug to administer to asthmatics in extremis?

> (ii) Did Ms Masson's condition render salbutamol a preferred or equally acceptable option to adrenaline?

> (iii) Was the non-administration of adrenaline at the time of the initial treatment contrary to the QAS asthma guideline?[44]

The key summative points and conclusions on each breach issue are provided in Justice Henry's words below:

Breach of issue 1 …

> The events of present concern occurred 16 years ago. The focus in some of the expert evidence on the lack of scientifically proved justification for the traditional preference seemingly diverted attention from any detailed exploration of the timing and degree of the shift in preferences in clinical practice. Nonetheless, while there were doubtless credible views in 2002 favouring the equivalent utility of salbutamol for asthmatics in extremis, it may reasonably be inferred from the whole of the expert evidence that the practising medical

profession's traditional view in favour of ordinarily administering adrenaline to asthmatics in extremis was then likely a predominant view in the profession.

That said, such a view was hardly binding and could at best have been be no more than a default starting point, for the mere characterisation of a patient being extremis is to say nothing of the broader detail of the patient's condition. The traditional view would not have precluded the administration of salbutamol in preference to adrenaline if that was medically appropriate having regard to the discrete aspects of the patient's condition.

Illustrating the relevance of discrete conditions, it is clear from the expert evidence that adrenaline is and likely was regarded as preferable to salbutamol for administration to asthmatics in extremis when suffering cardiac arrest or anaphylactic reaction. Further, salbutamol would have been regarded then, as now, as unlikely to assist with bradycardia, decreased perfusion and decreased cardiac output, whereas adrenaline may. This demonstrates the significance of the discrete detail of the patient's condition. Here of course cardiac arrest or anaphylactic reaction were not known to be present at the time of initial treatment. It was unknown whether Ms Masson's asthma was the product of anaphylaxis and at the time of initial treatment she was not in cardiac arrest. She was apparently perfused, with a high blood pressure and cardiac output, indeed she was tachycardic, not bradycardic. As will be seen, whether her high heart rate and blood pressure were conditions mitigating against the administration of adrenaline is a relevant issue here.

The above conclusions derive from the expert opinions of medical practitioners rather than ambulance officers, the opinions of the two expert ambulance officers adding nothing material in this context. However, it is reasonable to expect the approach of ambulance services in the training and guidance of their officers would be informed by widely accepted medical opinion.

Breach of issue 2 …

I conclude that there would have existed a responsible body of opinion in the medical profession in support of the view that Ms Masson's high heart rate and high blood pressure, in the context of her overall condition, provided a medically sound basis to prefer the administration of salbutamol to the administration of adrenaline at the time of initial treatment.

This conclusion heralds obvious difficulty for the plaintiff's case.

Breach of issue 3 …

The treatment which was administered did not fall below the standard of care to be observed by ambulance officers and was not contrary to the QAS asthma guideline. No breach of the duty of care has been established and the claim must fail.[45]

Causation

Justice Henry then helpfully assessed liability from the causative sense by completing the negligence loop despite not being required to do so. His Honour stated:

Lest I be wrong in that conclusion I should for completeness address causation, on the premise, contrary to my view that the non-administration of adrenaline did result from a breach.

Causation issue 1: Would timely administration of adrenaline have avoided the injury?

…

In the robust drawing of inferences called for in the present process I infer, by reason of Ms Masson's past positive responses to the administration of adrenaline in the 1997 and 2000 episodes, it was more likely than not that the timely administration of adrenaline would have avoided Ms Masson's injury. In the present case though there was no opportunity for a 'timely' administration of adrenaline. There was a material intervening period before the arrival of ambulance officers.

Causation issue 2: Was the time of initial treatment too late for the injury to be avoided by administering adrenaline?

…

While the issue is finely balanced, I conclude that if, contrary to my findings, there was a breach by reason of a failure to administer adrenaline during the initial treatment, that breach was likely a material contributing cause of Ms Masson's injury. Put differently and aided by information the ambulance officers did not have, I conclude on the balance of probabilities that it was not too late at the time of initial treatment for Ms Masson's injury to be avoided by administering adrenaline.[46]

Comments on the findings

Justice Henry segmented the breach of duty analysis into three discrete inquiries. It was a typical medical negligence case with duelling expert witnesses ranging on both sides from emergency physicians to intensive-care paramedics and educators. The differentiation of the breach of duty questions into three distinct, but intertwined, inquiries provides a wealth of information in analysing prospective liability in these, and potentially future, circumstances.[47]

In answering the questions that he posed, Justice Henry undertook a detailed analysis of the evidence provided by the treating paramedic, the vast array of expert witnesses, and a meticulous assessment of the *QAS Clinical Practice Manual* (CPM) and the specific asthma guideline. This allowed a range of relevant conclusions to be reached, which were then weighed against an assortment of considerations, including the lapse of time, what the paramedic knew and did not know about the patient's condition, the state of knowledge and practice in this particular clinical area at the time, and even the specific wording of the 'guideline', which differentiated between the application of treatment regimens when dealing with a 'protocol'.

While each case is assessed and reasoned on its individual facts in reaching sound conclusions, under our common law system these specific facts must be overlayed with the guiding principles derived from the fundamental tenet of precedent. This case is a good example of these two tensions at play.

After an exhaustive hearing over 9 days in the Supreme Court of Queensland, Justice Henry reached the conclusion that the paramedic was not negligent in his treatment because he had acted as a reasonable paramedic would in the circumstances. This *appeared* to be a straightforward legal finding.

The plaintiff appealed the findings, and on 10 May 2019 the Queensland Court of Appeal handed down its decision in *Masson v State of Queensland* [2019] QCA 80. McMurdo JA (with whom Fraser JA and Boddice J agreed) allowed the appeal. The court found that the state of Queensland was liable for the negligence of the Queensland Ambulance Service (QAS) as the vicarious principal of the paramedic.

Justice McMurdo undertook a further analysis of the facts while also relevantly placing great emphasis on the application and adherence to the asthma CPM. Her Honour concluded that the standard of care expected of a paramedic was to administer treatment guided by the *Clinical Practice Manual*, stating:

> For the appellant, it was contended that the case which was presented to the officers was within the first of the 'diamonds', headed 'Imminent Arrest', with the consequence that Ms Masson was to be treated in the way set out in the shaded section opposite that alternative. The officers were to 'Consider adrenaline I.V./ETT, I.M.' The appellant's case was that this meant that adrenaline had to be administered, with the officers to consider only how that was to occur: intravenously ('I.V.'), by an endotracheal tube ('ETT') or intramuscularly ('I.M.').
>
> For the respondent, it was argued that this was not a case within the diamond which was highest on the page, because not every circumstance which was there listed, most particularly bradycardia, was present. Ms Masson was not bradycardic, instead she was tachycardic. Further, had the circumstances been within the first diamond, it was argued that the ambulance officers had to consider whether to administer adrenaline, rather than being directed to administer it.
>
> The trial judge accepted the appellant's argument that this was a case of 'Imminent Arrest' which was within the first diamond, because not every circumstances there listed had to be present. It was sufficient that the GCS was under 12. However, the judge rejected the appellant's argument as to the meaning of '[c]onsider adrenaline', holding that this required the officers to consider whether to administer adrenaline (and if so how), rather than compelling its administration in some form in every case of imminent arrest.
>
> In my view, the trial judge's interpretation, in each respect, was correct.[48]

Her Honour concluded on this point when stating:

> … it would not be consistent with the exercise of reasonable care and skill for an ambulance officer to depart from the guidance of the CPM. A substantial issue in this appeal is the scope of the discretion, provided by the flowchart, to 'consider adrenaline'. The exercise of reasonable care required that such consideration actually occur, but consistently with the guidance provided by the CPM. A departure from that guidance, with the grave risk that the patient would not avoid serious injury or death, could not be easily justified upon the basis that the officer believed that there was a responsible body of medical opinion which supported that course. Unlike the medical specialist, the ambulance officer does not have the requisite competence to make their own professional judgment about the merits of competing views within a field of specialised medical practice.[49]
>
> Dr Michael Eburn, writing on his highly regarded *Australian Emergency Law* site, reviewed the Court of Appeal's decision in great detail and offered a range of pertinent observations and comments on the findings and the relevance for paramedic practice. Dr Eburn stated:

Compare the decisions in the trial court and the court of the appeal. The trial judge took the view that Mr Peters considered adrenaline but ruled it out because of the risk of adverse side effects and with the knowledge of contests of ideas of when and which drug to use. That is he found, and accepted as not negligent, that there was an exercise in professional decision making.

The Court of Appeal found that the trial judge had misunderstood the evidence. That Mr Peters did not make the sort of judgement described, rather seeing that all the symptoms in the first diamond were not present, he took the view that he was not permitted to administer adrenaline. Further there was no dispute in medical opinion. If that's correct, so be it. If the judge misunderstood the evidence and if Mr Peters misunderstood the CPG then that was, in the Court of Appeal's view, negligent. But the Court of Appeal went further. A paramedic is not expected to know or understand the science behind the treatment guidelines or issues in contest within the science. Further he or she is not expected to make decisions other than to assess the symptoms to identify what guideline applies and then apply that guideline.

Although this case was decided in 2019, the treatment given to Ms Masson was delivered in 2002. Paramedicine has come a long way since 2002 including the now almost universal requirement for new paramedics to have degree qualifications and the recognition of paramedic professionalism as shown by registration of paramedics under the *Health Practitioner Regulation National Law* since December 2018. There is no discussion of any evidence about developments in paramedic practice and it would not have been relevant as the question was whether the treatment delivered in 2002 meet the standard of reasonable care to be expected from a paramedic in 2002. But whether a court would take the same view of treatment in 2019 remains to be seen.

Perhaps Mr Peters did not exercise sufficient imagination in this case, seeing that this patient did not have bradycardia he concluded that she was not at risk of imminent arrest even though she was in fact in respiratory arrest. He was, according to the court, expected to take a more wholistic view of the patient's presentation and identify that [cardiac] arrest was imminent and therefore the only treatment called for was adrenaline, not salbutamol. I'll leave that to others to decide if that was reasonable and how you would read the QAS (CPM) flow chart.[50]

Comments on this case

Dr Eburn's observations and conclusions give rise to a number of interesting and challenging points in a sector that has evolved in a steady and strategic fashion over the past 20 years through its increasing professionalism, as exhibited by educational and regulatory advancements, which now manifest into a sector with its own body of knowledge and relative independence of practice.

Is this decision, with its requirement of rigid adherence to clinical guidelines, a case of 'one step forward and two steps back' for the profession? Time will tell.

At the time of writing, the defendant may have an appeal opportunity to the High Court of Australia but the narrowness of potential grounds may be a hindrance to this option.

Negligence case study 3

The case of *Neal v Ambulance Service of New South Wales* [2008] NSWCA 346 (Case 6.6) provides an interesting extension to the earlier cases analysed.

In this scenario—again, an all too familiar one in ambulance practice—the patient was able to sustain a claim in negligence against the Ambulance Service and the paramedics

Case 6.6 *Neal v Ambulance Service of New South Wales* [2008] NSWCA 346

Mr Neal was a 45-year-old man. On the night of 27 July 2001, Mr Neal (the initial plaintiff and now appellant in these proceedings) suffered a serious blow to the head while walking alone in Newcastle. Police discovered him and called an ambulance. He rejected assistance from the ambulance officers. Since he was clearly inebriated, the police took him into custody under the *Intoxicated Persons Act 1979* (NSW). The following morning, his condition was observed to deteriorate and, being unable to rouse him easily, the police had him taken to the Mater Hospital. A CT scan done at the Mater Hospital showed an extradural haematoma with a fracture to the skull. The plaintiff was transferred to the John Hunter Hospital for surgery to drain the extradural haematoma.

The plaintiff suffered different ongoing disabilities following the assault. Some, particularly his right-sided weakness (hemiparesis), were allegedly caused by the failure to take him to hospital when the police found him in the street.

He brought proceedings in the District Court for negligence against the state (it being responsible for the police's alleged negligence) and the Ambulance Service of New South Wales. He was successful only against the Ambulance Service, recovering damages assessed on the basis of a 'loss of a chance' of a better outcome. He appealed against the trial judge's findings with respect to the state's liability and damages. The Ambulance Service cross-appealed in relation to its liability.

The case created significant complications, because the court had to assess whether any further damage had been caused by the delay (the District Court found this to be 8 hours) between the first possibility of being taken to hospital after the police took control of the plaintiff and the actual time he initially received treatment at hospital. A number of experts were called to give evidence on the connection between the injuries the plaintiff was claiming, the initial blow and the delay in receiving treatment.

The plaintiff initially received nearly $100,000 for a range of damages, including past and future economic loss, care services and medical expenses.

because the court found that their performance had fallen below the standard of care required. Although the case did find a breach of duty by the paramedics, the appeal court overturned the lower court's decision on the ground that causation was not sustainable when the patient's condition and predicted behaviour were taken into account.

The case review will assess the scenario through the lower court's initial finding and the appeal court's alternative decision, and then analyse the decision in light of this problematic area of ambulance practice.

The negligence of the paramedics

The case was an interesting one from a number of negligence perspectives. The paramedics did not actually provide any active treatment to the patient in the way of care and transport; therefore, this was potentially a case of negligence by omission, or what they did not do.

The court noted the comments of the paramedic when stating:

> If the plaintiff had been willing to go to hospital they probably would have taken him because he had a laceration and a bump on his head. She was aware that there was a risk of a haematoma and that any head injury could be a significant head injury.[51]

The District Court gave this summary of what was assessed:

- As against the Ambulance Service, there are two relevant bases on which the plaintiff claims it was negligent through the actions of the ambulance officers.
- First, they should have spent longer trying to persuade the plaintiff to permit a full examination and/or be taken to hospital.
- Secondly, the ambulance officers should have informed the police officers that they had been unable to complete their examination of the plaintiff, there was a possibility of a serious injury and he needed to be taken to hospital to have the head injury thoroughly checked.[52]

The initial case revolved around the need for the paramedics to inform the police that the patient should either be taken directly to hospital or be taken should they see signs of deterioration, such as an altered conscious state or vomiting.

Conclusion as to the paramedic's negligence

The District Court concluded:

> I am satisfied that the ambulance officers breached their duty of care to the plaintiff in failing to inform the police officers:
>
> 1 Of the possible consequences of their inability to fully examine the plaintiff.
> 2 That the plaintiff should be taken to a hospital to be medically assessed. I do not consider however that the evidence establishes that the ambulance officers spent insufficient time trying to persuade the plaintiff to co-operate in the examination and/or go with them to a hospital. They continued trying until they formed the view that the plaintiff's attitude was unlikely to change.[53]

Comments on the district court judgment

This case study is in contrast to *Ambulance Service of NSW v Worley* (Case 6.4), because it involves an omission as distinct from a negligence allegation based on active treatment, and the manner in which the case was argued gives us more guidance on how to avoid negligence actions in an ambulance context.

It sets out the way in which patients who refuse transport should be handled when delivered to a third party for care or custody; in this instance, the further care or custody of the police.

The appeal to the NSW Supreme Court of Appeal

The plaintiff, Mr Neal, appealed the decision to the NSW Supreme Court of Appeal on the basis that his 'loss of chance' of a better outcome should be extended and his damages were inadequate. He was dramatically, and rather surprisingly, unsuccessful, because his appeal points were not even considered, due to a cross-appeal by the Ambulance Service of New South Wales, which was successful on the key negligence element of causation.

The Court of Appeal reviewed evidence from the earlier case, summarised the position, and focused on the next step in the analysis of negligence when stating:

> For present purposes, nothing is gained by asking, in the abstract, whether ambulance officers owed the plaintiff a duty of care: the only relevant question is whether the ambulance officers owed the plaintiff a duty which required them to advise the police that the plaintiff needed to be conveyed to hospital.[54]

The Court of Appeal then reconsidered numerous aspects of the initial case, while accepting the earlier court's decision that the paramedics breached their duty of care by not fully advising the police officers that Mr Neal required medical assessment due to his potential for greater injury, despite his lack of consent to treatment and his unwillingness to cooperate. The Court of Appeal said:

> The plaintiff contended that the ambulance officers should have been alert to the need for a medical assessment at hospital, something the police officers would not have appreciated. If properly advised, however, the police should have taken him to hospital themselves.[55]

Mr Neal's case came down to causation. Did the negligence of the paramedics cause his injury? The court concluded:

> With respect to the liability of the ambulance officers, accepting that they should have informed the police of the plaintiff's need for medical assessment and accepting that the police would have taken him to hospital, the plaintiff would still have failed to establish liability on the part of the Ambulance Service unless he satisfied the Court that he would have accepted medical assessment and treatment from a hospital. That question was not addressed in terms by the trial judge. Without an affirmative finding on that issue, the claim against the ambulance officers should have failed.[56]

> The only available inference is that he would not willingly have gone to hospital and submitted to medical assessment, whether taken by the police (which was itself improbable) or in an ambulance. It follows that he failed to establish, affirmatively, that he would have accepted medical assessment and treatment. Any breach of duty on the part of the ambulance officers was therefore not shown to have caused the delay in obtaining treatment and hence liability was not established. The cross-appeal should be upheld and the judgement in favour of the plaintiff set aside.[57]

The difficulties associated with intoxicated and/or non-compliant patients are highlighted when a paramedic is aware, as they were in this case, that an underlying injury or illness may be possible but the patient refuses treatment. The issues of patient autonomy, consent and restraint all arise in this scenario, but paramedics must operate within their designated guidelines.

In fact, the plaintiff's lawyers initially claimed negligence by the paramedics on the grounds that they did not forcibly restrain the patient and transport him to hospital, but this was withdrawn before it could be tested.

What the finding does tell us is that all care must be taken to persuade a patient who obviously requires hospital attention to go to hospital (as these paramedics were found to have done adequately, although they were unable to convince the patient to go to hospital), and, if the patient remains in the care of a third party, to inform that third party that they should take the patient to hospital and/or what they should do if certain events occur in relation to the patient's condition.

The case does not tell us whether the patient was asked to sign as a 'refused transport'. It is an all too familiar situation in the field that must be carefully assessed on each occasion.

While the Ambulance Service, as the authority ultimately responsible for the actions of the paramedics, was arguably fortunate on this occasion because causation was not established in the analysis, the case does provide paramedics and their employers with guidance in this area of the law.

A hypothetical negligence case

Case 6.7 was introduced at the beginning of this chapter.

This case should be considered in light of the elements of negligence and potential defences.

Case 6.7 Negligence

A paramedic has been called to the scene where a man has had a fall and suffered a non-life-threatening head injury that will require hospital treatment for suturing of a wound. When the paramedic arrives, the patient behaves aggressively, appears intoxicated and refuses transport, despite continued requests to take him to the hospital for treatment. The patient then leaves the scene after the paramedic has bandaged his head wound. He is later struck by a car and sustains significant injuries.

He sues the ambulance service for negligence, on the basis that his treatment was below the required standard in two areas: first, that he should have been convinced to go to hospital; and, secondly, that the bandage applied was not adequately secured, and slid down over his face, which obscured his vision and caused him to be struck by the car.

The elements are:
* duty of care
* breach of duty
* damage
* causation
* defences.

Duty of care Paramedics will always owe a patient a duty of care when acting in their professional capacity. Therefore, this element will be fulfilled—see *Neal v Ambulance Service of New South Wales* [2008] NSWCA 346.

Breach of duty Various factors are considered in the civil liability Acts when assessing a breach of duty, while noting that the fundamental question of whether *a person acted with reasonable care in avoiding foreseeable injury to others in the circumstances* is the essence of whether a breach of duty has occurred in a given fact situation.

This case gives rise to two assessments. First, should more have been done to ensure the patient was transported to hospital when the paramedics were aware that treatment was required, and, secondly, was the treatment that was provided below the standard expected of a reasonable paramedic in the circumstances?

On the first point, we are told that 'the patient behaves aggressively, appears intoxicated and refuses transport despite continued requests'. Although more information may be required, it would appear that the paramedics have done all that is possible in the circumstances to convince the patient to go to hospital, to no avail. The paramedics, in all of the circumstances, have not fallen below the required standard of care.

The extension in this scenario—similar to *Neal v Ambulance Service of New South Wales*—is whether a third party, such as the police, should have been involved to facilitate transport of the patient to hospital.

The second enquiry is whether the patient was adequately treated through the application of a bandage to his head. On the surface, it would appear that the bandage was applied in an inadequate manner because it did not stay in place; however, a detailed analysis of whether the paramedics had acted reasonably in the circumstances would take place to ascertain whether they had actually breached their duty. Further influencing factors could centre on the broader notions of patient autonomy and personal responsibility, with Australian courts over the past decade placing a greater emphasis on an individual's accountability for their own actions in negligence claims.

Although the initial finding *could* establish that the paramedics had fallen below the requisite standard of care, further analysis of the elements of negligence and defences would relieve the paramedics of liability.

Damage The facts inform us that the potential plaintiff has suffered 'significant' injuries. Therefore, we can assume that he meets the threshold requirements for damage.

Causation Causation requires an analysis of 'factual causation' and the 'scope of liability'.

Therefore, did the defendant's negligence *cause* the damage, or was it too *remote* to be blamed on the defendant in the circumstances? Although it would be in the balance as to whether liability would be found on the second point, causation principles can be applied to both inquiries. Factual causation would potentially be established if the paramedics were found to have breached their duty of care because it would be *reasonably foreseeable* that an intoxicated plaintiff with a head injury would be struck by a car if a bandage were to be inadequately applied. The scope of liability or remoteness of damage would also possibly be established because the actual injuries would, again, be reasonably foreseeable in the circumstances.

Further, in a similar fact scenario in *Neal v Ambulance Service of New South Wales*, the court found that causation was not sustainable because the plaintiff could not prove that, even if he was advised and treated at the required standard, he would not have accepted the care and transport. Applying this case to the facts, causation would not be established.

Defences The defence of contributory negligence and the statutory factors around intoxication would be highly relevant in this scenario, but would come into play only if all of the elements of negligence were upheld.

Focusing on the key defence of contributory negligence, the assessment is an objective test as to whether the plaintiff did what a reasonable person in that given situation would have, or should have, done. Applying this principle to the facts, the patient's aggressive and non-complying approach, which arguably contributed significantly to his injuries, would negate any breach of duty to a considerable degree and potentially by 100%, which is now possible under a number of civil liability Acts.

Conclusion on this case

This case has shown how a negligence action would progress in a typical ambulance scenario. The result would invariably see the paramedics exonerated from a negligence claim, due, initially, to doubts on the numerous aspects of causation, and, ultimately, to the patient's own actions.

From a number of perspectives, scenarios such as this exhibit the ease with which difficulties for paramedics can arise, even after they have dealt with a case and they are no longer in direct contact with the patient. Ensuring all of the relevant protocols and procedures are followed in every case is always a paramount consideration. The practical tip from this scenario is: when issues of intoxication and cognisance arise, ensure that all of the information possible is made available to the patient, and consider third-party intervention when your professional judgement identifies potential dangers to a patient who refuses transport.

Conclusion

The aim of this chapter was to introduce the important common law and statutory principles that are required to establish a negligence action, while reviewing a number of the issues that paramedics may encounter in the field when faced with problematic situations.

We identified the elements of negligence through an introduction to the duty of care and an assessment of the various aspects of breach of duty, then briefly examined causation and remoteness of damage, and rounded off the analysis by reviewing the two key defences that are available in a negligence action.

The relationship of the paramedic's employer through the window of vicarious liability was discussed, while also assessing the personal and professional responsibilities of the paramedic when acting in different capacities.

The chapter concluded by reviewing two relevant cases that applied the key elements of negligence in an ambulance/paramedical environment to contextualise our examination of negligence laws.

Review Questions

1 What are the elements of negligence, and which are the most problematic in ambulance practice?
2 What piece of legislation codifies the common law principles of negligence in your personal jurisdiction?
3 How might the defence of contributory negligence apply in common ambulance practice situations?
4 Do you agree with the NSW Court of Appeal in *Ambulance Service of NSW v Worley* [2006] NSWCA 102, where it was stated:
   a) Ambulance officers are not medical practitioners, let alone specialists in emergency medicine. Their training is by no means insignificant, but it does not equip them with the theoretical knowledge which would permit a fine evaluation of alternative treatments.
5 In *Neal v Ambulance Service of New South Wales* [2008] NSWCA 346, the court found that the paramedics were negligent because, despite their reasonable attempts to persuade the patient to go to hospital, they had failed to inform a third party (the police, in this instance) of the possible consequences of their inability to fully examine the plaintiff and that the plaintiff should be taken to a hospital to be medically assessed. Discuss how you might alleviate this danger in practice.

Endnotes

1 Mendelson, D. (2014) *The New Law of Torts*, 3rd ed. South Melbourne: Oxford University Press, p. 4.
2 Kerridge, I., Lowe, M. and Stewart, C. (2015) *Ethics and Law for the Health Professions*, 4th ed. Sydney: The Federation Press, p. 74.
3 Ipp, D., Cane, P., Sheldon, D. et al. *Review of the Law of Negligence—Final Report*. Canberra: Commonwealth of Australia. Available: https://static.treasury.gov.au/uploads/sites/1/2017/06/R2002-001_Law_Neg_Final.pdf (accessed 3 November 2018).
4 See *Wrongs Act 1958* (Vic), s 47.

5   Sappideen, C., Vines, P. and Watson, P. (2016) *Torts, Commentary and Materials*, 3rd ed. Pyrmont, NSW: Lawbook Co, p. 193.

6   *Donoghue v Stevenson* [1932] AC 562.

7   Ibid., at 580.

8   Stickley, A. (2016) *Australian Torts Law*, 4th ed. Chatswood, NSW: LexisNexis Butterworths, p. 151.

9   *Civil Liability Act 2002* (NSW), s 5B(1); *Civil Liability Act 2002* (Tas), s 9; *Wrongs Act 1958* (Vic), s 48; *Civil Law (Wrongs) Act 2002* (ACT), s 42; *Civil Liability Act 2003* (Qld), s 9; *Civil Liability Act 1936* (SA), s 31; *Civil Liability Act 2002* (WA), s 5B(1).

10 *Civil Liability Act 2002* (NSW), s 5B(2); *Civil Liability Act 2002* (Tas), s 11; *Wrongs Act 1958* (Vic), s 48(1); *Civil Law (Wrongs) Act 2002* (ACT), s 43; *Civil Liability Act 2003* (Qld), s 9; *Civil Liability Act 1936* (SA), s 32; *Civil Liability Act 2002* (WA), s 5B(2).

11 *Civil Liability Act 2002* (NSW), s 5B(2); *Civil Liability Act 2002* (Tas), s 11; *Wrongs Act 1958* (Vic), s 48(2); *Civil Law (Wrongs) Act 2002* (ACT), s 43; *Civil Liability Act 2003* (Qld), s 9; *Civil Liability Act 1936* (SA), s 32; *Civil Liability Act 2002* (WA), s 5B(2).

12 Mendelson, *The New Law of Torts.*

13 *Civil Liability Act 2002* (NSW), s 50; *Civil Liability Act 2003* (Qld), s 22; *Civil Liability Act 2002* (Tas), s 22; *Wrongs Act 1958* (Vic), s 59; noting that, in other states and territories, the common law will apply.

14 Kerridge, I., Lowe, M., and Stewart, C. *Ethics and Law for the Health Professions.*

15 Note that this is a codification of a common law principle that would be likely to apply in other jurisdictions.

16 *Wrongs Act 1958* (Vic), s 58; *Civil Liability Act 1936* (SA), s 40.

17 *Rogers v Whitaker* (1992) 175 CLR 479.

18 Mendelson, *The New Law of Torts.*

19 Ibid.

20 See *Wrongs Act 1958* (Vic), s 28LF.

21 *Civil Law (Wrongs) Act 2002* (ACT), s 45; *Civil Liability Act 2002* (NSW), s 5D; *Civil Liability Act 2003* (Qld), s 11; *Civil Liability Act 1936* (SA), s 34; *Civil Liability Act 2002* (Tas), s 13; *Civil Liability Act 2002* (WA), s 5C; *Wrongs Act 1958* (Vic), s 51; noting that the Northern Territory has no equivalent provision and the common law therefore applies.

22 Mendelson, *The New Law of Torts.*

23 *Civil Liability Act 2002* (NSW), s 57; *Civil Liability Act 2002* (Tas), s 35B; *Wrongs Act 1958* (Vic), s 31B; *Civil Law (Wrongs) Act 2002* (ACT), s 5; *Civil Liability Act 1936* (SA), s 74; *Civil Liability Act 2002* (WA), s 5AD; *Personal Injuries Act 2003* (NT), s 8; *Civil Liability Act 2003* (Qld), s 27.

24 See *Civil Liability (Wrongs) Act 2002* (ACT), s 5(4)(c).

25 See *Civil Liability (Wrongs) Act 2002* (ACT), s 3(c); *Civil Liability Act 1936* (SA), s 74(1)(c); *Personal Injuries Act 2003* (NT), s 8(4)(c).

26 *Civil Liability Act 2002* (NSW), s 50(1).

27 *Wrongs Act 1958* (Vic), s14(G)(2)(a) and (b).

28 Mendelson, The New Law of Torts.

29 *Civil Liability Act 2002* (NSW), s 5R; *Civil Liability Act 2002* (Tas), s 23; *Wrongs Act 1958* (Vic), s 48; *Civil Law (Wrongs) Act 2002* (ACT), s 47; *Civil Liability Act 1936* (SA), s 44; *Civil Liability Act 2002* (WA), s 5K; *Personal Injuries Act 2003* (NT), s 16; *Civil Liability Act 2003* (Qld), s 23.

30 Eburn, M. (2010) *Emergency Law—Rights, Liabilities and Duties of Emergency Workers and Volunteers*, 3rd ed. Leichhardt, NSW: The Federation Press.

31 Mendelson, *The New Law of Torts.*

32   Ibid.
33   *Wrongs Act 1958* (Vic), s 54(1).
34   Ibid., s 54(2)(a).
35   Ibid., s 53(1) and (2).
36   *Consumer and Competition Act 2010* (Cth), s 139A.
37   See section 5K of the *Civil Liability Act 2002* (NSW), where 'dangerous recreational activity' means a recreational activity that involves a significant risk of physical harm.
38   *Civil Liability Act 2002* (NSW), s 5L.
39   *Ambulance Service of NSW v Worley* [2006] NSWCA 102, at [60].
40   Ibid., at [72].
41   Ibid., at [29]–[30].
42   Ibid., at [96].
43   Ibid., at [154].
44   *Masson v State of Queensland* [2018] QSC 162, at [35], [38].
45   Ibid., at [56]–[59], [93]–[94], [155].
46   Ibid., at [156], [167], [182].
47   They should be read in their entirety to fully contextualise the findings to contemporary paramedic practice.
48   *Masson v State of Queensland* [2019] QCA 80, at [20]–[23].
49   Ibid., at [149].
50   Australian Emergency Law at https://emergencylaw.wordpress.com/.
51   *Neal v Ambulance Service of NSW and The State of New South Wales* [2007] NSWDC 123, at [11].
52   Ibid., at [11], [25].
53   Ibid., at [11], [40].
54   *Neal v Ambulance Service of New South Wales* [2008] NSWCA 346, at [24].
55   Ibid., at [16].
56   Ibid., at [33].
57   Ibid., at [49].

Chapter 7
End-of-life care

Ruth Townsend

Learning objectives

After reading this chapter, you should be able to:

- identify the legal requirements and mechanisms that allow patients to make an advance care directive (ACD) in each Australian jurisdiction
- understand the difference between the withdrawal and/or withholding of life-sustaining treatment from competent as opposed to incompetent adults
- understand the role of a substitute decision-maker in the end-of-life decision-making process
- determine the significance of the doctrine of double effect and how it applies in end-of-life care
- understand the paramedic's role in end-of-life care.

Definitions[1]

'Euthanasia' is Greek for 'good death'. However, because the term is associated with death, it holds great power to evoke an emotional response in people upon hearing it. What do you think of when you hear the term 'euthanasia'? Due to the lack of clarity of the definition of the terms used in end-of-life discussions, it is best to set out what the various terms used in this chapter mean.

Adult A person who has reached the age of 18 years of age in Australia, and 20 years in New Zealand, and has full legal capacity. In South Australia, an adult is someone 16 years or over for medical purposes.[2]

Advanced care directive A document that expresses a person's wishes in relation to medical treatment in the event of becoming incapacitated, and must relate to the condition at hand. It must have been signed by the patient.

Capacity See 'competence'.

Competence In the healthcare context, and in particular in end-of-life decision-making, a person is competent or has decision-making capacity if they are able to understand the nature, purpose and consequences of a decision. This is demonstrated when the patient

---

can 'comprehend, retain and weigh up relevant information', make a decision regarding their future healthcare treatment, and then communicate that decision to others. There is a presumption of competence in adults; it is a matter for healthcare staff to demonstrate otherwise.

Euthanasia A deliberate act or omission undertaken with the intention of causing the death of another person in order to relieve that person's suffering. Euthanasia can be voluntary, involuntary or non-voluntary.

Futile treatment Treatment that would offer no reasonable benefit to the patient or achieve a better outcome for the patient.

Involuntary euthanasia When the person concerned may possess the capacity to consent, but their life is terminated against their will.

Life-sustaining treatment Treatment that includes cardiopulmonary resuscitation (CPR), assisted ventilation, artificial nutrition and hydration, but *does not* include blood transfusions.

Non-voluntary euthanasia When a patient is incapable of forming an opinion on euthanasia or is unable to communicate any such opinion.

Substitute decision-maker A person appointed to make decisions on behalf of another who lacks the requisite mental capacity to make decisions for themselves. A person may be appointed to the role formally through an instrument (e.g. enduring guardianship form) or by order of a court or tribunal; or they may be appointed informally via a hierarchy of decision-makers as noted in guardianship legislation (e.g. *Guardianship Act 1987* (NSW), s 33A).

Terminal illness An illness or condition that is likely to result in death. The 'terminal phase' of such an illness is defined as 'the phase of the illness reached when there is no real prospect of recovery or remission of symptoms (on either a permanent or temporary basis)'.[3]

Urgent treatment Treatment urgently needed by a patient to save that patient's life, or to prevent serious damage to the patient's health, or to prevent the patient from suffering or continuing to suffer significant pain or distress.[4]

Voluntary euthanasia When euthanasia is carried out at a competent patient's request. For example, a person's life is ended through the withdrawal or withholding of medical treatment at the patient's request (*passive euthanasia*).

An introductory case

The dying patient

You are called to a case of 'patient unwell'. On arrival, you find a young female, aged around 30, lying on her bed, the phone beside her and a piece of paper on her chest.

Continued

An introductory case continued

She is semi-conscious, and when she sees you she says, 'Good, you're here. I don't want to be saved. Here are my directions', and passes you the paper from her chest. On the table beside the bed is an empty bottle of ethylene glycol (otherwise known as antifreeze). Her letter says the following:

To whom it may concern, if you attend to me because I have overdosed or made an attempt on my life, I do NOT want any life-saving treatment to be given. I would appreciate medicine to relieve my discomfort. I understand that refusing life-saving treatment may result in my death. I refuse life-saving treatment knowing this. If I survive the initial attempt but have resultant kidney failure, I do NOT consent to dialysis being commenced.

I only called the ambulance so that they could take me to hospital and make me comfortable. I would also prefer to die in hospital and not at home alone. Thank you for respecting my wishes.

(Adapted from Inquest into the death of Kerrie Wooltorton, unrep, Norfolk County Coroner's Court, Armstrong J, 28 September 2009.)

This chapter will introduce you to one of the key legal and ethical issues faced by paramedics in their practice: end-of-life decision-making.

Introduction

A percentage of patients who feel burdened with pain and suffering consider ending their lives.[5] In addition, there is a percentage of patients who have not experienced pain and suffering yet, but understand that if they wait until that point they may physically require the assistance of someone else to help them to relieve their suffering, and so seek to end their own lives prematurely, thus avoiding the involvement of any other person in their death.[6]

It is well understood that the bulk of individual healthcare spending occurs in the last few months of an individual's life.[7] According to a study by Lowthian et al.,[8] people aged over 85 accounted for 13.6% of ambulance transportations in 2007/08, and this was projected to increase substantially over the coming years. Katelaris argues that it is time to re-think how we manage the care of the elderly, and proposes some alternative models of care in the pre-hospital environment that would assist in the better management of both patients and resources.[9] One way in which this management can be facilitated is to allow individuals to make known their wishes regarding their end-of-life care. In an attempt to encourage this behaviour and to sanction it, state and territory governments have introduced legislation and guidelines that enable the patient's wishes, with regard to the care and treatment they do not want, to be acknowledged and upheld by health practitioners. However, state and federal laws differ with regard to the regulation in this area. This chapter will provide a comparative overview of Australian law, and will examine the paramedic's role in end-of-life decision-making. This chapter will also integrate the ethical considerations that accompany any discussion on the end of life.

Background

In 1995 the Northern Territory became the first jurisdiction in the world to permit doctor-assisted suicide. The *Rights of the Terminally Ill Act 1995* (NT) provided legal authority for a doctor to end the life of a terminally ill patient at their request. The law has been described as 'neither an unqualified "licence to kill" nor an unqualified affirmation of a competent adult patient's right to assistance in dying'.[10]

The first person to try to rely on the Act was 66-year-old Max Bell, who was suffering from terminal stomach cancer. He travelled from his home in Broken Hill to Darwin to die. The Act stipulated that he had to find three doctors to verify his eligibility to utilise the provisions of the Act, but he was able to find only one. Max returned home to Broken Hill to die of natural causes. Max Bell's case highlights the difficulties of implementing such an Act even if one were to be reintroduced into Australia. (The Northern Territory law was repealed by the federal government in 1997.)[11]

A further attempt to reintroduce pro-euthanasia laws in Australia was the South Australian *Criminal Law Consolidation (Medical Defences—End of Life Arrangements) Amendment Bill* 2011;[12] however, this Bill was defeated in the South Australian Parliament. Another attempt was made by New South Wales in 2017 with the *Voluntary Assisted Dying Bill 2017*, which was described as 'An Act to establish the right of persons who are terminally ill to request assistance from medically qualified persons to voluntarily end their own lives; and for related purposes.' Despite overwhelming support by the whole Australia community,[13] both the New South Wales government and the opposition parties declined to support the Bill.

However, in October 2017 Victoria introduced the *Voluntary Assisted Dying Bill*. It was passed through both houses of parliament after a marathon debate. The law is set to take effect in 2019, and will be Australia's first assisted-dying legislation since the Northern Territory law two decades ago. Unlike with the earlier law, the Commonwealth will have no power to repeal Victoria's law. The law will permit a terminally ill person with only 6 months to live, or 12 months for those with neurodegenerative conditions, such as motor neurone disease, multiple sclerosis and Alzheimer's disease, and who has lived in Victoria for at least 12 months, and who is suffering in a way that 'cannot be relieved in a manner the person deems tolerable' to obtain a lethal drug if they are approved following two independent medical assessments. They must be over the age of 18, competent and able to administer the drug themselves. A doctor may be able to assist with administration in special cases. There are some issues with placing time limits on estimating when a person will die, because those timeframes are usually 'arbitrary and difficult to accurately predict'. Some have argued that 'they can also lead to people taking harmful steps to fall inside them [the timeframes], such as starving themselves'.[14]

Although Victoria will permit assisted dying in 2019, it will only be under strictly prescribed circumstances. The law essentially remains that the deliberate taking of a life, or assisting another person to die, even when that person gives their consent, is a crime in all Australian jurisdictions.

A study conducted in 1997 found that 1.8% of all Australian deaths involved active voluntary euthanasia and physician-assisted suicide.[15] The study also revealed that the decision not to treat, with the objective of quickening death or not extending a patient's life, occurred in an estimated 24.7% of all Australian deaths, and 14.3% of such deaths were preceded by a medical decision. Of great concern is that only a tenth of these decisions were made at the patient's request.[16] There is little evidence to suggest that much has changed, because the area remains unregulated, and the results of this study highlight the dangers inherent within the relatively unregulated system, which is more open to abuse than a regulated, ethical voluntary euthanasia scheme.

Apart from highlighting the power that doctors have to engage in such behaviour and not be sanctioned for it, it suggests that a more strongly regulated and transparent euthanasia scheme might allow patients to make better choices with regard to their end-of-life care, while at the same time providing protection to those who do not wish to die. In addition, it would offer some protection to practitioners working in this area. The community largely favours the terminally ill having the right to choose a medically assisted death.[17] A 2016 survey revealed that 75% of Australians support legalising euthanasia.[18] However, there is a segment of the community that remains reluctant to support it, and this includes the Australian Medical Association and various religious groups.[19]

As a result of acknowledging that (1) there is a segment of the community that wants to have some control over the time and way in which they die, but that their choices in this area are currently limited, and (2) healthcare resources are finite, there has been a move in recent years to increase the use of advance care directives (ACD) to inform health practitioners about a patient's preferences with regard to end-of-life care. Indeed, case law suggests that, particularly in those cases where a patient is refusing life-sustaining treatment and has a valid and applicable advance directive, the court will prioritise upholding the autonomy of the patient over the preserving of a life.[20]

ACDs offer an opportunity for competent adults to outline their wishes with respect to what healthcare they refuse to consent to at some future time when their capacity may be lost. The legal authority for ACDs comes out of the common law, and is now also found in much legislation.[21] Despite legislation facilitating written and oral advance directives, government-funded research projects and a plethora of official policies promoting them, very few elderly or terminally ill patients make advance directives in Australia.[22] However, ACDs offer some choices to people regarding their end-of-life care, and at the very least promote discussion of these difficult issues within families and communities.

Advance care directives and advance care plans

There are statutory provisions in six Australian states and territories that set out the requirements of a valid advance directive. The purpose of legislating this area is captured in the South Australian Act, which sets out the objects of the law as follows:

(a) to make certain reforms to the law relating to consent to medical treatment—
    (i) to allow persons of or over the age of 16 years to decide freely for themselves on an informed basis whether or not to undergo medical treatment; and
    (ii) …
    (iii) to provide for the administration of emergency medical treatment in certain circumstances without consent; and

(b) to provide for the medical treatment of people who have impaired decision-making capacity; and

(c) to allow for the provision of palliative care, in accordance with proper standards, to people who are dying and to protect them from medical treatment that is intrusive, burdensome and futile.[23]

The Victorian, Western Australian and Australian Capital Territory[24] laws allow refusal for any treatment, but, although Queensland, the Northern Territory and South Australia have advance planning laws, the laws can apply only to a patient who is terminally ill or permanently unconscious and/or they do not permit euthanasia.[25]

New South Wales currently lacks any formal legislation relating to end-of-life decisions, but it does have non-binding guidelines that indicate that an ACD should be considered as sufficient authority for a medical treatment decision, provided that it is specific to the disease or injury relevant to the decision, is current and is made by a competent individual.[26]

NSW Health's *End of Life Care and Decision-Making—Guidelines* provide healthcare practitioners with the tools to navigate the processes with patients and their families. For example, the Ambulance Service of New South Wales has produced a palliative care instruction sheet regarding treatment options to guide patients, treating clinicians and family members in the event that the patient suffers a cardiac arrest. However, the document places the onus for completion, and validating, on the treating medical officer, prior to submission to the Ambulance Service of New South Wales, for it to be processed. This procedure is problematic, because: if there are processing delays (which may be more pronounced if the form is incomplete), then the patient's wishes may be disregarded and, contrary to their wishes, treatment initiated; the Ambulance Service of New South Wales cannot dictate that the treating medical officer has the responsibility for validating the ACD, given the 2009 decision of the New South Wales Supreme Court in *Hunter and New England Area Health Service v A* [2009] NSWSC 761, that if the ACD is signed by the patient it should be assumed to be valid.[27]

To date, Tasmania has not legally attempted to address the topic of ACDs, and so possesses no legislation allowing directives either to be made or followed.

In essence, there are two key requirements for an advance directive to be considered valid.[28] They are:

1 The maker of the directive must be competent. (The elements of competence were discussed in Chapter 5, 'Consent and refusal of treatment'.)

2 The maker of the directive must make the direction freely.

The introductory case, 'The dying patient', gives us the opportunity to explore some of the issues likely to be faced by paramedics in this area. For example, you might consider the following:

1 Should we uphold the patient's request as it is listed in her directive?

2 Is the directive the patient has given you 'legal' or 'legally enforceable'?

3 What would happen if you did uphold it and the patient died?

4 What would happen if you didn't uphold it and saved the patient's life?

These are all valid and sensible questions to ask. Question 1 captures well the ethical problem at the heart of this case, as discussed in the PRECARE decision-making model introduced in Chapter 3, 'PRECARE—an ethical decision-making model for paramedics'. And the answers to questions 2, 3 and 4 are facts a paramedic would ideally uncover as part of the reconnaissance stage of the PRECARE model.

Competence

If we assume that Ms Wooltorton, from the introductory case in this chapter, was legally competent when we arrived and she stated to the paramedics 'I don't want to be saved. Here are my directions', the question of the validity of the directive is essentially irrelevant, because the patient (1) is presumed to be competent, and (2) has stated that she does not want treatment. Therefore, her wishes should be upheld. It should be noted that paramedics may encounter patients who, unlike Ms Wooltorton, are not able to give verbal directions as to the care they refuse to consent to, because capacity has already been lost. This is where a written directive would come into effect.

You will recall from the section on 'Consent' in Chapter 5 that an adult patient is presumed to be competent, and the onus is on the health practitioner to demonstrate that the patient is not. In the case of an advance directive, the patient must have had competence at the time of writing it, and the directive applies only once the patient loses competence. If the paramedics were to treat Ms Wooltorton under these circumstances, they may be guilty of committing the tort of trespass, assault and battery. This tort stands between the individual and others with respect to individual bodily inviolability, and upholds the principles of the autonomy of the person, personal security, physical integrity, dignity, control and self-determination.[29] That is, a person must seek consent before touching another, or else be guilty of trespassing upon that person. If the latter has occurred, it is a course of action that the patient would have to pursue at some later time post-recovery, as Mrs Schloendorff did in Case 7.1.

Case 7.1 *Schloendorff v Society of New York Hospital*[30]

Mary Schloendorff consented to having a fibroid tumour examined under an anaesthetic at New York Hospital. She did not consent to having the tumour removed. The doctor making the examination found the tumour to be malignant and proceeded to remove it. Mrs Schloendorff brought a case against the doctor for battery. After finding the doctor had committed a battery, the judge deciding the matter, Justice Cardozo, stated:

Every human being of adult years and sound mind has a right to determine what shall be done with his own body; and a surgeon who performs an operation without his patient's consent commits an assault for which he is liable in damages. This is true except in cases of emergency where the patient is unconscious and where it is necessary to operate before consent can be obtained.

Directive made voluntarily

Paramedics commonly operate under high pressure, time-critical conditions. In these circumstances it is not always possible to verify the veracity of documentation provided by patients, their family or carers. In other words, determining whether or not the directive was made voluntarily is virtually impossible. Again, the case law provides us with some indication of how we should proceed here. In the New South Wales case of *Hunter and New England Area Health Service v A*, a patient had completed a document called a 'worksheet'. This document was not signed, but it contained a refusal of consent to undertake renal dialysis. He was later admitted to hospital with kidney failure and placed on dialysis. The hospital brought the case to court to ascertain whether or not it could or should withdraw that treatment in light of the contents of the 'worksheet'. Justice McDougall took the view that the document should be followed, saying that there should not be 'an over-careful scrutiny'[31] of the language used, and to do so may undermine the autonomy of the patient. Justice McDougall also said 'that the individual acted freely and voluntarily, and intended his or her decision to apply to the situation at hand', and as such the refusal should be followed.[32]

New South Wales does not have legislation prescribing the form of the ACD as other jurisdictions do, but nevertheless the statutory provisions contained therein do not extinguish the patient's common law right to make a contemporaneous refusal of treatment. In other words, there is no requirement that a refusal has to be written or made in advance. If, for example, Ms Wooltorton had allowed the paramedics to treat her but on arrival at the hospital had decided to withdraw her consent for treatment, this refusal would have had to be respected by the treating staff unless they could demonstrate that she had lost capacity. Likewise, the legislation does not make the advance directive binding. It can be revoked at any time.

Liability of staff

There is justifiably concern among healthcare staff surrounding the ambiguity of their position with regard to upholding (or not) an ACD. This is particularly acute in New South Wales and Tasmania, where no legislation exists to protect staff,[33] and has been compounded by case law that has found that healthcare staff may be liable for treating a person who has refused consent for treatment,[34] and liable for not treating a patient who was refusing treatment but was not competent to do so.[35] The ACT law[36] says that if a health professional, or a person acting under the direction of a health professional, makes a decision that they believe on reasonable grounds complies with the Act, or honestly acts to withhold or withdraw treatment from a person based on a reliance on a decision made by that person, the withholding or withdrawing of treatment is not a breach of professional etiquette or ethics or a breach of a rule of professional conduct, and no civil or criminal liability will be incurred.

Victoria[37] provides protection for health practitioners who act in good faith on the reliance of a refusal of treatment certificate, but who are not aware that the certificate has been cancelled.

The South Australian Act only specifies protection for medical practitioners. It says:

A medical practitioner responsible for the treatment or care of a patient, or a person participating in the treatment or care of the patient under the medical practitioner's supervision, incurs no civil or criminal liability for an act or omission done or made—

(a) with the consent of the patient or the patient's representative or without consent but in accordance with an authority conferred by this Act or any other Act; and

(b) in good faith and without negligence; and

(c) in accordance with proper professional standards of medical practice; and

(d) in order to preserve or improve the quality of life.[38]

Western Australia has no protection written into the legislation. Queensland's *Powers of Attorney Act 1998* says:

(1) This section applies if a health provider has reasonable grounds to believe that a direction in an advance health directive is uncertain or inconsistent with good medical practice or that circumstances, including advances in medical science, have changed to the extent that the terms of the direction are inappropriate.

(2) The health provider does not incur any liability, either to the adult or anyone else, if the health provider does not act in accordance with the direction.

(3) However, if an attorney is appointed under the advance health directive, the health provider has reasonable grounds to believe that a direction in the advance health directive is uncertain only if, among other things, the health provider has consulted the attorney about the direction.[39]

The Australian judicial system has been reluctant to engage in a dialogue addressing the uncertainties that still exist within much of the current law on end-of-life decisions,[40] and so informing paramedics about how they should approach this difficult area of their practice in a definitive way is not possible, but, in general terms, a paramedic should rely on their clinical guidelines.

Clinical practice guidelines

In the *Wooltorton* case, there was no question as to the validity of the directive, because the paramedics could determine that the patient was competent and refusing consent by talking with her. They had the additional benefit of the written directive to confirm her wishes. If they were in doubt as to the validity of the directive (e.g. did she in fact write it, was she free from undue influence while writing it, was she competent at the time, has she since revoked it or changed her mind?), the legislation provides a relief from liability for 'health professionals' who have acted in accordance with it on the assumption that it is valid or have acted against it because they formed a reasonable belief that the directive had been revoked or does not comply with the relevant law.[41] All paramedics in Australia are now registered with the Paramedicine Board of Australia under the *Health Practitioner Regulation National Law Act 2009* (Qld). This provides statutory recognition of paramedics as healthcare providers/professionals, and as such they fall under the protection of the legislation, provided they act within the legislative framework of their respective jurisdictions.

The Paramedicine Board of Australia's *Interim Code of Conduct* also acknowledges the role paramedics play in end-of-life care and of the patient's right to refuse treatment.[42] If a paramedic conscientiously objects to a patient refusing care, who will die without such care, then the paramedic must be prepared to justify any decision not to uphold the patient's wishes to the Paramedicine Board and any other authority (e.g. employer) that may question that decision.

Ambulance Victoria also makes it clear in its clinical practice guideline how a case like this should be handled. It says:

> A paramedic may provide or withhold treatment based upon the patient's wishes as recorded on an Advance Care Directive that is sighted by them or paramedics may accept, in good faith, the advice from those present at the scene of the patient's wishes and that this supporting documentation exists.[43]

In summary, a competent adult has the lawful right to refuse medical treatment, even if it will result in their death. To treat in the face of a refusal is to commit an offence. In Ms Wooltorton's case it was determined that she had exercised her right as a competent adult to refuse treatment knowing that it would result in her death, and this decision was respected by the health practitioners who attended her.

However, if Ms Wooltorton had not been competent and the paramedics were uncertain as to the validity of the directive, or had no way of establishing her wishes, or if there was no surrogate decision-maker available to consult and there was a requirement to act urgently in order to save her life and prevent further harm, the paramedics should have treated her.

Lack of capacity and surrogate decision-makers

Another method by which the patient can exercise their autonomy with regard to medical treatment decision-making is via a surrogate decision-maker, power of attorney or guardian. These terms—like the terms referring to advance directives—differ depending on which jurisdiction you are in. South Australia, Victoria and the Australian Capital Territory have laws that enable a competent adult ('the principal') to execute an enduring power of attorney, under which the principal appoints another adult ('an agent' or 'enduring guardian') to make decisions about the principal's medical treatment in the event that the principal becomes incompetent. Thus, through the agent the principal effectively has a legal means of refusing medical treatment, with the caveat that the refusal is consistent with the wishes of the principal and does not conflict with any instructions provided by the principal or embodied in the legislation in the power of attorney document while they were competent.[44] In effect, the power of attorney legislation facilitates the indirect decision-making of the principal prospectively. Notably, the legislation does not displace the competent principal's capacity to give other forms of binding anticipatory refusal for undesired medical treatment.

What happens if no 'default decision-maker' has been appointed?

There are occasions where no guardian or health attorney has been appointed by a person to make healthcare decisions on their behalf once they become incompetent to do so themselves. The subjective needs of an individual are difficult to evaluate in situations where a patient is incapable of giving consent to medical procedures, particularly by healthcare staff who do not know the patient and what their wishes might be with regard to their healthcare treatment. Healthcare staff also have limited legal authority to act to treat (or refuse to treat) a patient without the patient's consent. The law therefore has allowed for the authority regarding the healthcare decision-making of an incompetent person to be transferred to a person who is more likely to have a better understanding of what the patient's wishes might be. In Australia, legislation in different states and territories generally requires that health practitioners approach a hierarchy of next-of-kin to act as a surrogate decision-maker to act in the best interests of the patient if one has not been appointed by the patient. It is thought that this role is best undertaken by someone who knows the patient well and can act as a 'surrogate' decision-maker; who, in effect, can make decisions as the principal would have if they were still competent to do so. This 'default decision-maker' is generally the 'first person reasonably available and willing to act from a statutory list of people'.[45]

The parliaments have passed laws that allow authority to be transferred under conditions where a person loses competence. In these circumstances, the law in New South Wales defers to the *Guardianship Act 1987* (NSW), which applies to incapable persons above the age of 16.[46] It functions by providing for proxy consent by an appointed guardian or, where one is not available, another 'person responsible'.[47] The 'default decision-maker' is determined by a descending hierarchy of suitable persons. Priority is given to a spouse where there is a strong, long relationship, then the carer, and, where no carer or spouse is available, the role is assigned to a close relative or friend.[48]

This statutory scheme permits the person responsible to make decisions on the principal's behalf only where there is a positive action of consent to medical treatment. *Prima facie* it fails to be a device by which refusal or discontinuation of treatment can be used, and so, arguably, cannot be utilised as a form of advance care directive achieved via previous communication in the course of a relationship. In *WK v Public Guardian* [2006] ADT 93, it was identified that another means of recourse, by which the guardian might be granted the power of refusal or discontinuation of treatment on behalf of their charge, would be through an application to the New South Wales Supreme Court for an assessment of the patient's best interests under *parens patriae* jurisdiction.[49] The Supreme Court's *parens patriae* jurisdiction allows the court to make decisions on behalf of those who cannot make decisions for themselves. *Parens patriae* is Latin for 'parent of the people'.

Victorian common law is somewhat more liberal than that of New South Wales. This can be seen in *Gardner; re BWV* [2003] VSC 173, where the court ruled that it was the parliamentary intention of the Victorian *Guardianship and Administration Act 1986* (Vic) that refusal of treatment for a ward be a power that the guardian is authorised to give. *Gardner* also restated the common law position supporting the authority of a doctor to legally withdraw nutrition and hydration where it is considered to be in the patient's best interests.[50]

Qumsieh v Guardianship and Administration Board [1998] VSCA 45 was one case that sought to resolve the dilemma of guardians possessing the authority to override patient ACDs for the refusal of specific treatment.[51] As there was no definitive ruling from the court on this issue, the authority of the guardian to override an ACD remains unsettled.

Paramedics may come into contact with a surrogate decision-maker who has not been appointed via a formal instrument or document. This person has become the decision-maker as a result of circumstance and, most commonly, falls under the authority of the relevant *Guardianship Act*. Guardianship is discussed further in Chapter 5, 'Consent and refusal of treatment'.

What is the difference between passive euthanasia and withdrawing treatment, voluntary euthanasia and aiding and abetting a suicide, and involuntary euthanasia, and why should paramedics know it?

There can be confusion over the terms used when describing end-of-life care. *Euthanasia* is an all-encompassing term that is often used to describe legal and illegal behaviour, and so is not particularly helpful when discussing the law at the end of life. We already know that a patient can refuse lifesaving treatment provided they are competent to make that decision, or a proxy decision-maker can be authorised to make decisions regarding an incompetent patient's healthcare. An ACD refusing lifesaving treatment is an example of a competent patient committing suicide, which, as we have discussed, is lawful. *Passive euthanasia* is the withdrawal or withholding of treatment that results in the patient's death, and this may be as a result of following a patient's ACD, or it may be as a result of doctors determining that further treatment is futile (this is discussed in more detail later in this chapter). In short, both of these mechanisms are lawful.

Voluntary euthanasia is a competent person requesting to be killed, which is unlawful because aiding and abetting a suicide is unlawful, so any provision of assistance to die is illegal. *Involuntary active euthanasia* is also known as manslaughter or murder, and attracts criminal liability in all states and territories of Australia. Each state and territory of Australia has legislation to the effect of it being 'unlawful to kill any person unless such killing is authorised or justified or excused by law'.[52] The specific elements of *murder* include that the conduct engaged in is intentional, or there exists reckless indifference to human life, and the death of another occurs.[53] *Manslaughter* is a residual homicide charge available if murder is not satisfied on the facts, or where the requisite intention is lacking, or where the death results by way of reckless or negligent conduct.[54] In short, paramedics are not able to assist a patient to die even if the patient is requesting that type of assistance (active) unless that patient competently refuses to consent to treatment by paramedics (passive).

Pain relief and hastening death

Paramedics should be conscious of the fact that studies show patients are routinely administered respiratory depressive opioids by health practitioners as 'pain relief'. These drugs have the potential to hasten death.[55] Some health practitioners are reluctant to administer these doses of opiates because they believe their action will result in the patient's death, for which they do not want to be held accountable. The issue to be considered here is the intention of the health professionals behind their act. Providing a patient with pain relief that has the primary intention of relieving pain but may have the incidental effect of depressing respiratory function is considered ethical, and is commonly justified via reliance on the 'doctrine of double effect'. In short, the *doctrine of double effect* means that an action is arguably ethical if it produces a harm as a result of an attempt to limit a greater harm. So, for example, if a patient had a gangrenous leg that needed to be amputated to save the patient's life, the amputation would produce a harm to the patient. But if the leg was not amputated, the patient would be subject to the greater harm of death.

Some jurisdictions have legislated for the provision of palliative care with protection against liability for carers even though an incidental effect of the treatment is to hasten the death of the patient. For example, with regard to the care of people who are dying, the South Australian Act says that no civil or criminal liability will be incurred by a doctor or 'a person participating in the treatment or care of the patient' under a doctor's supervision, when administering 'medical treatment with the intention of relieving pain or distress', provided it is administered in 'good faith' and 'without negligence' and 'in accordance with proper professional standards of palliative care' and 'with the consent of the patient or the patient's representative'.[56]

A problem arises when the primary intention is not to reduce pain and suffering, but rather to kill the patient either with or without the patient's consent. Studies like Kuhse et al.'s demonstrate that some doctors administer this form of 'pain relief' with the primary purpose of assisting the patient to die. This is unlawful, whether or not the practitioner has the patient's permission. Kuhse et al. found that many staff were administering this treatment without even bothering to discuss it with the patient and/or their guardian first. This is homicide, and it is unlawful.[57]

Mercy killing

Mercy killing is an act of non-voluntary euthanasia. It differs from aiding and abetting a suicide because it is involuntary; that is, it is not consented to by the patient. In other words, it is a form of homicide, but it is usually carried out by someone close to the victim. The Australian courts have been inconsistent in relation to mercy killing crimes. In *R v Maxwell* [2003] VSC 278[58] and *R v Hood* [2002] VSC 123,[59] both defendants received suspended sentences. Coldrey J, who presided over both cases, commented:

> The law may be seen as life-affirming and not life-denying and directed at discouraging suicide as a response to the emotional vicissitudes of life.

> The degree of moral blame attributable to a person who assists or encourages an act of suicide may vary greatly from case to case. At one end of the spectrum may be placed a person who assists or encourages a person to commit suicide in order to inherit property or for some other ulterior motive; at the other end, there is the individual who supplies potentially lethal medication to a terminally ill person, perhaps a loved one who is in extreme pain and who wishes to end that suffering at the earliest possible opportunity.[60]

He went on to say that there existed such situations where 'justice may be tempered with mercy', such that minimal punishment might be imposed where the act is performed out of kindness.[61]

Aid, abet and assist suicide

The common law of Australia has transitioned from seeing suicide as indicative of mental illness to accepting it as a situation where possible psychiatric or psychological issues may exist, but not necessarily to the extent that testamentary capacity is extinguished.[62] This shift in thinking facilitated the move to have suicide decriminalised in all states and territories.[63] Queensland, Tasmania and Western Australia's criminal legislation and codes omit suicide as an offence.

However, Western Australia and Queensland hold that aiding suicide is a crime where 'a person procures, aids or counsels to induce another to kill themselves'.[64] The Tasmanian *Criminal Code* is more succinct in the language, finding it a crime for either instigating or aiding another to kill themself.[65] South Australia, New South Wales, Victoria and the Australian Capital Territory use near-identical discourse in finding an indictable offence where a person 'aids, abets or counsels the suicide of another, or an attempt by another to commit suicide'.[66] However, South Australia takes the offence one step further, in finding that actions of 'fraud, duress or undue influence' that procure suicide or an attempted suicide are crimes of murder or attempted murder, depending on the circumstance.[67] The Northern Territory legislation is much like that of New South Wales and the ACT; however, it omits the language of 'abetting' or 'counselling', and complicates the offence by requiring that the accused has intended their conduct to assist the other to commit suicide.[68]

As paramedics, you might be asked by our patients to assist them to die, or you might believe that the patient would be better off dead. This is simply not something that you can lawfully assist your patients with, no matter whether you feel compassion towards your patients and wish to relieve their pain and suffering; no matter that the patient is terminally ill and will die anyway and, thus, your actions are only hastening the inevitable or imminent; and no matter that the patient is competent, is informed of the benefits and risks of their choice, and is making the choice voluntarily (i.e. without coercion). None of those factors is relevant according to Australian law. Remember, the competent patient's rights to self-determination with regard to ending their life only go as far as:

- committing suicide themselves, alone, unaided, unassisted and without support from others; and
- refusing medical treatment that they have been given that may have the effect of extending their lives, but, once withdrawn, will have the effect of ending their lives—medical treatment includes artificial ventilation, hydration and nutrition, and cardiopulmonary resuscitation.

Regardless of the language used, all legislation prohibits a healthcarer from taking active steps to intentionally bring about a patient's death. Such actions attract a criminal penalty from 5 years' to life imprisonment.

Consider Case 7.2. In this case it is necessary for the paramedic to determine a number of things. What can you lawfully do in this situation? What does your duty of care extend to? Who has the legal authority to make decisions with regard to the patient and his care? What are the potential consequences of the action or inaction for paramedics?

Case 7.2 'I want him to die'

You are called to a nursing home where you find an elderly woman sitting beside a bed with a man in it. She says it is her husband. The man is groaning and is in obvious respiratory discomfort. You know that you could administer morphine to relieve his discomfort and ease his breathing. His wife says, 'I want him to die.'

Futile treatment

Most ambulance services have clinical guidelines that state when treatment can be withheld from a patient. For example, resuscitation need not be commenced on a patient with injuries that are incompatible with life (e.g. decapitation). For example, Ambulance Victoria CPG A0203 outlines the guidelines for 'withholding and/or ceasing pre-hospital resuscitation'. It says that resuscitation may not be given where injuries are incompatible with life, but also where an adult (18 years or older) is found by paramedics in asystole, the time since collapse and paramedic arrival is greater than 10 minutes and there is no other clinical reason to continue (e.g. hypothermia, drug overdose or a family member/bystander requests continued efforts). This mirrors the position at law that there is no obligation on the state or their servants to treat a patient where treatment would be futile—'where there are no reasonable prospects of a return to a meaningful quality of life'.[69]

For example, there is no obligation on a paramedic to give a patient morphine merely because the patient demanded it when there was no clinical indication for it.

An example of futile treatment is given in Case 7.3.

Some senior Australian doctors still refuse to make not-for-resuscitation orders despite manifest and accepted futility of treatment for the patient in question, owing to irrational fears of legal liability.[70] If treatment is declared clinically futile and is withdrawn or withheld, the cause of the patient's death is noted on the medical record and death certificate as the disease process or injury that was the underlying causative factor. The South Australian legislation says the following:

17—The care of people who are dying

(1) A medical practitioner responsible for the treatment or care of a patient in the terminal phase of a terminal illness, or a person participating in the treatment or care of the patient under the medical practitioner's supervision, incurs no civil or criminal liability by administering medical treatment with the intention of relieving pain or distress—

(a) with the consent of the patient or the patient's representative; and

(b) in good faith and without negligence; and

(c) in accordance with proper professional standards of palliative care, even though an incidental effect of the treatment is to hasten the death of the patient.

(2) A medical practitioner responsible for the treatment or care of a patient in the terminal phase of a terminal illness, or a person participating in the treatment or care of the patient under the medical practitioner's supervision—

Case 7.3 Futile treatment

Mr Isaac Messiha was a 75-year-old man with a history of chronic obstructive pulmonary disease, a history of cardiac surgery, and a hospital admission following a cardiac arrest in early 2004. In October 2004 he suffered an out-of-hospital asystolic cardiac arrest. It was estimated that Mr Messiha was without oxygen for up to 25 minutes prior to the arrival of paramedics. Mr Messiha had no advance directive, so paramedics commenced cardiopulmonary resuscitation. Mr Messiha was admitted to the intensive care unit of St George Hospital. Over the following days, his Glasgow coma score did not climb above 5. An electroencephalograph (ECG) showed the complete absence of cortical activity. The patient was mechanically ventilated, required constant suctioning, was incontinent of faeces, had an indwelling catheter and was being fed via a nasogastric tube. Mr Messiha's family were told by the medical director of the intensive care unit, Dr Theresa Jacques, that there was no reasonable prospect of Mr Messiha returning to a meaningful quality of life, and that it was in the best interests of the patient that treatment be withheld. The 'treatment' to be withdrawn and withheld included removal from the ventilator, no further pharmacological treatment, and a 'do not resuscitate' order in the event of a cardiac or respiratory arrest. The relatives believed that Mr Messiha was making meaningful eye movements, and sought an order from the Supreme Court that the withdrawal of treatment be stayed. The court agreed with the doctors and treatment was withdrawn.[71]

(a) is under no duty to use, or to continue to use, life sustaining measures in treating the patient if the effect of doing so would be merely to prolong life in a moribund state without any real prospect of recovery or in a persistent vegetative state (whether or not the patient or the patient's representative has requested that such measures be used or continued); and

(b) must, if the patient or the patient's representative so directs, withdraw life sustaining measures from the patient.

(3) For the purposes of the law of the State—

(a) the administration of medical treatment for the relief of pain or distress in accordance with subsection (1) does not constitute an intervening cause of death; and

(b) the non-application or discontinuance of life sustaining measures in accordance with subsection (2) does not constitute an intervening cause of death.[72]

What is the definition of 'death', and what happens to a dead body?

Death is defined by law as the:

• irreversible cessation of all function of the person's brain, or
• irreversible cessation of circulation of blood in the person's body.[73]

There is a requirement under all state and territory laws that notification of the death of a person be made to the relevant authority. In the case of a 'reportable' death, the death must be reported to the police, who will then report to the coroner.[74] The body should be transported by the coroner, or, if in a rural setting, the body may need to be transported to the local morgue by ambulance. If the death is not unexpected, then the paramedic should endeavour to contact the patient's doctor to ask whether they will sign a death certificate. Once the certificate is signed, the body can be released to the funeral director for collection. If the doctor is unwilling or unable to sign a death certificate, the death should be reported to the police for them to follow up.

End-of-life decision-making and the freedom to choose— food for thought

Broader issues on the relief of suffering, the right to die, the role of religion and the limits of the state's authority in these matters were considered by Ronald Dworkin, an American legal philosopher, in his book *Freedom's Law: The Moral Reading of the American Constitution*.[75] Dworkin considers the case of Nancy Cruzan, who was involved in a car accident that left her in a permanent vegetative state. She was fed and hydrated through tubes, and her parents and husband continued to hope that she would recover. When it became apparent that she would likely remain in this state for the rest of her life, some 30 years or more, her parents as her legal guardians asked that the tubes be removed and she be allowed to die. The hospital refused to do so without a court order. The court granted the order, on the basis that it was in Cruzan's best interest that she 'be permitted to die with dignity now rather than to live on in an unconscious state'.[76] The decision was overruled by a superior court, who found that unless Cruzan herself had provided 'clear and convincing' evidence that she would not have wanted to continue to live as she was, they could not withdraw the treatment.

Her parents appealed to the United States Supreme Court, where Chief Justice Rehnquist, joined by Justices Kennedy and White, wrote that for the purposes of the *Cruzan* case, they assumed that there was a hypothetical right to die, but that there was still a question as to whether 'even a competent person's freedom to die with dignity could be overridden by a state's own constitutional right to keep people alive'. Rehnquist wrote that a 'living will' would embody the rights of the competent person to make such decisions for themself, but that it was legitimate for states to regulate the requirements of a valid will. It was also noted that some people prefer to nominate a surrogate decision-maker instead of scribing their wishes, and this, too, was recognised as a valid instrument to convey an incompetent person's end-of-life wishes. With respect to religion and faith, Justice Stevens, in dissent, examined the religious basis of the Missouri Supreme Court's decision, and said, 'Not much may be said with confidence about death unless it is said from faith, and that alone is reason enough to protect the freedom to conform choices about death to individual conscience.'[77]

Dworkin concluded by saying that one reading of the US constitution allows for individuals to make their own decisions with regard to this issue, as it is at the core of liberty, further arguing, 'making someone die in a way others approve, but he believes contradicts his own dignity, is a serious, unjustified, unnecessary form of tyranny'.[78] The balance is in ensuring that the law protects those who may be abused by this system, but also enables those individuals who wish to exert it the authority and process by which they can make their own choices regarding their own death.

Conclusion

This chapter examined the various mechanisms by which end-of-life issues are discussed and decisions authorised under various Australian state and territory laws. This is an area that will continue to grow in importance as the population increases and places more pressure on limited healthcare service resources, including ambulance care. It is vital that paramedics have a solid understanding of their legal authority to act under the law that applies to their practice with regard to these issues in order that they uphold the law, but, perhaps more importantly, that they uphold the autonomous choices of their patients with regard to their end-of-life care.

Review Questions

1 Can a patient refuse treatment that will lead to their death?
2 Is assisting suicide unlawful?
3 Can patients/families demand treatment when treatment is futile?
4 Can paramedics accelerate the dying process?
5 What is the legal definition of 'death'?

Endnotes

1 Butt, P. and Hamer, D. (eds) (2011) *Concise Australian Legal Dictionary*, 4th ed. Chatswood: Lexis Nexis.

2 *Consent to Medical Treatment and Palliative Care Act 1995* (SA), s 6.

3 Ibid., s 4.

4 *Guardianship and Administration Act 1990* (WA), s 110ZH.

5 Emanuel, E., Fairclough, D. and Emanuel, L. (2000) Attitudes and desires related to euthanasia and physician-assisted suicide among terminally ill patients and their caregivers. *Journal of the American Medical Association* 284(19), 2460–2468; consider also the number of patients who seek to end their own lives using 'right-to-die' laws, including the now repealed *Rights of the Terminally Ill Act 1995* (NT), according to which four people chose to end their lives, with one of the essential criteria for eligibility being 'pain and suffering'.

6 See also Stewart, G., Cutrer, W., Demy, T. et al. (1998) *Basic Questions on Suicide and Euthanasia: Are They Ever Right?* Grand Rapids, MI: Kregel Publications.

7 Katelaris, A. (2011) Time to rethink end-of-life care. *Medical Journal of Australia* 194(11), 563. Available: https://www.mja.com.au/journal/2011/194/11/time-rethink-end-life-care (accessed 29 November 2018).

8 Lowthian, J., Cameron, P., Stoelwinder, J. et al. (2011) Increasing utilization of emergency ambulances. *Australian Health Review* 35(1), 63–69.

9 Katelaris, A. (2011) Time to rethink end-of-life care, at p. 563

10   Cica, N. (1996) *Euthanasia: The Australian Law in an International Context*. Parliament of Australia Research Paper 3. Online. Available: http://www.aph.gov.au/About_Parliament/Parliamentary_ Departments/Parliamentary_Library/pubs/rp/RP9697/97rp3 (accessed 29 November 2018).

11   *Euthanasia Laws Act 1996 (Cth)*, passed by the Senate on 24 March 1997.

12   *Criminal Law Consolidation (Medical Defences – End of Life Arrangements) Amendment Bill 2011*. Online. Available: https://www.legislation.sa.gov.au/LZ/B/ARCHIVE/CRIMINAL%20LAW%20 CONSOLIDATION%20(MEDICAL%20DEFENCES%20-%20END%20OF%20LIFE%20 ARRANGEMENTS)%20AMENDMENT%20BILL%202011_HON%20STEPH%20KEY%20MP/B _AS%20INTRODUCED%20IN%20HA/CRIMINAL%20ARRANGEMENTS%20 AMENDMENT%20BILL%202011.UN.PDF (accessed 29 November 2018).

13   Blumer, C. (2016, 26 May). Vote Compass: Aussies want it, but euthanasia still a 'great untouched issue'. *ABC News*. Online. Available: http://www.abc.net.au/news/2016-05-25/vote-compass-euthanasia/7441176 (accessed 24 February 2019).

14   Castro, J. (2017, 21 July) Victoria may soon have assisted dying laws for terminally ill patients. *The Conversation*. Online. Available: https://theconversation.com/victoria-may-soon-have-assisted-dying-laws-for-terminally-ill-patients-81401 (accessed 24 February 2019).

15   Kuhse, H., Singer, P., Baume, P. et al. (1997) End-of-life decisions in Australian medical practice. *Medical Journal of Australia* 166(4), 191–196.

16   Ibid.

17   *Rights of the Terminally Ill (Euthanasia Laws Repeal) Bill 2008*.

18   Blumer, Vote Compass: Aussies want it, but euthanasia still a 'great untouched issue'.

19   Australian Medical Association (AMA) (2016) *AMA Position Statement on Euthanasia and Physician Assisted Suicide*, s 3. Barton, ACT: AMA. Online. Available: https://ama.com.au/system/tdf/documents/ AMA%20Position%20Statement%20on%20Euthanasia%20and%20Physician%20Assisted%20 Suicide%202016.pdf?file=1&type=node&id=45402 (accessed 29 November 2018).

20   *Re B (Adult: Refusal of Medical Treatment)* [2002] 2 All ER 449, at 456.

21   *Powers of Attorney Act 1998* (Qld), s 36; *Advanced Care Directives Act 2013* (SA); *Guardianship and Administration Act 1990* (WA), Pt 9B; *Medical Treatment (Health Directions) Act 2006* (ACT); *Advance Personal Planning Act 2013* (NT); *Medical Treatment Planning and Decisions Act 2016* (Vic).

22   White, B., Willmott, L., Trowse, P. et al. (2011) The legal role of medical professionals in decisions to withhold or withdraw life-sustaining treatment: Part 1 (New South Wales). *Journal of Law and Medicine* 18(3), 498–522.

23   *Consent to Medical Treatment and Palliative Care Act 1995* (SA), s 3.

24   *Medical Treatment Planning and Decisions Act 2016* (Vic); *Medical Treatment (Health Directions) Act 2006* (ACT); *Guardianship and Administration Act 1990* (WA).

25   *Powers of Attorney Act 1998* (Qld), s 36; *Advanced Care Directives Act 2013* (SA), s 4; *Advance Personal Planning Act 2013* (NT), s 51.

26   NSW Health. *End of Life Care and Decision-Making—Guidelines*. Online. Available: https:// www1.health.nsw.gov.au/pds/ActivePDSDocuments/GL2005_057.pdf (accessed 29 November 2018); NSW Health. *Using advance care directives*. Online. Available: https://www1.health.nsw.gov.au/pds/ ActivePDSDocuments/GL2005_056.pdf (accessed 29 November 2018).

27   If the ACD is signed by the patient, it is assumed to be valid because the patient had capacity when the document was signed. The treating clinician cannot override the patient's wishes by authorising the paramedic to implement treatment. As a health practitioner, the paramedic is bound by the law even if it contradicts their employer. A professional paramedic has a duty to raise anomalies in their employer's policies and procedures with their employer when they become aware of them, so that both the paramedic and the employer are compliant with the law. It should be noted that any policy that places the onus

on the treating medical clinician to direct a paramedic to enact a treatment plan that does not comply with the paramedic's legal obligations will not provide any form of legal protection to the paramedic. That is, the paramedic cannot rely on the 'I was just following orders' defence.

28 *Powers of Attorney Act 1998* (Qld); *Consent to Medical Treatment and Palliative Care Act 1995* (SA); *Advance Personal Planning Act 2013* (NT); *Guardianship and Administration Act 1990* (WA); *Medical Treatment (Health Directions) Act 2006* (ACT); *Medical Treatment Planning and Decisions Act 2016* (Vic).

29 *Secretary, Department of Health and Community Services (NT) v JWB and SMB* (1992) 175 CLR 218 *(Marion's case)*.

30 *Schloendorff v Society of New York Hospital* 105 NE 92 (NY 1914).

31 *Hunter and New England Area Health Service v A* (2009) 74 NSWLR 88, at [36].

32 Ibid., at [37].

33 Townsend, R. and Giles, D. (2006) End of life decision and the NSW *Guardianship Act*: a square peg in a round hole? The law and clinical practice. *Australian Health Law Bulletin* 15(1), 4–7.

34 *Malette v Shulman* (1990) 67 DLR (4th) 321.

35 *Re T (Adult: Refusal of Medical Treatment)* [1992] 4 All ER 649.

36 *Medical Treatment (Health Directions) Act 2006* (ACT), s 16.

37 *Medical Treatment Planning and Decisions Act 2016* (Vic).

38 *Consent to Medical Treatment and Palliative Care Act 1995* (SA), s 16.

39 *Powers of Attorney Act 1998* (Qld), s 103.

40 Stewart, C. (2000) *Qumsieh's case*, civil liability and the right to refuse medical treatment. *Journal of Law and Medicine* 8(1), 56–67; Faunce, T.A. and Stewart, C. (2005) The *Messiha* and *Schiavo* cases: third-party ethical and legal interventions in futile care disputes. *Medical Journal of Australia* 183(5), 261–263.

41 *See Medical Treatment (Health Directions) Act 2006* (ACT).

42 Paramedicine Board of Australia. (2018) *Interim Code of Conduct for Registered Health Practitioners*, at 3.2. Melbourne: Australian Health Practitioner Regulation Agency. Online. Available: https://www .paramedicineboard.gov.au/professional-standards/codes-guidelines-and-policies/code-of-conduct.aspx (accessed 3 December 2018).

43 Ambulance Victoria. (updated 2018, 13 March) *Clinical Practice Guideline A0203: Withholding or Ceasing Resuscitation*. Doncaster: Ambulance Victoria. Available: https://www.ambulance.vic.gov.au/wp-content/ uploads/2018/07/Clinical-Practice-Guidelines-2018-Edition-1.4.pdf (accessed 24 March 2018).

44 *Guardianship and Administration Act 1990* (SA); *Medical Treatment Planning and Decisions Act 2016* (Vic); *Medical Treatment (Health Directions) Act 2006* (ACT).

45 White, B., Willmott, L. and Then, S. (2010) Adults who lack capacity: substitute decision-making. In: B. White, F. McDonald and L. Willmott (eds), *Health Law in Australia* (pp. 149–207). Sydney: Thomson Reuters.

46 *Guardianship Act 1987* (NSW).

47 Ibid.

48 Stewart, C. (1997) Who decides when I can die? Problems with proxy decisions to forego life-sustaining treatment. *Journal of Law and Medicine* 4, 386–401; Fidler, D.P. (2008) Global health jurisprudence: a time of reckoning. *Georgetown Law Journal* 96(2), 393–412.

49 *WK v Public Guardian* [2006] ADT 93.

50 *Re BWV, Ex parte Gardner* [2003] VSC 173.

51 Stewart, *Qumsieh's case*, civil liability and the right to refuse medical treatment.

52 *Criminal Code Act 1913* (WA), s 268.

53 *Crimes Act 1900* (NSW), s 18.

54 *Criminal Code* (NT), s 160.

55 Kuhse et al., End-of-life decisions in Australian medical practice; Kinzbrunner, B.M., Weinreb, N.J. and Pouczer, J.S. (2001) *20 Common Problems in End-of-Life Care.* New York: McGraw Hill.

56 *Consent to Medical Treatment and Palliative Care Act 1995* (SA), s 17.

57 Kuhse et al., End-of-life decisions in Australian medical practice.

58 *R v Maxwell* [2003] VSC 278.

59 *R v Hood* [2002] VSC 123.

60 *R v Maxwell*, at [32]–[33].

61 Ibid., at [41].

62 *Stuart v Kirkland-Veenstra* [2009] HCA 15; (2009) 237 CLR 215. Online. Available: http://www.austlii.edu.au/au/cases/cth/HCA/2009/15.html (accessed 28 November 2018).

63 *Crimes Act 1900* (NSW), s 31A; *Criminal Law Consolidation Act 1935* (SA), s 13A(1); *Crimes Act 1958* (Vic), s 6A; *Criminal Code* (WA), s 288; *Criminal Code* (Qld), s 311; *Criminal Code* (Tas), s 163.

64 *Criminal Code* (WA), s 288; *Criminal Code* (Qld), s 311.

65 *Criminal Code* (Tas), s 163.

66 *Criminal Consolidation Act 1935* (SA), s 13A; *Crimes Act 1900* (NSW), s 31C; *Crimes Act 1958* (Vic), s 6B2b; *Crimes Act 1900* (ACT), s 17.

67 *Criminal Code* (SA), s 13A.

68 *Criminal Code* (NT), s 162(2).

69 *Messiha v South East Health* [2004] NSWSC 1061.

70 *Medical Treatment Planning and Decisions Act 2016* (Vic); *Medical Treatment (Health Directions) Act 2006* (ACT).

71 *Messiha v South East Health.*

72 *Consent to Medical Treatment and Palliative Care Act 1995* (SA), s 17.

73 *Transplantation and Anatomy Act 1978* (ACT), s 45; *Human Tissue Act 1983* (NSW), s 33; *Transplantation and Anatomy Act 1979* (NT), s 23; *Transplantation and Anatomy Act 1979* (Qld), s 45; *Human Tissue Act 1985* (Tas), s 27A; *Human Tissue Act 1982* (Vic), s 41.

74 *Coroners Act 2003* (Qld), s 8; *Coroners Act 2009* (NSW), s 6; *Coroners Act 2008* (Vic), s 4; *Coroners Act 2003* (SA), s 28; *Coroners Act 1996* (WA), s 17; *Coroners Act* (NT), s 12(1); *Coroners Act 1995* (Tas), s 19; *Coroners Act 1997* (ACT), s 2.

75 Dworkin, R. (1999). *Freedom's Law: The Moral Reading of the American Constitution.* Oxford: Oxford University Press.

76 Ibid., at p. 130.

77 Ibid., at p. 133.

78 Ibid., at p. 146.

Chapter 8
Protective jurisdiction

Stephen Bartlett

Learning objectives

After reading this chapter, you will:

- be familiar with the issues of domestic violence, child maltreatment and elder abuse, and how these issues intersect with paramedic care
- understand child protection reporting responsibilities in Australia and New Zealand
- be familiar with the laws on domestic violence and child protection in Australia and New Zealand
- be aware of the needs of other vulnerable members in communities: cultural and linguistic differences (CALD), and people with developmental disabilities who require paramedics to advocate on behalf of their health needs.

Definitions

Age of majority The age at which a person reaches full legal capacity (18 years in all Australian states and territories, and 20 years in New Zealand).

Capacity The ability to understand the nature, purpose and consequences of a decision. All people of the age of majority are presumed to have capacity unless demonstrated otherwise. Minors do not have capacity at law, although exceptions can be made based on whether a child can demonstrate sufficient maturity and understanding to grant them the right to choose or refuse proposed healthcare: *Gillick v West Norfolk and Wisbech Area Health Authority*,[1] *Secretary, Department of Health and Community Services (NT) v JWB and SMB*.[2]

Child Generally, a child is a person under 18 years old. Some jurisdictions are responsible for slight differences in relation to the general definition. The English case of *Paton v Trustees of the British Pregnancy Advisory Service*[3] established that, in order for a child to have legal status and therefore immutable rights conferred on it, a child must demonstrate spontaneous respiratory and cardiac output, and no longer rely on the mother for life support. This is recognised as the point of 'life' beginning. Appendix 8.1 provides the legal definition of a child in Australia[4] and New Zealand.[5]

Continued

Child maltreatment or child abuse and neglect One or more of the following: physical abuse, sexual abuse, psychological and emotional abuse, and neglect. For the purposes in this chapter, exposure to domestic violence (EDV) is also considered an example of child maltreatment.

Mandatory reporting The law generally phrases mandatory reporting in this way: if personnel have reasonable grounds for suspecting or believing that a child has been abused, or is at risk of being abused, the person must, as soon as practicable, notify a prescribed child welfare authority of his or her suspicion and the basis for the suspicion.[6]

An introductory case

The challenging environment

You are a newly recruited qualified paramedic who has achieved all of your graduate competencies. It is your first shift as an unsupervised qualified paramedic, and you are working with another paramedic who is coming to the end of their graduate-entry program. It is 22:35 on a fairly busy Friday night. You have both overheard on the radio, dispatch encouraging crews to clear from the hospital as quickly as possible due to the number of emergency calls still waiting response.

You are dispatched under emergency conditions to a somewhat isolated property. The call is to a 31-year-old, insulin-dependent, hypoglycaemic female; she is breathing, but her level of consciousness is still being established by the call-taker. You arrive on scene within 7 minutes of the call being made. There is a short delay in gaining entry to the property, as there are four cars on the property blocking your access. A deep, loud voice shouts, 'The back! Come around to the back way.' You make your way to the back of the property. You are careful not to scrape the response kit you are carrying against any of the cars, which are parked tightly on the driveway.

Once at the back door, you are greeted by a male whose demeanour appears unnaturally relaxed and polite given the potentially grave circumstances of the call. He leads you from the porch, through the kitchen, down a short, poorly lit hallway and into an unkempt and rather compact bedroom at the front of the house. Your crewmate follows a short distance behind. In there you find a female. She is alert and, without offering a greeting, says, 'It's 3.2 … I'm getting better. I'm beginning to feel better.'

To the right of the patient's bed there is a young child sitting on the floor, playing what appears to be a box-building, character-slaying video game. He wears thick glasses, and his face is scarcely an arm's length from the television screen, which is propped up on top of two cardboard boxes. Your arrival does nothing to distract him from his game. You

An introductory case continued

turn your attention to your female patient and commence your assessment and standard cares.

All the while, the male who greeted you stands in the door jamb between the hallway and the bedroom. The size of the bedroom and the male in the doorway prevent your colleague from getting into the bedroom and helping you treat your patient. The man leans to the left against the door jamb, his left arm propped above his head, and the thumb of his right hand runs through the belt loop of his jeans. There are fresh abrasions on the knuckles of his right hand. His presence can be felt despite his silence. During your assessment, you glance around at various items in the bedroom.

Answers to your questions on how the patient came to be hypoglycaemic are vague and guarded. The patient claims to have been feeling 'under the weather' for the past 3 days. Her temperature and other vital signs are normal. Following intervention, the patient's blood glucose level returns a reading of 4.6 mmol/L. Feeling happy that her health is steadily improving, your crewmate asks you to make your excuses and leave the patient for a short time.

You both walk out the way you came in, and without saying anything your crewmate points to a door to a larder in the kitchen. The door is caved in and is broken in several places. There appears to be fresh blood smeared on the broken remnants of the door. Various jars, which you hadn't noticed on the way in, lie in pieces on the ground. You exchange glances with your colleague before returning to the patient. You tell her that you would like her to be checked up at hospital; the reason for her hypoglycaemic episode needs to be explored fully. The male protests, while at the same time attempting to gain your favour. The patient consents to transport to hospital. The man's disapproval fades.

The patient asks to walk out to the ambulance. As you move past the first car, she whispers, 'I don't want him to come.' 'Who? Your child? Or your partner?' you reply. 'Him' is all she says. When you ask, 'Is your child safe?', she asks whether her son can come in the ambulance, too. You agree, and your colleague goes to collects him as well as some night things for them both. You are concerned that some disturbance could break out at this point. None does.

A short time later, with everyone safely in the ambulance and the trip to hospital commenced, your patient begins to sob. 'I only did it to escape! I only did it to escape! I've tried to break free; I've tried to leave, but it keeps coming back to this. I had no other option but to do it!'

Continued

> ## An introductory case continued
>
> *This chapter will provide you with some context in which to consider and reflect on this case. It also aims to provide students and paramedics alike with information to raise awareness of domestic abuse and child protection, as well as other health and social issues that intersect with paramedic care. It will provide some assistance and guidance where examples of relationship-specific community violence are suspected.*

Introduction

This chapter examines the paramedic's role and response to suspected child maltreatment, domestic violence and elder abuse through the lens of community violence. Paramedics, as frontline health professionals, have an important role to perform. They are well-positioned to advocate and intervene on behalf of people whose lives are blighted by violence, fear and intimidation.[7] The patient's environment, when read and surveyed by paramedics, is an incredibly helpful and revealing tool. This chapter also emphasises the importance of non-judgemental practice, notwithstanding the suspected existence of certain cultural practices, and their compliance with Australian criminal law. The chapter explains the paramedic's role in responding to domestic violence and children affected by domestic violence. Each state and territory in Australia has its own dedicated domestic violence and child protection statutes, as does New Zealand. The paramedic's role in relation to elder abuse will also be explored.

Community violence: an overview

Child maltreatment, domestic violence and elder abuse can be committed by anyone, against anyone, no matter their background, socioeconomic status (SES), ethnicity, cultural identity and so on. It is unacceptable to view child maltreatment in terms of issues that affect only certain groups within a community.[8] That said, it cannot be overlooked that first peoples can have poorer outcomes compared with their European or Asian counterparts, and are disproportionally represented in child protection systems in Australia and New Zealand.[9] Paramedics must remain alert to their own biases and practise their profession without judgement.

Perpetrators of community violence like child maltreatment and domestic violence do not fit into a single demographic, and they cannot be categorised. Anyone can be a perpetrator of child maltreatment. Similarly, any child can be the victim of child maltreatment. A significant challenge faced by paramedics working with suspected victims of child abuse is their confidence to know, in absence of an explicit disclosure, whether a child they are treating has been the victim of significant harm, is currently a victim of significant harm, or at serious risk of being a victim of significant harm.

Above all, paramedics must be alert to, and be aware of, the signs of child abuse and neglect. The secretive and insidious nature of abuse can make identification difficult.[10]

These difficulties do not relieve the paramedic of the legal[11] or moral obligation to report suspected incidences of child abuse and neglect. If anything, such challenges should focus the paramedic to work tirelessly to protect vulnerable members of the community from further harm and abuse.

This chapter will discuss the types of violence collectively termed *relationship-specific community violence*. The first section will examine domestic violence, and also discuss children's exposure to domestic violence. The next section will examine child maltreatment, as well as discuss reporting laws in relation to child maltreatment. This will be followed by examining the paramedic's role in responding to elder abuse in the community. The chapter will examine other vulnerable groups through domestic violence and child protection: people who identify as having cultural and linguistic differences (CALD) backgrounds.

Domestic violence

Domestic violence can include physical violence, sexual violence and psychological violence.[12] It also includes various forms of coercion and control. For example, it may involve preposterous limitations on the access to finances that a person is entitled to. The Australian Bureau of Statistics (ABS) Personal Safety Survey (PSS) in 2016 reported that 1 in 6 women had experienced physical abuse by a partner, and 1 in 4 women had experienced partner emotional abuse since they were 15 years old. The report also found that 1 in 17 men had experienced physical abuse by a partner, and 1 in 6 men had experienced partner abuse.[13] A woman is far likelier to be killed by a partner or former partner than a man is likely to be killed by a partner or former partner.

Governments in all of the states and territories in Australia, as well as the New Zealand government, have made efforts to address all forms of domestic and family violence. The following reports are examples of recent work on addressing domestic and family violence: *The National Plan to Reduce Violence against Women and their Children 2010–2022*; Queensland's *Not Now, Not Ever: Putting an end to domestic and family violence in Queensland*; Victoria's Royal Commission into Family Violence.

Until recently, ambulance services have been overlooked as a resource to respond to victims of domestic violence in comparison to other healthcare providers.[14] Paramedics are well placed to provide support to victims of domestic violence.[15] The pertinence of paramedic input is demonstrated when victims of domestic violence are not transported to hospital. Unless paramedics are trained to intervene, report and refer, opportunities to interrupt and eliminate violence may be lost. Domestic and family violence legislation for every state and territory in Australia, and in New Zealand, can be found in Appendix 8.2.

Domestic violence in pregnancy

Domestic violence is shown to feature during and following pregnancy.[16] Paramedics come into contact with patients with obstetric involvement. Although obstetric care is not an exclusive feature of paramedic care, paramedics respond to maternal health issues. It is not known whether paramedics make a connection between assessment of the pregnant patient and her likelihood of being a victim of domestic violence.[17] The literature supports more open discussion on pregnancy and domestic violence.[18] Paramedics should be encouraged to discuss appropriately the potential of domestic violence in patients who are, or may be, pregnant.[19]

Attempted strangulation

Attempted strangulation is considered an augur of significantly more serious repercussions due to domestic violence.[20] It has been found to be a cause of strokes in victims of domestic violence.[21] It is indicative of, and antecedent to, homicide from domestic violence.[22] Queensland, along with some other states and territories, has amended legislation codifying attempted strangulation as a criminal offence.[23] An example is the *Criminal Code Act 1899* (Qld). Section 315A introduced the offence of choking, suffocation or strangulation in a domestic setting. In late 2018, New Zealand introduced strangulation as a new criminal offence, similarly recognising its significance in domestic violence.

Paramedics may attend many cases of non-fatal strangulation without ever knowing that it was a feature in their patient's presentation.[24] Signs and symptoms of attempted strangulation may be missed: a hoarse voice may be dismissed as an upper respiratory tract infection rather than as the result of attempted strangulation.[25] Also, signs and symptoms of strangulation may not present until days after the initial assault.[26] There are numerous signs and symptoms associated with strangulation, and they can all be missed unless paramedics are encouraged to include them as part of their clinical matrix. Given the sequela that can develop following attempted strangulation, developing paramedical knowledge of this subset of abuse needs to be undertaken through training and education.

Child abuse and neglect

In 1989, the *United Nations Convention on the Rights of the Child (CROC)* set out in article 19(1) the signatory nations' responsibilities to children.[27] Children at risk of abuse will always require adults to safeguard them from abuse, harm and non-accidental injury. Due to their unique privilege of being able to observe patients in their homes, paramedics are well-placed to protect the safety and wellbeing of children. They are trusted with sensitive personal information, which is sometimes presented with unguarded honesty. Perpetrators of abuse may still be in the process of formulating responses to how a child in their care came to be physically injured. The evidence to support a paramedic's suspicion may not be as easily cloaked due to the environments in which paramedics operate.

It can be difficult to determine the distinction between physical discipline and child abuse, but an examination of the law assists in clarifying the distinction. However, a defence available to the accused is that the person assaulted the child as a form of 'reasonable chastisement' or 'lawful correction'. Parents or legal guardians—but not anyone else—are permitted to discipline their children if it is deemed to be in the child's best interests; for example, if the child is going to come to some harm. Others may have a defence against assaulting another person (including a child) if they are able to demonstrate that they had a 'lawful excuse' for doing so; for example, playing contact sport, colliding with another on a busy street, or when acting in self-defence or out of necessity (pushing someone to prevent a harm coming to them). An example of 'reasonable chastisement' or 'lawful correction' in the case of a child would be if a child was about to place their hand on a hot stove and a parent hits the child's hand away. This may be considered an assault *but for* the parent's intention to prevent a greater harm from ensuing. What would not meet a 'reasonable chastisement' test is a hard blow with a closed fist or tying a child to a tree.

In the Victorian case of *R v Terry*,[28] the action of an adult needed to be 'moderate and reasonable' and 'by way of correction not retribution' and carried out with a 'reasonable means or instrument' to avoid a charge of assault. In New South Wales, lawful correction is limited to reasonable force, and any force applied to the head or neck of the child is considered unreasonable, as is an action that could harm the child for more than a 'short period'. (Note, however, that 'short' is not defined in section 61AA(2)(b) of the *Crimes Act 1900* (NSW).) New Zealand introduced 'anti-smacking' legislation in 2007, but this was challenged by a citizen-initiated referendum in 2009 asking the question: 'Should a smack as part of good parental correction be a criminal offence in New Zealand?' Despite problems with the question, including the linking of 'good' and 'criminal offence', New Zealanders answered a resounding 'no' with 87% of the vote. However, Parliament did not act on the vote, and the 'anti-smacking' legislation remains under the *Powers of discipline*.[29]

Responding to suspected child maltreatment is complex. Paramedics spend typically short amounts of time on-scene. Making on-scene assessments about child safety at the same time as treating and caring for members of the community is a challenge. Transport to hospital and time to offload can be prolonged; it is during these times that paramedics develop rapport with their patients. If patients are going to reveal deeply personal information, it can be during a natural lull from intensive clinical activity—in the event the patient is transported—before arrival at hospital. Paramedics can make use of this time to get to understand the challenges their patients are living with. Irrespective of the abuse their patients are receiving—whether it be child maltreatment or other forms of abuse, like elder abuse or domestic violence—this unique time spent in the safe boundaries of the ambulance should be used by paramedics to better understand their patient and how to advocate on their behalf.

History of child protection

The history of child maltreatment is as old as civilisation itself. However, over 70 years have passed since its rediscovery.[30] In 1962, Dr Henry Kempe coined the term 'battered child'.[31] Prior to this, the legal system, including medicine,[32] had been reluctant to interfere and/or intervene on behalf of children. Over time, as the acknowledgment that children are vulnerable to exploitation and abuse has been made, there has been a concerted effort made through health, legal and social policies to improve the safety of children. However, there have been times when children have been let down by the policy put in place to protect them.[33] However, although failures do still occur, there have been considerable improvements within child safety and protection services, particularly in knowledge and the understanding of the devastating effects that child maltreatment can have on child development.[34]

Child protection should be considered a shared responsibility, and not be left up to individuals, individual groups or governments to manage alone. It should be an all-of-community response. Paramedics can play an important role by increasing their own awareness and understanding of the legal responsibilities and issues pertaining to child protection, so that they are better equipped to disseminate that information to the community and act in the child's best interest.

Who is a child in need of protection?

Legally, a child would be considered in need of protection when a child has suffered, or is likely to suffer, significant harm, caused either directly or indirectly that is detrimental to the health, safety and wellbeing of the child. The federal government in Australia defines abuse in relation to a child in section 4 of the *Family Law Act 1975* (Cth). Legislation is framed around what is believed to be in the best interests of the child. In Victoria, section 10 of the *Child, Youth and Families Act 2005* (Vic) details underpinning principles that seek to ensure that the best interests of children remain paramount. Each state and territory in Australia is responsible for its own child protection legislation. The statutes, along with New Zealand legislation on child protection, are detailed in Appendix 8.3. The legislative provisions on what triggers state intervention on behalf of a child suspected of being maltreated—also referred to as the *threshold for intervention*—are listed in Appendix 8.4.

The challenge for paramedics is to know what constitutes significant harm, and therefore serves as a catalyst for protective measures to be implemented by services. For example, where a toddler has a soiled nappy with obvious sign of dermatitis and pruritus, is it a deliberate attempt by a parent to withhold care and attention, or is it down to a more fundamental reason, like post-natal depression or the state of being impecunious? Knowing the legislative provisions is one step in helping paramedics make informed decisions about vulnerable patients.

The role of the paramedic in identifying abuse

It takes a multidisciplinary team approach to protect at-risk children. Child maltreatment tends not to occur in isolation within vulnerable families. Associated issues, such as alcohol or drug dependency, may also be present. The reasons that child abuse occurs are numerous, and arise out of frustration, anger, an inability to cope, or simply because the parent has no knowledge of good parenting skills and lacks support. Evaluating the history and mechanism of either physical or psychological injury is the predominant concern for the treating paramedic. The patient is the paramedic's chief focus, and care should of course be the priority. However, the paramedic has an important role to play here, and can assist in determining whether the stated events caused the presenting injury. In doing so, the paramedic needs to consider whether:

1 The injury has been caused by another person and is considered to have been inflicted.

2 The injury is adequately explained by the circumstances of the injury event provided (by the carer or other witness).

3 The injury is self-inflicted—has been caused by the child's own behaviour as a result of normal childhood activity (with no other person actively involved).

4 The mechanism or sequence of events leading to the injury remains indeterminate or unclear.[35]

Considering these four issues will allow the paramedic an opportunity to alert authorities to the at-risk child if they develop a 'reasonable' level of suspicion. The relevant authorities are listed in Appendix 8.5. Paramedics can locate further information on where and what to report in each jurisdiction.

Even among people tasked in the role of child protection, it is widely believed that workers fail to identify abuse because they choose to believe it is not actually happening.[36] They would rather believe that people are not capable of committing atrocious acts against children. This sentiment is born out of self-preservation, and is a structured coping mechanism.[37] It is a form of psychological self-defence; it may be formed on the basis of misguided preconceived beliefs. Education services can prevent profligate anecdotes from masquerading as fact.

Being aware of undue optimism and its role in causing professionals to discount the likelihood of significant harm will help people who may encounter abused children through the course of their work.[38] An advanced awareness of the subjective nature of the situation, as well as of the pitfalls and possible prejudices associated with suspected abuse and neglect, will help paramedics treat and support their patients appropriately. Knowing what to do with the information and the responsibilities associated with reporting child abuse are critical to paramedical practice. Understanding our personal responses and unspoken prejudices through self-reflection is a pillar of sound clinical practice.

The ambulance service has changed in recent years to incorporate more solo responders. The traditional ambulance dual-crewed ambulance (frequently 3 if an undergraduate paramedic student is also staffing the ambulance) remains a common sight on the roads. Having the benefit of working with a qualified colleague provides an opportunity to discuss areas of their work where issues and outcomes are not completely clear. In these cases, the opportunity to discuss with someone also on-scene, and witnessing the same events, can help paramedics make decisions on how best to intervene appropriately on behalf of someone they suspect is being abused.

Mandatory reporting of suspected child abuse and neglect

Paramedics are not explicitly mentioned as mandatory reporters of child abuse in Australia and New Zealand, unlike doctors, nurses and midwives. However, a careful reading of legislation reveals that paramedics in some states and territories are required by law to report some or all suspected forms of child abuse. Appendix 8.6 reveals the states and territories that require paramedics by law to report. Appendix 8.7 reveals the laws on the voluntarily reporting of suspected child maltreatment.[39] Irrespective of the legal duty imposed, all people are encouraged to report suspected child maltreatment. Non-mandated reporters contribute to reporting suspected child maltreatment, and should not be overlooked as a valuable asset in combatting all forms of child maltreatment.[40]

Paramedics have surveillance opportunities not available to other clinicians due to the point-of-care delivery. Ambulance services can improve training on identifying and responding to child abuse and neglect within their clinical matrix, as well as other forms of abuse, including domestic violence and elder abuse (discussed below).

Types of abuse

Child abuse or child maltreatment is a construct that is not defined equally across all jurisdictions.[41] The direction adopted in this chapter is that child abuse is inflicted through:

1 physical abuse

2 sexual abuse

3 psychological and emotional abuse

4 neglect.[42]

Exposure to domestic violence (EDV) and *fabricated or induced illness by carers (FII)* are also distinct examples of child maltreatment, and will be discussed. Children can be victims of multiple types of abuse. Poly-victimisation describes children who are recipients of several types of abuse. Many children who are exposed to domestic violence are also victims of sexual abuse,[43] as well as other forms of abuse.[44] Although no one form of abuse is easier to identify or suspect than any other, physical abuse causes injuries. Covering up injuries and inconsistent explanations are features of this type of abuse, but consider the child's age and their mobility factor when assessing for cause. Of the four types of abuse stated above, there may be indications that they are not carried out in isolation of one another. A child may experience physical abuse as part of sexual abuse, as well as emotional and psychological abuse.

Children are very prone to manipulation, and the imbalance of power between an adult and a child can be taken to horrifying extremes. This means that the abuse may pass undetected for a very long time because of the influence the perpetrator has over the child victim. Perpetrators use many methods to protect themselves from being discovered, and these include the abuser engendering fear in the child, which might include threats against people or animals that the child loves, or the threat of the removal of items that are valuable to the child, as well as many other forms of coercion.[45] The perpetrator may be so deceptive that the abused child may not perceive what is, by objective standards, actually abuse.[46] There will be varying degrees of harm. It is imperative that ambulance services and paramedics work towards raising their own levels of awareness on the signs and presentations associated with child abuse and how to spot them.

Physical abuse

Children, particularly pre-school children, will often have bruises that are consistent with normal, healthy experiences during childhood (e.g. climbing trees, falling over, running into objects). These marks are usually located in areas of the body that would correspond with the mechanism of injury. For example, falling over while running would result in bruises and abrasions on the knees. Injuries sustained as a result of abuse tend to be located in unusual areas that can be easily covered; for example, the upper arm, the back of the thighs, and the back. Appendix 8.8 and Appendix 8.9 list possible causes of accidental and non-accidental injuries, and are designed to help paramedics determine whether the injuries they observe are appropriate to the child's age and level of mobility, or whether they have been inflicted intentionally to cause harm.

Appendices 8.8 and 8.9 are not designed to be definitive, but rather to act as a guide; they provide a point of reference to assist paramedics examining physical injuries, such as whether there are numerous bruises and what stages of healing they are at. Injuries may not indicate that harm has occurred for any reason other than accidentally, but they may provide justification for the paramedic to report their suspicions to child protection services should there be doubt. Some injuries will be more obvious than others in terms of the purpose of their infliction. For instance, a scalding could have a justifiable explanation, but a cigarette burn would not, even if it were accidental.

Compounding the difficulties associated with the above is balancing the right, discussed earlier, of the parent to be able to reasonably chastise their child.[47] The stage at which reasonable chastisement crosses the line towards physical abuse is not always obvious or clear. Another challenge to identifying physical abuse is that the signs of abuse can be caused by other conditions that are not the result of abuse. For example, many skin conditions could mimic the signs of abuse, and the paramedic should remain cautious about differential reasons that could also account for presentations that can appear like physical abuse. For example, among the relatively benign conditions that can be mistaken for physical abuse is parvovirus B19, also known as 'fifth disease' or 'slapped cheek syndrome'; it gets this last name because the erythema seen on some children's cheeks mimics the mark left by being slapped across the cheek, so can be mistaken for physical abuse. Another skin condition that can mimic the signs of abuse is Mongolian blue spots, which are common in some ethnicities. It can be mistaken for bruising, especially in children who have not become fully mobile, but the skin pigmentation is a birthmark and not a bruise.

Despite the challenges attributed to differential findings, paramedics should be neither overly cautious nor too dismissive. Paramedics must learn to develop confidence in identifying certain anomalies in the children they assess, and also develop appropriate strategies when investigating unfamiliar presentations.

Sexual abuse

Sexual abuse is a distinct category of child maltreatment; it is carried out for the sexual gratification of the perpetrator. Abuse of a child can be perpetrated when children are not even present; for example, the accessing of child pornography on the internet. The makers, the distributors and the viewers of this material are nevertheless committing a criminal offence.[48] For the victim, issues of shame and confusion can arise even when they experience normal, healthy feelings of arousal. This can lead to a fear of disclosure of abuse, because the child mistakenly believes that their own arousal somehow negates the abuse. Although the child may ultimately determine that the action being carried out against them is wrong, it may take many years not only for the abuse to stop, but for the memories of the abuse to surface. This period ideally requires considerable support and therapeutic intervention for the benefit of the victim/survivor.

The sexual abuse of a child provokes intense reactions in members of society who view the fetishisation of children as unacceptable. Paramedics are no exception to experiencing feelings of revulsion. As healthcare professionals it is essential, in the event that child sexual abuse is suspected, for paramedics to not challenge children or any other person present about their concerns. The role of the paramedic is to gather history, perform assessments, document findings, and be extremely supportive of children suspected of being abused.

If disclosure regarding abuse is made to the paramedic, it is of extreme importance to let the child know that they are believed, that attending paramedics will take the allegation seriously, and will respond professionally and appropriately. At a fundamental level this will make the child feel safe and protected. Paramedics must also be aware that children making a disclosure will use language relative to their age and understanding. That is, children of a certain age will lack the sophistication to articulate a disclosure clearly, and so signals relating to abuse may be missed, although the description may seem clear to the child.[49] Conversely, inappropriate sexualised behaviour and language may be a flag that the child has been exposed to acts or images of a sexual nature. Paramedics need to be sensitive to this, and will need to employ skills of comprehension pertinent to the child's level of understanding.

Paramedics should be aware of their feelings toward certain events and circumstances that they could, in all likelihood, encounter as part of their practice. Through an awareness of these emotions, the paramedic will be able to respond professionally until such time as they are able to seek appropriate support.

It is inappropriate to examine a child's genitals or anus in the absence of a stated clinical need. However, if the child is complaining of pain and discomfort associated with genitalia or the anus, and/or pain on urination and/or bleeding/discharge from the anus, vagina or penis, examination would be justifiably indicated. This, however, is a highly challenging area for paramedics, and one that needs to be addressed through training and education.[50]

If paramedics feel that an examination is necessary prior to arriving at hospital, they must not undertake an examination on their own, and if possible they should have someone the child trusts with the child at the time. Alternatively, police or community service staff trained in dealing with abused children could be called to assist. Like physical abuse, suspected sexual abuse can have differential findings. Pain associated when voiding the bladder may be due to a urinary tract infection, which can commonly affect younger children. Factually documenting and sharing findings with child health specialists, and remaining supportive of the child patient, are vital in responding to and combatting child sexual abuse and exploitation.

As the child ages into adolescence, taking an interest in sex and sexual exploration is a normal part of growing up. Children mature at different times. Paramedics need to be aware of the laws on ages young people can consent to sexual relations in their specific country, state or territory. Being under the age of consent does not absolutely preclude a person from having or wanting sexual relations. Appendix 8.10 summarises the law with regard to consent. Familiarity with this legislation will help paramedics when responding to minors and sexual health matters.

The majority of the jurisdictions recognise an offence when sexual relations have occurred with anyone under the age of 16. If two people who are both below the lawful age of consent for a particular jurisdiction have engaged in sexual intercourse and a paramedic becomes aware of it, referral may be appropriate. This will allow the parties involved to receive appropriate sexual health advice. However, if there is less than 2 years of age difference between them, and the sex is irrefutably consensual, it is unlikely that there will be a need to report. The paramedic should consider offering public health advice about safe sex practices and sexual health. Young people, of similar age and on the cusp of being able to provide lawful consent to sexual relations, should be supported, helped and advised as a way of educating them about their sexual health.

Psychological and emotional abuse

Emotional and psychological abuse covers a very broad range of practices; it is challenging to define, which makes for uncertainty when attempting to measure rates of prevalence.[51] Whereas in cases of physical and sexual abuse there are signs and symptoms that can be used to confirm suspicions and determine prevalence, in instances of emotional and psychological abuse there are not always tangible examples of abuse. It can be challenging to connect observable behaviours to fit definitions of psychological or emotional harm.[52] Akin to physical and sexual abuse, the long-term deleterious effects of such abuse are significant, and the effects may be hidden for years into adulthood.

This type of abuse can be characterised by the following examples:

- withholding love and affection
- isolating and ignoring the child
- making the child feel worthless
- providing a constant barrage of baseless criticism
- using fear as a punitive measure
- referring to the child as something non-specific and gender-neutral, not by their name.[53]

Paramedics, in the course of their normal response, must remain alert, especially when dealing with children. Paramedics should refrain from being put off by challenging or disruptive behaviour exhibited by a child, no matter how discourteous. This needs to be reinforced whether the child is a patient or part of another patient's social context. As with all types of suspected child abuse, it is not for the paramedic to confront or challenge, but simply to identify it. Paramedics must remain supportive in their role, and, in so doing, they may create a window of opportunity for the recipient of alleged abuse to request help.

Paramedics may be able to observe the relationship between the caregiver and the child.[54] Such observations may be sufficient, and, in this way, emotional/psychological abuse differs from sexual abuse due to the covert nature of sexual abuse. Paramedics should understand that this type of suspected abuse could be the product of parental coping in a given set of circumstances, rather than an act of malice. It may be that a parent or caregiver requires suitable support to allow them to parent effectively. Paramedics alert to this fact could use their observations to help intervene and support families affected by emotional and psychological abuse.

Neglect

Ideally, all children should be brought up in a loving, safe, nourishing and supportive environment. With positive parenting, children will hopefully, although not exclusively, go on to develop into well-adjusted, dependable and contributing members of society.

Neglect may occur without malicious intent: the death of a parent, the loss of parental income, health issues related to one or more carers, additional siblings introduced into an already over-stretched family unit, or ineffective parenting can all contribute to a child being neglected. It could also be due to environmental factors, such as a result of natural disasters and the loss of personal possessions leading to a period of displacement and disruption. Conversely, a child may be neglected maliciously or abandoned when adult care is available.

The signs of neglect may become apparent in many ways. Similar to other forms of child abuse, the harm caused by the neglect may filter into other forms of child abuse. For instance, if a child is not being provided with adequate clothing or their clothing is too small, too big or is very dirty, this can impact psychologically on the child, and therefore merge with emotional abuse due to possible exposure to ridicule by the child's peers at school. Neglect therefore shares some similarities with emotional abuse and psychological harm. Neglect will usually manifest itself physically, based on failure to thrive, which can lead to presentations considered inappropriate for the child's age.[55] It can also occur when the child is unwell and medical intervention is not summoned, which will lead to the child's health or condition deteriorating. Questions that the attending paramedic may seek to ask themselves as part of their patient history-taking are:

- Is the child not putting on weight because the carer is refusing to feed the child?
- Is the child not putting on weight because the carer is unable to feed the child effectively due to the carer's own developmental, mental health or socioeconomic issues?
- Is the child not putting on weight despite adequate feeding and attention from the carer, due to the patient having a medical problem (e.g. worms), where medical intervention has not been sought due to the carer's limited understanding of the situation?

Paramedics may be more likely to observe neglect than report it. Additional observations may need to be made and facts found to support a decision to notify that a child is suspected of being a victim of neglect. Prejudices and bias may creep in and sway a paramedic away from, or towards, notifying agencies that a child is suspected of being neglected. All people hold prejudices and are biased. It is what makes human beings sapient, and gives us the ability to reason empirically.

Paramedics observe patients in their environments, and they are capable of identifying squalor. However, conflating squalor and poverty with neglect is not an entirely accurate method of identifying neglect. Paramedics need to be aware of their own prejudices and biases, and how their views impinge upon their decision to report and refer suspected cases of neglect. Challenging prejudices is a continual struggle, but is one that must be undertaken to prevent paramedics from becoming jaded and fatigued by exerting compassion. Remaining alert to abuse through objective observation is central. Paramedics must ensure that reports are made accurately, reasonably and honestly to raise the prospect that notifications will be substantiated during investigation by child protection services and/or the police.

Exposure to domestic violence

Doubt remains, and debate continues, whether exposure to domestic violence (EDV) should be classified as a type of child maltreatment.[56] The reports and commission of inquiry on violence against woman and children—when read in conjunction with legislation on domestic and family violence from Australia and New Zealand—support the contention that EDV is a form of harm which can have damaging outcomes for children exposed to it.

EDV occurs when a child witnesses any form of domestic violence. It is not limited to viewing the violence; hearing is sufficient, as is witnessing the aftermath of domestic violence. Any act held to be domestic violence and observed by a child is EDV. Legislation on domestic and family violence is found in Appendix 8.2. Not all children suffer harm as a result of witnessing domestic violence, but many do go on to suffer significant health and social consequences.[57] Witnessing domestic violence can contribute to child witnesses experiencing depression, anxiety, drug and alcohol abuse, and antenatal harm later in life.[58] It can also contribute to social and legal issues, such as aggression and poor social outcomes, including low academic achievement.[59] Although paramedics may not routinely inquire about a child's experience of domestic violence, there is opportunity for them to develop and become more involved with children who do experience violence within the family home.

The Australian Bureau of Statistics (ABS) Personal Safety Survey (PSS) of 2016 reported that 1.2 million of the study's female participants had witnessed violence against their mother by partners, and 440,900 had witnessed violence against their father by partners.[60] The study reported also that 896,700 male participants in the survey witnessed violence against their mothers, and 380,000 witnessed violence against their father by partners.

The mandatory reporting laws for child protection, found in Appendix 8.6, vary from state to state. Not all states and territories place an obligation on paramedics to report a child's exposure to domestic and family violence. Despite not being explicitly referred to by their profession, paramedics in New South Wales, the Northern Territory and Tasmania are required by law to report children whom they know to have been exposed to domestic violence to the agencies responsible for child protection.

Raising EDV with paramedics and encouraging an integrated approach with other services could lead to reduced service demand, with the resulting early intervention reducing acute presentations from the fallout from EDV. The variety of offences that can be attributed to domestic violence may mean that a paramedic will be more likely to acknowledge explicit cases. Evidence of physical battery against an intimate partner, or disclosure by a victim, is a sufficient indicator to warrant response and intervention from paramedics.

To confirm EDV, a paramedic needs to only be aware that children are on scene of a domestic violence incident or have witnessed the aftermath. This combined knowledge makes for relatively straightforward identification, compared to identifying other examples of child maltreatment. Abusers and perpetrators are not loyal to one form of abuse over another. This is an important feature for paramedics, and could galvanise them when working in environments that are grounded in domestic violence and exposure to domestic violence. This is called poly-victimisation, and is explored in the next section.

Poly-victimisation

Poly-victimisation is a cluster of abuse types. It is not restricted to types of maltreatment, but can include other forms of victimisation, such as property crime or robbery.[61] However, poly-victimisation in the context of child maltreatment is important to consider, particularly in conjunction with EDV. Reporting and referring EDV can help facilitate the early identification of other abuse manifestations that would otherwise continue unreported.[62] Raising awareness of the co-occurrence of abuse, rather than focusing on an incident of abuse as an isolated event,[63] should encourage paramedics to report and refer all forms of suspected abuse, but particularly EDV. Compared to other forms of child maltreatment, it can be identified without too much inquiry on the part of paramedics. Involving paramedics in protective community care acknowledges that paramedical care is not exclusively clinical. Paramedical care intersects with health and social care,[64] and ambulance services must take responsibility for leading the way in designing interventions that reflect the needs of the community.

Child maltreatment and the toxic trio

Child maltreatment is not identified solely through the assessment and examination of children. The constellation of parental mental health issues, parental substance abuse and parental violence—the so-called *toxic trio*—are sentinel signs of increased risk of child maltreatment.[65] Paramedics are increasingly tasked with responding to mental health concerns, and drug and alcohol abuse in the community. During assessment and history-taking, if it is revealed that a parent or parents have a history of mental health issues combined with drug and alcohol abuse, this should raise the prospect that child maltreatment is co-occurring. Mental health, substance misuse and domestic violence were at play in the death of Daniel Pelka, whose vulnerability was overlooked by the people tasked with keeping him safe.[66] Parental characteristics can be a helpful addition to the early identification of child maltreatment by paramedics.[67] Paramedics are encouraged to look beyond the presenting complaint and address whether there is any factor or combination of factors that point to an increased risk of harm to children within the family unit.

Fabricated or induced illness by carers

A less exact and controversial type of child maltreatment is fabricated or induced illness by carers (FII), which also goes by the term *Munchausen syndrome by proxy*. It occurs when a carer creates events or reports anecdotally that a child is unwell or injured in order to receive therapeutic treatment. The child could also suffer physical abuse, not merely from the infliction of injury as a punitive measure, but also in order to receive medical help and attention.

In this context, the paramedic needs to be aware of age-inappropriate intentional injuries versus, for example, accidental poisoning. They should remain alert to carers who access multiple healthcare providers—'doctor shopping'[68]—as a way of inflicting abuse and avoiding detection. Professor Sir Roy Meadow identified FII and its potential progression:

1 false illness story alone
2 false illness story plus fabrication of signs
3 induced illness.[69]

Each is harmful, but how the harm affects the child differs. The first may involve limited school attendance or unnecessary medical tests (such as taking blood) and needless painful procedures. The second may involve the carer withholding treatment to ensure the child does not improve, changing details on doctors' letters, or interfering with medical samples to falsify results. The third could involve the carer over-medicating the child to the point of toxicity, or inflicting injury to actually generate the need for medical attention.

The paramedic must be sensitive in the management of incidents where FII is suspected. In no way should they challenge the carer about the child's presentation. It is important to treat the patient objectively and report the findings at an appropriate level. Carers may be extremely shrewd about medical matters, and will be suspicious of a health professional's interference, which they may view as an attack. It is therefore vital that appropriate supportive pre-hospital measures are implemented, such as notifying the receiving facility staff without raising the suspicion of the carer who may be responsible for the alleged fabrication.

Child maltreatment and cultural diversity

Pluralism exists in all parts of the developed world, and it is important to celebrate people's cultural heritages and their beliefs. Paramedics, therefore, need to be culturally aware, safe, sensitive and competent.[70] Multiculturalism stems from migration. Immigration can be the result of social choices, or of people seeking asylum or refugee status on the basis of human rights abuses. The reasons for migration are multifactorial, and cannot be categorised as a single type. To people born or brought up outside of Australia and New Zealand, the cultural transition to a new country, its language and its laws takes time and requires support.

Some immigrants may hold views and carry practices that are contrary to the predominant culture that exists within their currently domiciled country. Some practices that are considered acceptable and sometimes even positively encouraged in their country of origin may be contrary or unlawful if practised in Australia and New Zealand. At this intersection lies the need to balance the rights of the individual with the right of the state to govern and implement laws that it considers appropriate and equitable.[71] The question of cultural issues regarding child protection is worthy of a text of its own, but, for reasons of space, cannot be included here in detail.

However, one area that requires special mention is the practice of female genital cutting (FGC), female circumcision or female genital mutilation (FGM). While the practice is considered culturally acceptable and is practised in many countries,[72] in Australia and New Zealand it is unlawful, irrespective of whether a person consents to it or not. Nor is it lawful for a person who is a resident or citizen of Australia and New Zealand to leave the country to have the procedure carried out. The terms for these procedures themselves are highly problematic, because they feature within the designation labels that the recipient of such a procedure may not welcome. A recipient of an ethnically performed clitoridectomy will not welcome the implication that they have been mutilated.[73] By the same token, a society that outlaws the abuse of such a procedure will feel compelled to use the weightiest language possible to decry the abuse.

Generally, though not exclusively, this practice occurs before the age of puberty;[74] hence, the topic is featured as part of this chapter on child protection. Despite its unlawful nature, the practice may still be observed by some groups who subscribe to this procedure as part of their cultural identity. Due to migration from countries where the practice is held to be most prevalent, the procedure may be carried out without knowledge of the state—akin to what is euphemistically known as a 'back-street procedure'—and therefore may possibly not be performed aseptically. Paramedics may be called to respond to patients who have become septic following the removal of the clitoris or one of the other permutations of this act. This will be a highly challenging area for many paramedics to respond to. Not only will the attending paramedics treat the patient, they will also need to consider filing a report to the organisation responsible for child protection within their state, territory or country.[75]

A less extreme example of cultural difference is in relation to putting a child down to rest at night. There are many cultural and social differences on child-rearing practices. To minimise the risk of sudden infant death syndrome, current policy is for the newborn baby to be placed on its back, in its own cot, next to the parental bed for the first year of the child's life.[76] Some cultural groups may prefer and recommend that the child sleep in the parental bed. It is important to mention that, if parents choose to share their bed with their newly born, it does not mean that they are providing substandard care by not following popular guidance. Parents are informed by cultural beliefs and practices. However, a real and significant danger exists where two people share their bed with an infant and one or both adult persons have consumed alcohol and/or drugs (be they recreational or prescribed sedatives), as they might roll, while asleep, onto the infant. The most common effect of the alcohol or drugs with respect to this example will be to desensitise the intoxicated person to the infant's movements underneath them, risking crush injuries, asphyxiation and death.[77]

Elder abuse and abuse of other vulnerable groups

Elder abuse is generally held to include physical abuse, sexual abuse, psychological abuse, financial abuse and neglect.[78] Prevalence rates of elder abuse differ between community and institutional settings. A recent study suggests that 141 million elderly people are victim to abuse globally.[79] This figure is held to be an underestimation of the full extent of elder abuse.[80] Elder abuse in institutional settings is believed to be just as high as it is in the community.[81] A power imbalance can develop as we age, and infirmity and cognitive deterioration can cause reduced agency. The elderly often require people whom they can trust to advocate on their behalf, be it as a power of attorney or a health advocate, and to make decisions on their behalf in the event that they no longer have the capacity to do so.

As with domestic violence and child maltreatment, paramedics are supremely well placed to identify elder abuse in community and institutional settings, such as aged-care facilities.[82] However, their ability to do so depends on their knowledge, confidence and abilities to not only identify elder abuse, but also to report it. Unlike domestic and family violence, and child maltreatment, there are no specific legislative instruments in Australia and New Zealand, instead relying on existing criminal and civil legislation to protect the elderly from abuse and neglect. The abuse of the elderly and infirm is an under-reported area.

Mean mortality rates are dropping,[83] and more and more people are living longer, with multiple and involved care needs. Our ageing population, with its multiple care needs, requires not only reactive frontline health services, but proactive services as well: clinicians who can identify and help prevent poorer health outcomes for an ageing population. This includes being aware of non-organic causes for particular presentations, especially among patients who are not able to advocate for themselves. Being alert to the suspicion that someone who appears to be caring for an elderly person is in fact abusing them is challenging. A paramedic's initial reaction can be to think the best of a situation, disabuse their self of any notion that harm is occurring, and subsequently miss an opportunity to intervene on behalf of someone lacking agency who is being abused.

These situations are not limited to the elderly. The same applies to people with developmental challenges such as autism, people with traumatic brain injuries, people with consuming depression and anxiety, people with motor neuron disease or dementia—the list is long. Identifying abuse in people with significant and substantial health issues is challenging, particularly as baseline observations in these patient groups may not be straightforward to determine. Paramedics should not assess 'what is normal?', but instead assess 'what is normal for this patient?'

A key feature of paramedic work is vigilance. Paramedics need to remain attentive and observant to the subtle cues given by their patients—cues that if picked up could lead to suspicions of abuse being substantiated, and a considerable improvement for the patient and others affected by a perpetrator's actions.

Conclusion

The purpose of this chapter has been to address the challenges faced by paramedics when working with vulnerable patients. Relationship-specific community violence is an understudied area of ambulance work.

By now you should understand:
- the need to involve paramedics in responding to relationship-specific community violence, which could include domestic violence, child maltreatment, elder abuse and abuse of individuals affected by infirmity or disability
- that a child is generally any person under 18 years for the purposes of child protection
- one aspect of child abuse rarely occurs in isolation; there may be other factors present that increase the risk of exposure to child abuse and neglect
- detection and disclosure can be highly problematic, but the obstacles are not insurmountable
- the types of child abuse consist of:
  - physical abuse
  - sexual abuse
  - emotional/psychological abuse
  - neglect
- child maltreatment also includes:
  - exposure to domestic violence
  - fabricated or induced illness

- cultural sensitivities are important with respect to child protection
- each jurisdiction discussed legislates for a threshold to intervention
- thinking the best of a situation may, on some occasions, allow the abuse to be perpetuated
- reports and referrals must be objective and devoid of emotion, no matter how upsetting the situation is
- challenging and disruptive behaviour by a child may be a coping mechanism due to abuse they have suffered—it is important not to overlook this; adopting an alternative perspective to the situation may ensure that the child's needs, unique to them, are met.

Review Questions

1 What are paramedics' responsibilities for reporting all of the various forms of child maltreatment in Australia and New Zealand? Do you think mandatory reporting laws for healthcare professionals should be harmonised in Australia? Do you think mandatory reporting laws should be introduced into New Zealand? Give reasons for your answers.

2 Why is it important to remain professional should you become aware of child maltreatment, or in the event a disclosure of child abuse is made to you?

3 What examples of domestic violence do you think could be misinterpreted as other clinical presentations? Review the introductory case if you are unsure. Why is it important to be vigilant?

4 Although the child is not physically injured, is witnessing domestic or intimate partner violence a form of child abuse? If so, why? Would you ever ask a patient of any age whether they had experienced exposure to domestic violence? What do you think this could tell you about the relationship, if there is one, between EDV and other pathology?

5 What role do you think ambulance services could develop in the future to help eliminate relationship-specific community violence?

Text continued on p. 208

Appendix 8.1 Legislation defining 'child and young person'			
Jurisdiction	**Legislation**	**Article/Section**	**Definition**
International convention	*Convention on the Rights of the Child (CROC)*	art 1	Every human being below the age of 18 years
Australian Commonwealth	*Family Law Act 1975* (Cth)	s 4	A person who is under 18

Appendix 8.1	Legislation defining 'child and young person' continued			
Jurisdiction	**Legislation**	**Article/Section**	**Definition**	
New Zealand	*Vulnerable Children Act 2014*	s 5	A person who is under 18	
Australian Capital Territory	*Children and Young People Act 2008* (ACT)	s 11	Child	under 12 years
		s 12	Young person	12–18 years
New South Wales	*Children and Young Persons (Care and Protection) Act 1998* (NSW)	Section 3	A person who is under 16	
		s 221(1)(a)	A person who is under 15 (Children's employment)	
Northern Territory	*Care and Protection of Children Act 2007* (NT)	s 13	A person less than 18 years of age	
Queensland	*Child Protection Act 1999* (Qld)	s 8	An individual under 18 years	
South Australia	*Children's Protection Act 1993* (SA)	s 6	A person under 18 years of age	
Tasmania	*Children, Young Persons and Their Families Act 1997* (Tas)	s 3	A person under 18 years of age	
Victoria	*Child Wellbeing and Safety Act 2005* (Vic)	s 3	A person who is under the age of 18 years	
Western Australia	*Children and Community Services Act 2004* (WA)	s 3	A person who is under 18 years of age	

Appendix 8.2	Laws in Australia and New Zealand on domestic and family violence
Jurisdiction	**Legislation**
Australian Commonwealth	Section 4AB *Family Law Act 1975* (Cth)
New Zealand	*Domestic Violence Act 1995*
Australian Capital Territory	*Family Violence Act 2016* (ACT)
New South Wales	*Crimes (Domestic and Personal Violence) Act 2007* (NSW)
Northern Territory	*Domestic and Family Violence Act 2007* (NT)
Queensland	*Domestic and Family Violence Act 2012* (Qld)
South Australia	*Intervention Orders (Prevention of Abuse) Act 2009* (SA)
Tasmania	*Family Violence Act 2004* (Tas)
Victoria	*Family Violence Act 2008* (Vic)
Western Australia	*Restraining Orders Act 1997* (WA) *Domestic Violence Orders (National Recognition) Act 2017* (WA)

Appendix 8.3 Child protection legislation in Australia and New Zealand		
Jurisdiction	**Principal act**	**Other relevant legislation**
New Zealand (www.legislation.govt.nz) Oranga Tamariki—Ministry for Children (www.orangatamariki.govt.nz)	*Vulnerable Children Act 2014*	*Oranga Tamariki Act 1989*
Australian Capital Territory (www.legislation.act.gov.au) Office for Children, Youth and Families (www.communityservices.act. gov.au/ocyfs)	*Children and Young People Act 2008* (ACT)	*Human Rights Act 2004* (ACT)
		Human Rights Commission Act 2005 (ACT)
		Family Law Act 1975 (Cth)
New South Wales (www.legislation.nsw.gov.au) Family and Community Services (www.facs.nsw.gov.au)	*Children and Young Persons (Care and Protection) Act 1998* (NSW)	*Children (Protection and Parental Responsibility) Act 1997* (NSW)
		Child Protection (Offenders Registration) Act 2000 (NSW)
		Crimes Act 1900 (NSW)
		Ombudsman Act 1974 (NSW)
		Family Law Act 1975 (Cth)
Northern Territory (www.legisaltion.nt.gov.au) Territory Families (www.territoryfamilies.nt.gov.au)	*Care and Protection of Children Act 2007* (NT)	*Information Act 2006* (NT)
		Disability Services Act 2004 (NT)
		Criminal Code Act 2006 (NT)
		Family Law Act 1975 (Cth)
Queensland (www.legislation.qld.gov.au) Department of Child Safety, Youth and Women (www.csyw.qld.gov.au)	*Child Protection Act 1999* (Qld)	*Education (General Provisions) Act 2006* (Qld)
		Public Health Act 2005 (Qld)
		Family Law Act 1975 (Cth)
South Australia (www.legislation.sa.gov.au) Department for Child Protection (www.childprotection.sa.gov.au)	*Children's Protection Act 1993* (SA)	*Young Offenders Act 1993* (SA)
		Children and Young People (Safety) Act 2017 (SA)
		Children's Protection Regulations 2010 (SA)
		Family and Community Services Act 1972 (SA)
		Family Law Act 1975 (Cth)

Appendix 8.3 Child protection legislation in Australia and New Zealand continued

Jurisdiction	Principal act	Other relevant legislation
Tasmania (www.legislation.tas.gov.au) Department of Health and Human Services (www.dhhs.tas.gov.au/children)	*Children, Young Persons and their Families Act 1997* (Tas)	*Family Law Act 1975* (Cth)
Victoria (www.legislation.vic.gov.au) Department of Health and Human Services (www.services.dhhs.vic.gov.au/ child-protection)	*Children, Youth and Families Act 2005* (Vic)	*Child Wellbeing and Safety Act 2005* (Vic)
		Children, Youth and Families (Consequential and Other Amendments) Act 2006 (Vic)
		Charter of Human Rights and Responsibilities Act 2006 (Vic)
		Family Law Act 1975 (Cth)
Western Australia (www.legislation.wa.gov.au) Department for Child Protection and Family Support (www.dcp.wa.gov.au)	*Children and Community Services Act 2004* (WA)	*Family Law Act 1975* (Cth)

Appendix 8.4 Threshold of intervention for child protection in Australia and New Zealand

Jurisdiction	Legislation	Section	Threshold for intervention[84] (overview)	
New Zealand	*Oranga Tamariki Act 1989*	s 14(1)(a)	Is being, or is likely to be, harmed, ill-treated, abused, or seriously deprived	
Australian Capital Territory	*Children and Young People Act 2008* (ACT)	s 345	(1)(a)(i)	Has been abused or neglected
			(1)(a)(ii)	Is being abused or neglected
			(1)(a)(iii)	Is at risk of abuse or neglect
New South Wales	*Children and Young Persons (Care and Protection) Act 1998* (NSW)	s 23(1)(a)–(f)	At risk of significant harm	
Northern Territory	*Care and Protection of Children Act 2007* (NT)	s 20(a)–(d)	Suffered or is likely to suffer harm or exploitation	
Queensland	*Child Protection Act 1999* (Qld)	s 10	(a)	Has suffered significant harm, is suffering significant harm or is at unacceptable risk of suffering significant harm
			(b)	Does not have a parent able and willing to protect the child from the harm

Continued

Appendix 8.4 Threshold of intervention for child protection in Australia and New Zealand continued

Jurisdiction	Legislation	Section	Threshold for intervention[84] (overview)	
South Australia	*Children's Protection Act 1993* (SA)	s 6	(2)(aa)	Significant risk of serious harm (physical, psychological or emotional wellbeing)
			(2)(a)	Has been, or is being abused or neglected
Tasmania	*Children, Young Persons and Their Families Act 1997* (Tas)	s 4(1)(a)	The child has been, is being, or is likely to be, abused or neglected	
Victoria	*Children, Youth and Families Act 2005* (Vic)	s 162(1)(a–f)	Has suffered or is likely to suffer significant harm due to absence of parental care, physical injury, sexual abuse, emotional or psychological harm, neglect	
Western Australia	*Children and Community Services Act 2004* (WA)	s 28	Has suffered, or is likely to suffer, harm that is significant in nature as a result of physical abuse, sexual abuse, emotional abuse or neglect	

Appendix 8.5 Statutory child protection authorities

Jurisdiction	Responsible authority	Website
New Zealand	Oranga Tamariki—Ministry for Children	www.orangatamariki.govt.nz
Australian Capital Territory	Office for Children, Youth and Families	www.communityservices.act.gov.au/ocyfs
New South Wales	Family and Community Services	www.facs.nsw.gov.au
Northern Territory	Territory Families	www.territoryfamilies.nt.gov.au
Queensland	Department of Child Safety, Youth and Women	www.csyw.qld.gov.au
South Australia	Department for Child Protection	www.childprotection.sa.gov.au
Tasmania	Department of Health and Human Services	www.dhhs.tas.gov.au/children
Victoria	Department of Health and Human Services	www.services.dhhs.vic.gov.au/child-protection
Western Australia	Department for Child Protection and Family Support	www.dcp.wa.gov.au

Appendix 8.6	Child protection mandatory reporting laws		
Jurisdiction	**Legislation**	**Health profession mandated reporters**	**What is reported**
Australian Capital Territory	*Children and Young People Act 2008* (ACT), ss 342, 356	Doctor, dentist, nurse, enrolled nurse and midwife	Physical abuse, sexual abuse, emotional abuse, domestic violence (s 342(d)(i)–(iii)), neglect
New South Wales	*Children and Young Persons (Care and Protection) Act 1998* (NSW), ss 23, 27	Health care professionals	Physical abuse, sexual abuse, psychological harm, ill-treatment; domestic violence, neglect
Northern Territory	*Care and Protection of Children Act 2007* (NT), ss 15, 16, 26	Health practitioners	Physical abuse, psychological abuse, emotional abuse, sexual abuse, neglect, exploitation, exposure to physical violence (domestic violence)
Queensland	*Child Protection Act 1999* (Qld), s 13E	Doctors, registered nurses	Physical abuse, sexual abuse
South Australia	*Children's Protection Act 1993* (SA), ss 6, 11 (*Intervention Orders (Prevention of Abuse) Act 2009* (SA) s 7(1)b) describes EDV)	Medical practitioner, pharmacist, registered nurse, enrolled nurse, dentist, psychologist, any other person that provides health services	Sexual abuse, physical abuse, emotional abuse, neglect
Tasmania	*Children, Young Persons and Their Families Act 1997* (Tas), ss 3, 14 *Family Violence Act 2004* (Tas) ss 4, 7	Medical practitioner, registered nurse, enrolled nurse, midwife, dentist (including therapists and hygienists), psychologists, any other person that provides health services	Sexual abuse, physical injury or abuse, emotional injury or abuse, neglect, family violence
Victoria	*Children Youth and Families Act 2005* (Vic), ss 162, 182 *Family Violence Protection Act 2008* (Vic), s 5	Registered medical practitioner, nurse, midwife, registered psychologist	Physical injury, sexual abuse, emotional harm, psychological harm (see s 5(1)(a)(ii) and (b) *Family Violence Protection Act 2008* (Vic)), neglect
Western Australia	*Children and Community Services Act 2004* (WA), s 124B(1)(a)	Doctor, nurse, midwife	Sexual abuse
New Zealand	New Zealand does not have mandatory reporting laws for suspected child abuse and neglect		

Appendix 8.7 Laws on voluntarily reporting child protection

Laws in Australia and New Zealand on voluntarily reporting a child in need of protection (where paramedics are not mandated to report child maltreatment)

New Zealand	*Oranga Tamariki Act 1989*, s 15
Australian Capital Territory	*Children and Young People Act 2008* (ACT), s 354
New South Wales	
Northern Territory	
Queensland	*Child Protection Act 1999* (Qld), s 13A
South Australia	
Tasmania	
Victoria	*Children Youth and Families Act 2005* (Vic), s 183
Western Australia	No legislative provision made for the voluntary reporting of suspected child maltreatment

Appendix 8.8 Possible accidental injuries

Infant			Child		
Area of body	Type of injuries	Possible causes	Area of body	Type of injuries	Possible causes
Forehead Nose Chin	Minor cuts Bruises Grazes	Impacting with furniture as mobility improves	Head Eyes Nose Chin	Minor cuts Bruises Grazes	Running Tripping Play-fighting Climbing
Elbows	Bruises Grazes	Furniture or carpet friction	Elbows	Bruises Grazes	Running Tripping Play-fighting Climbing
Hands	Grazes	Furniture or carpet friction	Hands	Grazes Cuts	Through normal exploration of outdoor environment
Fingers	Cuts Marks left through catching fingers	Caught in unsecured doors or toys with hinges and hard flaps	Fingers	Cuts Bruises	As a result of practising fine-motor skills such as using an age-appropriate knife or scissors General play
Knees	Bruises Grazes	Furniture or carpet friction	Hips	Bruises Grazes	Running into furniture
			Knees	Cuts Bruises Grazes	Running Tripping General play
			Shins	Bruises	Falling or hitting hard objects while running

Appendix 8.9	Possible non-accidental injuries				
Infant			**Child**		
Area of body	Type of injuries	Possible causes	Area of body	Type of injuries	Possible causes
Head	Significant laceration Fractures Internal haemorrhaging	Striking with an object Shaking Throwing	Head	Lacerations Internal haemorrhaging	Striking
Eyes	Bruises Cuts	Striking	Eyes	Bruises Cuts	Striking
Nose	Cuts	Striking	Nose	Damaged cartilage	Striking
Cheek	Bite marks	Biting	Cheek	Burns	Applying lit cigarette
Mouth	Torn fraenulum	Forcing pacifier/ feeding bottle into mouth	Mouth	Cuts Bruises	Striking
Neck	Bruises	Forceful pressure Attempted asphyxiation	Neck	Bruises	Forceful pressure Attempted asphyxiation
Shoulders	Bruises	Forceful direct pressure	Shoulders	Bruises	Forceful direct pressure
Arms	Bruises Fractures Bite marks	Striking Twisting Biting	Arms	Bruises Fractures Bite marks	Striking Twisting Biting
Chest	Burns Scalds Bruising	Grasping Applying lit cigarette	Chest	Bruises	Striking
Anus	Cuts Bruising	Sodomy	Anus	Cuts Bruising	Sodomy
Genitals	Bruises	Sexual abuse	Genitals	Bruises	Sexual abuse
Buttocks	Burns Bruises	Immersion burns Forcing child to sit on hot stove Kicking	Buttocks	Bruises	Kicking
Legs	Abnormal-shaped bruising patterns Scalds Fractures	Twisting Striking Applying hot iron	Legs	Bruises Fractures	Striking Kicking
Feet	Scalds	Immersion burns	Feet	Burns	Applying lit cigarette

Appendix 8.10 Age of consent laws			
Jurisdiction	**Legislation**	**Section**	**Definition**
New Zealand	*Crimes Act 1961*	s 134	Age of consent is 16
Australian Capital Territory	*Crimes Act 1900* (ACT)	s 55	Age of consent is 16 It is a defence if one participant was above the age of 10 and the other participant was no more than 2 years older than them and the parties consented
New South Wales	*Crimes Act 1900* (NSW)	s 66C	Age of consent is 16
Northern Territory	*Criminal Code Act 1983* (NT)	s 127	Age of consent is 16
Queensland	*Criminal Code Act 1899* (Qld)	s 215	Age of consent is 16
South Australia	*Criminal Law Consolidation Act 1935* (SA)	s 49	Age of consent is 17
Tasmania	*Criminal Code Act 1924* (Tas)	s 124	Age of consent is 17 It is a defence if one participant was above the age of 12 and the other participant was no more than 3 years older and the parties consented It is a defence if one participant was above the age of 15 and the other participant was no more than 5 years older and the consent is valid
Victoria	*Crimes Act 1958* (Vic)	s 45	Age of consent is 16
Western Australia	*Criminal Code Act Compilation 1913* (WA)	s 321	Age of consent is 16

Appendix 8.11 Useful websites
International
http://www.inpea.net/
http://www.kempe.org/
http://www.who.int/ageing/projects/elder_abuse/en/
http://www.who.int/news-room/fact-sheets/detail/violence-against-women
http://www.who.int/violence_injury_prevention/violence/child/en/
http://www.workingtogetheronline.co.uk/
https://safeandtogetherinstitute.com/
https://www.ispcan.org/
https://www.nspcc.org.uk/
https://www.ohchr.org/en/professionalinterest/pages/crc.aspx
https://www.unicef.org/crc/
Commonwealth
http://www.circinfo.org/index.php
http://www.earlychildhoodaustralia.org.au/
http://www.familycourt.gov.au
http://www.unisa.edu.au/childprotection/
https://aifs.gov.au/
https://bravehearts.org.au/
https://dvcs.org.au/
https://toolkit.seniorsrights.org.au/toolkit/what-is-elder-abuse/
https://www.1800respect.org.au/
https://www.alrc.gov.au/publications/what-elder-abuse
https://www.anrows.org.au/
https://www.blueknot.org.au/
https://www.eapu.com.au/
https://www.humanservices.gov.au/individuals/families
https://www.legislation.gov.au/
https://www.myagedcare.gov.au/legal-information/elder-abuse-concerns
https://www.smartsafe.org.au/support/family-violence-related-services/national
https://www.whiteribbon.org.au/

Continued

Appendix 8.11 Useful websites continued
Australian Capital Territory
http://www.communityservices.act.gov.au/ocyfs/children
http://www.communityservices.act.gov.au/women/womens_directory/domestic__and__family_violence
http://www.legislation.act.gov.au/
https://form.act.gov.au/smartforms/csd/child-concern-report/
https://www.communityservices.act.gov.au/wac/ageing/elder-abuse
New South Wales
http://www.elderabusehelpline.com.au/
http://www.elderabusehelpline.com.au/for-professionals/responding-to-elder-abuse
http://www.keepthemsafe.nsw.gov.au/
https://childstory.net.au/
https://www.childwise.org.au/page/41/state-legislation-reporting-nsw
https://www.facs.nsw.gov.au/
https://www.legislation.nsw.gov.au
Northern Territory
https://legislation.nt.gov.au/
https://nt.gov.au/
https://nt.gov.au/law/crime/domestic-and-family-violence
https://territoryfamilies.nt.gov.au/
https://www.cotant.org.au/information/elder-abuse-information-line/
https://www.smartsafe.org.au/elder-abuse-information-line-territory
Queensland
https://noviolence.org.au/
https://stopdomesticviolence.com.au/
https://www.communities.qld.gov.au/
https://www.csyw.qld.gov.au/child-family/protecting-children
https://www.legislation.qld.gov.au/
https://www.qld.gov.au/seniors/safety-protection/elder-abuse
South Australia
http://www.sa.agedrights.asn.au/
https://publictrustee.sa.gov.au/news/elder-abuse-can-be-stopped/
https://www.childprotection.sa.gov.au/

Appendix 8.11 Useful websites continued
https://www.legislation.sa.gov.au
https://www.police.sa.gov.au/your-safety/child-safety
https://www.sa.gov.au/topics/family-and-community/safety-and-health/domestic-violence
www.sahealth.sa.gov.au
Tasmania
http://www.dhhs.tas.gov.au/children/child_protection_services
http://www.dhhs.tas.gov.au/disability/projects/elder_abuse/elder_abuse_resources/what_is_elder_abuse
http://www.dhhs.tas.gov.au/service_information/children_and_families/family_violence_counselling_and_support_service
http://www.dpac.tas.gov.au/safehomessafefamilies
http://www.police.tas.gov.au/what-we-do/family-violence/
https://www.legislation.tas.gov.au/
Victoria
http://dvvic.org.au/
http://www.legislation.vic.gov.au/
http://www.police.vic.gov.au/content.asp?Document_ID=48513
http://www.rcfv.com.au/
https://seniorsrights.org.au/
https://services.dhhs.vic.gov.au/
https://www.dpc.vic.gov.au
https://www.nari.net.au/
https://www.relationshipsvictoria.com.au/services/familyviolence/
https://www.safesteps.org.au/
https://www.vic.gov.au/familyviolence.html
https://www.vic.gov.au/health-community/children/child-protection.html
Western Australia
http://www.advocare.org.au/
http://www.dcp.wa.gov.au/Pages/Home.aspx
https://www.legislation.wa.gov.au/
https://www.police.wa.gov.au/Your-Safety

Continued

Appendix 8.11   Useful websites continued
New Zealand
http://www.areyouok.org.nz/
http://www.childmatters.org.nz/
http://www.jigsaw.org.nz/seeking-help-with-family-abuse/
http://www.legislation.govt.nz/
http://www.msd.govt.nz/what-we-can-do/families/index.html
http://www.strengtheningfamilies.govt.nz/
http://www.superseniors.msd.govt.nz/elder-abuse/
https://www.ageconcern.org.nz/ACNZPublic/Services/EANP/ACNZ_Public/Elder_Abuse_and_Neglect.aspx
https://www.healthnavigator.org.nz/health-a-z/a/abuse-elder/
https://www.justice.govt.nz/family/
https://www.justice.govt.nz/family/care-of-children/care-and-protection/
https://www.orangatamariki.govt.nz/

Endnotes

1   *Gillick v West Norfolk and Wisbech Area Health Authority* [1986] AC 112 (*Gillick's case*).

2   *Secretary, Department of Health and Community Services v JWB and SMB* (1992) 175 CLR 218 (*Marion's case*).

3   *Paton v Trustees of the British Pregnancy Advisory Service* [1979] QB 276.

4   *Family Law Act 1975* (Cth), s 4.

5   *Vulnerable Children Act 2014* (NZ), s 5.

6   Australian Institute of Family Studies (AIFS). (2017) *Mandatory reporting of child abuse and neglect.* Melbourne: AIFS. Online. Available: https://aifs.gov.au/cfca/publications/mandatory-reporting-child-abuse-and-neglect.

7   Markenson, D., Tunik, M., Cooper, A., et al. (2007) A national assessment of knowledge, attitudes, and confidence of prehospital providers in the assessment and management of child maltreatment. *Pediatrics* 119(1), e103–e108; Mason, R., Schwartz, B., Burgess, R. et al. (2010) Emergency medical services: a resource for victims of domestic violence? *Emergency Medicine Journal* 27(7), 561–564.

8   Raman, S. and Hodes, D. (2012) Cultural issues in child maltreatment. *Journal of Paediatrics and Child Health* 48(1), 30–37.

9   Campo, M. (2015) *Children's Exposure to Domestic and Family Violence: Key Issues and Responses.* CFCA Paper No. 36 2015. Melbourne: Australian Institute of Family Studies. Available: https://aifs.gov.au/cfca/sites/default/files/publication-documents/cfca-36-children-exposure-fdv.pdf; Macintosh, C. (2013) The role of law in ameliorating global inequalities in indigenous peoples' health. *Journal of Law, Medicine and Ethics* 41(1), 74–88.

10 *See Re H (Minors) (Sexual Abuse: Standard of Proof)* [1996] 2 WLR 8, per Lord Nicholls of Birkenhead, at 29.

11 Depending on which state or territory in Australia paramedics work in.

12 Ali, P.A., Dhingra, K. and Mcgarry, J. (2016) A literature review of intimate partner violence and its classifications. *Aggression and Violent Behavior* 31, 16–25.

13 Australian Bureau of Statistics (ABS). (2017) *Key findings. 4906.0—Personal safety, Australia, 2016.* Canberra: ABS. Online. Available: http://www.abs.gov.au/ausstats/abs@.nsf/mf/4906.0.

14 Edlin, A., Williams, B. and Williams, A. (2010) Pre-hospital provider recognition of intimate partner violence. *Journal of Forensic and Legal Medicine* 17(7), 359–362; Naidoo, N., Knight, S.E. and Martin, L.J. (2013) Conspicuous by its absence: domestic violence intervention in South African pre-hospital emergency care: original contributions. *African Safety Promotion* 11(2), 76–92.

15 Sawyer, S., Coles, J., Williams, A. et al. (2015) Preventing and reducing the impacts of intimate partner violence: opportunities for Australian ambulance services. *Emergency Medicine Australasia* 27(4), 307–311; Sawyer, S., Coles, J., Williams, A. et al. (2018) Paramedics as a new resource for women experiencing intimate partner violence. *Journal of Interpersonal Violence*, doi: 10.1177/0886260518769363; Sawyer, S., Parekh, V., Williams, A. et al. (2014) Are Australian paramedics adequately trained and prepared for intimate partner violence? A pilot study. *Journal of Forensic and Legal Medicine* 28, 32–35.

16 Gartland, D., Hemphill, S.A., Hegarty, K. et al. (2011) Intimate partner violence during pregnancy and the first year postpartum in an Australian pregnancy cohort study. *Maternal and Child Health Journal* 15(5), 570–578; Cooper, T.M. (2013) Domestic violence and pregnancy: a literature review. *International Journal of Childbirth Education* 28(3), 30–33.

17 Campo, *Children's Exposure to Domestic and Family Violence*.

18 Bacchus, L., Mezey, G. and Bewley, S. (2006) A qualitative exploration of the nature of domestic violence in pregnancy. *Violence Against Women* 12(6), 588–604.

19 Williams, H., Foster, D.D. and Watts, P. (2013) Perinatal domestic abuse: midwives making a difference through effective public health practice. *British Journal of Midwifery* 21(12), 852–858.

20 Glass, N., Laughon, K., Campbell, J. et al. (2008) Non-fatal strangulation is an important risk factor for homicide of women. *Journal of Emergency Medicine* 35(3), 329–335.

21 Milligan, N. and Anderson, M. (1980) Conjugal disharmony: a hitherto unrecognised cause of strokes. *British Medical Journal* 281(6237), 421–422.

22 Strack, G.B. and Gwinn, C. (2011) On the edge of homicide: strangulation as a prelude. *Criminal Justice* 26(3), 32–36.

23 Douglas, H. and Fitzgerald, R. (2014) Strangulation, domestic violence and the legal response. *Sydney Law Review* 36(2), 231–254.

24 Glass et al., Non-fatal strangulation is an important risk factor for homicide of women.

25 Faugno, D., Waszak, D., Strack, G.B. et al. (2013) Strangulation forensic examination: best practice for health care providers. *Advanced Emergency Nursing Journal* 35(4), 314–327.

26 Clarot, F., Vaz, E., Papin, F. et al. (2005) Fatal and non-fatal bilateral delayed carotid artery dissection after manual strangulation. *Forensic Science International* 149(2–3), 143–150.

27 '[all] … States' Parties shall take all appropriate legislative, administrative, social and educational measures to protect the child from all forms of physical or mental violence, injury or abuse, neglect or negligent treatment, maltreatment or exploitation, including sexual abuse, while in the care of parent(s) … or any other person who has the care of the child.': *United Nations Convention on the Rights of the Child*, art. 19(1).

28 *R v Terry* [1955] VLR 114, at 116.

29 *Crimes Act 1961*, s 59.

30 Caffey, J.I. (1946) Multiple fractures in the long bones of infants suffering from chronic subdural hematoma. In: A.C. Donnelly and K. Oates (eds), *Classic Papers in Child Abuse* (pp. 163–173). Thousand Oakes: Sage Publications.

31 Kempe, H.C., Silverman, F.N., Steele, B.F. et al. (1962) The battered-child syndrome. In: A.C. Donnelly and K. Oates (eds), *Classic Papers in Child Abuse* (pp. 437–439). Thousand Oaks: Sage Publications.

32 Van Haeringen, A.R., Dadds, M. and Armstrong, K.L. (1998) The child abuse lottery—will the doctor suspect and report? Physician attitudes towards and reporting of suspected child abuse and neglect. *Child Abuse and Neglect* 22(3), 159–169.

33 Marinetto, M., 2011. A Lipskian analysis of child protection failures from Victoria Climbié to 'Baby P': a street-level re-evaluation of joined-up governance. *Public Administration* 89(3), 1164–1181.

34 Leventhal, J.M. and Krugman, R.D. (2012). 'The battered-child syndrome' 50 years later. Much accomplished, much left to do. *Journal of the American Medical Association* 308(1), 35–36.

35 Skellern, C. and Donald, T. (2011) Suspicious childhood injury: formulation of forensic opinion. *Journal of Paediatrics and Child Health* 47(11), 771–775.

36 Haselton, M.G. and Nettle, D. (2006) The paranoid optimist: an integrative evolutionary model of cognitive biases. *Personality and Social Psychology Review* 10(1), 47–66.

37 Lazenbatt, A. and Freeman, R. (2006) Recognizing and reporting child physical abuse: a survey of primary healthcare professionals. *Journal of Advanced Nursing* 56(3), 227–236.

38 Johnson, D.D.P., Blumstein, D.T., Fowler, J.H. et al. (2013) The evolution of error: error management, cognitive constraints, and adaptive decision-making biases. *Trends in Ecology and Evolution* 28(8), 474–481.

39 In states and territories where paramedics are captured by the terms 'healthcare professional', 'health practitioner' and 'health service provider', the legislation on voluntarily reporting of suspected child maltreatment has been left blank deliberately in Appendix 8.7.

40 Mathews, B., Bromfield, L., Walsh, K. et al. (2015) *Child Abuse and Neglect: A Socio-legal Study of Mandatory Reporting in Australia. Report for the Tasmanian Department of Health and Human Services.* Brisbane: Queensland University of Technology.

41 Powell, A. and Murray, S. (2008) Children and domestic violence: constructing a policy problem in Australia and New Zealand. *Social and Legal Studies* 17(4), 453–473.

42 Healey, J. (ed.) (2014) *Children and Young People at Risk.* Thirroul, NSW: The Spinney Press.

43 Bidarra, Z.S., Lessard, G. and Dumont, A. (2016) Co-occurrence of intimate partner violence and child sexual abuse: prevalence, risk factors and related issues. *Child Abuse and Neglect* 55, 10–21.

44 Herrenkohl, T.I., Higgins, D.J., Merrick, M.T. et al. (2015) Positioning a public health framework at the intersection of child maltreatment and intimate partner violence: primary prevention requires working outside existing systems. *Child Abuse and Neglect* 48, 22–28.

45 Rufo, R.A. (2011) *Sexual Predators Amongst Us.* Bosa Roca: CRC Press.

46 Weiss, K.J. and Alexander, J.C. (2013) Sex, lies, and statistics: inferences from the child sexual abuse accommodation syndrome. *Journal of the American Academy of Psychiatry and the Law* 41(3), 412–420.

47 Rowland, A., Gerry, F. and Stanton, M. (2017) Physical punishment of children. *International Journal of Children Rights* 25(1), 165–195.

48 Gillespie, A.A. (2011) *Child Pornography: Law and Policy.* Abingdon: Taylor & Francis Group.

49 Lyon, T.D. and Ahern, E.C. (2011) Disclosure of child sexual abuse: implications for interviewing. In: J.E.B. Myers (ed.), *The APSAC Handbook on Child Maltreatment*, 3rd ed. (pp. 233–254). Los Angeles: Sage Publications.

50 Brady, M. (2018) UK paramedics confidence in identifying child sexual abuse: a mixed-methods investigation. *Journal of Child Sexual Abuse* 27(4), 439–458.

51 Stoltenborgh, M., Bakermans-Kranenburg, M.J., Alink, L.R.A. et al. (2015) The prevalence of child maltreatment across the globe: review of a series of meta-analyses. *Child Abuse Review* 24, 37–50.

52 Hibbard, R., Barlow, J. and Macmillan, H. (2012) Psychological maltreatment. *Pediatrics* 130(2), 372–378.

53 Hart, S.N., Brassard, M.R., Davidson, H.A. et al. (2011) Psychological maltreatment. In: J.E.B. Myers (ed.), *The APSAC Handbook on Child Maltreatment*, 3rd ed. (pp. 125–144). Los Angeles: Sage Publications.

54 Glaser, D. (2009) Emotional abuse. In: R. Meadow, J. Mok and D. Rosenberg (eds), *ABC of Child Protection*, 4th ed. (pp. 64–66). Hoboken: John Wiley and Sons.

55 Herrenkohl et al., Positioning a public health framework at the intersection of child maltreatment and intimate partner violence.

56 Edleson, J.L. (1999) Children's witnessing of adult domestic violence. *Journal of Interpersonal Violence* 14(8), 839–870; Edleson, J.L. (1999) The overlap between child maltreatment and woman battering. *Violence Against Women* 5(2), 134–154; Edleson, J.L., Gassman-Pines, J. and Hill, M.B. (2006) Defining child exposure to domestic violence as neglect: Minnesota's difficult experience. *Social Work* 51(2), 167–174; Humphreys, C. and Absler, D., 2011. History repeating: child protection responses to domestic violence. *Child and Family Social Work* 16(4), 464–473; Kimball, E. (2016) Edleson revisited: reviewing children's witnessing of domestic violence 15 years later. *Journal of Family Violence* 31(5), 625–637.

57 Graham-Bermann, S.A., Gruber, G., Howell, K.H. et al. (2009) Factors discriminating among profiles of resilience and psychopathology in children exposed to intimate partner violence (IPV). *Child Abuse and Neglect* 33(9), 648–660.

58 Adams, C.M. (2006) The consequences of witnessing family violence on children and implications for family counselors. *Family Journal* 14(4), 334–341; Bacchus et al., A qualitative exploration of the nature of domestic violence in pregnancy; Campo, *Children's Exposure to Domestic and Family Violence*.

59 Richards, K. (2011) *Children's Exposure to Domestic Violence in Australia. Trends and Issues in Crime and Criminal Justice No. 419.* Canberra: Australian Institute of Criminology. Available: https://aic.gov.au/publications/tandi/tandi419; Rivett, M., Howarth, E. and Harold, G. (2006) 'Watching from the stairs': towards an evidence-based practice in work with child witnesses of domestic violence. *Clinical Child Psychology and Psychiatry* 11(1), 103–125; Sousa, C., Herrenkohl, T.I., Moylan, C.A. et al. (2011) Longitudinal study on the effects of child abuse and children's exposure to domestic violence, parent–child attachments, and antisocial behavior in adolescence. *Journal of Interpersonal Violence* 26(1), 111–136.

60 Australian Bureau of Statistics, Key findings. *4906.0—Personal safety, Australia, 2016.*

61 Finkelhor, D., Ormrod, R.K. and Turner, H.A. (2009) Lifetime assessment of poly-victimization in a national sample of children and youth. *Child Abuse and Neglect* 33(7), 403–411.

62 Radford, L., Corral, S., Bradley, C. et al. (2013) The prevalence and impact of child maltreatment and other types of victimization in the UK: findings from a population survey of caregivers, children and young people and young adults. *Child Abuse and Neglect* 37(10), 801–813.

63 Bidarra et al., Co-occurrence of intimate partner violence and child sexual abuse.

64 Scott, D., Crossin, R., Ogeil, R. et al. (2018) Exploring harms experienced by children aged 7 to 11 using ambulance attendance data: a 6-year comparison with adolescents aged 12–17. *International Journal of Environmental Research and Public Health* 15(7), PMC6068488.

65 Middleton, C. and Hardy, J. (2014) Vulnerability and the 'toxic trio': the role of health visiting. *Community Practitioner* 87(12), 38–39.

66 Holt, A. (2013, 17 September) *Starved boy Daniel Pelka 'invisible' to professionals.* BBC News. Online. Available: http://www.bbc.com/news/uk-england-coventry-warwickshire-24106823.

67 Gonzalez-Izquierdo, A., Ward, A., Smith, P. et al. (2015) Notifications for child safeguarding from an acute hospital in response to presentations to healthcare by parents. *Child: Care, Health and Development* 41(2), 186–193.

68 Sansone, R.A. and Sansone, L.A. (2012) Doctor shopping: a phenomenon of many themes. *Innovations in Clinical Neuroscience* 9(11–12), 42–46.

69   Meadow, R. (2009) Fabricated or induced illness (Munchausen syndrome by proxy). In: R. Meadow, J. Mok and D. Rosenberg (eds), *ABC of Child Protection*, 4th ed. (pp. 67–70). Hoboken: John Wiley and Sons.

70   Laverty, M., McDermott, D.R. and Calma, T. (2017) Embedding cultural safety in Australia's main health care standards. *Medical Journal of Australia* 207(1), 15–16.

71   Nnamuchi, O. (2012) 'Circumcision' or 'mutilation'? Voluntary or forced excision? Extricating the ethical and legal issues in female genital ritual. *Journal of Law and Health* 25, 85–121.

72   Mathews, B. (2013) Legal, cultural and practical developments in responding to female genital mutilation: can an absolute human right emerge? In: R. Maguire, B. Lewis and C. Sampford (eds), *Shifting Global Powers and International Law: Challenges and Opportunities* (Chapter 13, pp. 207–227). London: Routledge.

73   Nyangweso, M. (2014) *Female Genital Cutting in Industrialized Countries: Mutilation or Cultural Tradition?* Westport: ABC-CLIO, LLC.

74   World Health Organization. (2018) *Female genital mutilation*. Online. Available: http://www.who.int/ news-room/fact-sheets/detail/female-genital-mutilation (accessed 3 July 2018).

75   Brady, UK paramedics confidence in identifying child sexual abuse.

76   Horne, R.S.C., Hauck, F.R. and Moon, R.Y. (2015) Sudden infant death syndrome and advice for safe sleeping. *BMJ*, 350.

77   Ibid.

78   Kaspiew, R., Carson, R. and Rhoades, H. (2016) *Elder Abuse: Understanding Issues, Frameworks and Responses. Research Report No. 35*. Melbourne: Australian Institute of Family Studies.

79   Yon, Y., Mikton, C.R., Gassoumis, Z.D. et al. (2017) Elder abuse prevalence in community settings: a systematic review and meta-analysis. *The Lancet Global Health* 5(2), e147–e156.

80   Yon, Y., Ramiro-Gonzales, M., Miktom, C.R. et al. (2019) The prevalence of elder abuse in institutional settings: a systematic review and meta-analysis. *European Journal of Public Health* 29(1), 58–67.

81   World Health Organization. (2018) *Elder abuse: key facts*. Online. Available: http://www.who.int/ news-room/fact-sheets/detail/elder-abuse (accessed 4 July 2018).

82   Rosen, T., Lien, C., Stern, M.E. et al. (2017) Emergency medical services perspectives on identifying and reporting victims of elder abuse, neglect, and self-neglect. *Journal of Emergency Medicine* 53(4), 573–582.

83   Australian Institute of Health and Welfare (AIHW). (2017) *Deaths in Australia. Cat. No. PHE 229*. Canberra: AIHW. Online. Available: https://www.aihw.gov.au/reports/life-expectancy-death/ deaths-in-australia/contents/trends-in-deaths (accessed 4 July 2018.).

84   For a definitive understanding of the legislation, please refer to the complete and up-to-date Acts.

Chapter 9
Mental illness and the law in the pre-hospital emergency care setting

Ramon Shaban and Ruth Townsend

Learning objectives

After reading this chapter, you will be able to:

- define 'mental illness'
- distinguish mental health emergencies from mental illness
- describe the contemporary ethical and legal challenges with respect to mental illness
- describe the relevant legislative obligations and professional frameworks that apply to paramedic practice and the care provided to the mentally ill.

Definitions

Mental health emergency A circumstance in which an individual's mental illness presents an immediate danger to the individual or others, often characterised by delusions, hallucinations, and/or serious disorders of the thought, mood, perception or memory.

Mental illness A clinically significant disturbance of thought, mood, perception or memory.

An introductory case

Acting strangly

You are dispatched to attend a male patient, Azim, who called for help, but is reported to be acting 'strange'. When you question Azim, he asks you and your partner in a whisper to step outside the house. He says he lives with his parents and he doesn't want to worry them. He keeps looking over his shoulder anxiously. He appears distracted and jumpy. It becomes apparent that he is unable to give you a coherent account of the past few days; the facts change often, and he can't remember what he has said previously. He says he has not slept for 'a couple of days', because 'I think he's going to

Continued

> ## An introductory case continued
>
> kill me.' He says that he has not been using any drugs, but you can see recent track marks on his arms, which would seem to contradict this. Azim also avoids answering any direct questions about suicidal ideation, saying only that his suicidal thoughts are 'no more than usual', and the only reason he called an ambulance was because he thought he was having a heart attack after feeling his 'heart beating through my chest'. After a few more minutes of questioning, Azim suddenly becomes quite verbally aggressive, and violently throws his cigarette lighter on the ground, shouting, 'They're going to kill me! If you're not going to help me, then you can just $*&% off!' Azim then storms back into his house.

Introduction

Paramedic and emergency department (ED) staff will encounter patients with mental health issues on a regular basis. Each state and territory in Australia has its own legislation with respect to the care and treatment of the mentally ill. The overall purpose of the law is to ensure that a mentally ill person will receive the best possible care and treatment in the least restrictive environment. This includes limiting any restriction or interference with their civil liberties, rights, dignity and self-respect to the minimum necessary to effectively provide care and treatment.

This chapter will set out the legal and ethical issues most commonly experienced in pre-hospital mental healthcare. It is by no means exhaustive, and readers are advised to supplement this chapter with a reading of the laws of the state or territory in which they practise. In general, the Mental Health Acts are jurisdictionally specific and prescriptive, and contain a lot of detail about what can and should be done to lawfully care for people who come under the protection of the Act. This chapter will provide you with the means to examine and determine important legal and ethical aspects of cases such as the one above, in the context of paramedic practice within Australia and New Zealand.

What is 'mental illness'?

Mental illness is a very broad term that incorporates a wide variety of conditions and disorders that vary in nature and severity. It is nonetheless a well-recognised global health problem.[1] Defined as a clinically significant disturbance of thought, mood, perception or memory,[2] mental illness is a significant cause of morbidity and comorbidity, and has a profound influence on the social determinants of individuals' and communities' health globally. In the contemporary setting, what constitutes mental illness within an individual depends on many factors that are contextual.[3] A small percentage (3%) of the total population lives with a serious psychiatric disorder at any one point in time.[4-8] Serious psychiatric disorders, such as schizophrenia, are characterised generally as a disturbance of thought, mood, perception or memory where the individual demonstrates a loss of connection with reality.

On average, 1 in 4 people experience mental illness worldwide, amounting to more than 450 million people with mental, neurological or behavioural problems at any one time.[9] Recent data suggests that the global burden of mental illness accounts for 32·4% of years lived with disability (YLDs) and 13.0% of disability-adjusted life-years (DALYs),[10] eclipsing many other diseases, such as cancer, heart disease, acquired immune deficiency syndrome (AIDS), tuberculosis and malaria combined.[11,12] At least 850,000 people die by suicide every year around the world.[13]

In Australia, mental illness is a national health priority.[14] Providing appropriate mental health services is at the forefront of the needs of Australians.[15,16] Approximately 1 in 5 Australians suffer from a mental illness, and 3% of the total population live with a serious psychiatric disorder at any one point in time,[17] and nationally carry the greatest burden of disability and illness than any other health problem.[18] The antecedents of mental illness are multidimensional.[19] People with mental illness are systematically subjected to social isolation, have a poor quality of life, and have increased mortality, all of which have staggering economic and social consequences.[20] Many cases of mental illness go unreported or unmanaged, or are concealed for a variety of social, political and economic reasons.[21]

In Western countries, mental illnesses are diagnosed according to a classification system outlined in the *Diagnostic and Statistical Manual of Mental Disorders, Fifth Edition Text Revision (DSM-V-TR)*[22] and the *International Classification of Diseases Tenth Revisions (ICD-10)*.[23] The DSM-V-TR provides a classification system for all mental health disorders in both children and adults, where the assessment of the mental illness occurs across five different axes. It provides key diagnostic criteria and other information, such as epidemiological data, guidelines for management, and key research findings.[24] Mental illness presents in many different forms and types, as listed in Table 9.1.

History of mental health and mental health law

Mentally ill or disordered patients are particularly vulnerable to abuse, and historically they have been abused. In the past they have had limitations placed on their rights, because society has wrongly believed that people with a mental illness were not capable of making decisions for themselves, and so a paternalistic approach to managing these patients has been taken instead. While this has been done with good intentions, the intention is, in and of itself, not enough to justify the limitation of a patient's rights to make decisions for themselves where they have the capacity to do so. There have also been examples where society, and the individuals responsible for the care of these vulnerable people, have not acted with good intentions, or have acted out of fear or ignorance or prejudice, and in so doing have harmed these patients.

Mental illnesses may can be acute and chronic, mild or significantly debilitating. They may also co-exist, where individuals experience more than one particular mental illness or they experience comorbid medical conditions that are a result of, or exacerbate, their mental illness. The diagnosis of mental illness has been a highly controversial practice for thousands of years. Historically, mental illness was associated with evil, criminality, and failures of religious faith and spiritualty. Within many cultures around the world, mental illness has been, and is, considered a consequential form of divine retribution for the individual's behaviour, which was considered to be socially unacceptable at the time.

Table 9.1 General classifications of mental illness

- Disorders usually first diagnosed in infancy, childhood or adolescence
- Delirium, dementia, and amnestic and other cognitive disorders
- Mental disorders due to a general medical condition
- Substance-related disorders
- Schizophrenia and other psychotic disorders
- Mood disorders
- Anxiety disorders
- Somatoform disorders
- Factitious disorders
- Dissociative disorders
- Sexual and gender identity disorders
- Eating disorders
- Sleep disorders
- Impulse-control disorders not elsewhere classified
- Adjustment disorders
- Personality disorders

Regulatory frameworks governing the management of those with mental illness were typically pejorative in their language and operation. Individuals where imprisoned in 'lunatic asylums' for 'mental hygiene'.

In some countries and cultures, there have been extensive revisions in what constitutes mental illness within psychiatry and other behavioural sciences. The revisions have been accompanied by reforms in policy, practice and law. Within Western countries, recent reforms have been influenced by the assertion of human rights for people with mental illness. The legislative response in some countries has reinforced the protection of individuals, attempted to shift public perceptions about mental illness, and emphasised governmental responsibility for vulnerable people.[25] For example, governments rewrote legislation and policy relating to people experiencing mental illness to reflect international conventions established by the United Nations, such as the *United Nations Principles for the Protection of Persons with Mental Illness and for the Improvement of Mental Health Care.*[26] At the centre of these reforms was the protection of vulnerable individuals. Despite this progress, many governments, medical authorities and cultures continue to deem various social behaviours to be mental illnesses. In some countries, people with mental illness are incarcerated with little or no treatment or intervention, violating their basic human rights.

The ethical challenges associated with providing quality mental healthcare are related in part to historical policies and the consequence of reforms in mental healthcare. These policies and systems, and the problems associated therein, are well-documented.[27,28–32] In Australia, the launch of the *National Mental Health Policy* by the Australian Health Ministers in 1992 provided the stimulus for significant changes to psychiatric services within the Australian health care system.[33–35] Decriminalisation of mental illness and the mainstreaming of services, whereby mental healthcare services shifted from specialist institutions to generalist health services in community settings, were the central features of these reforms. The policy of decentralisation of mental health services was central to the reform of mental healthcare in Australia and New Zealand in the 1990s. It was hoped that these reforms would address the longstanding problems associated with traditional psychiatric care service delivery.[36]

However, the outcomes of these reforms attracted criticism and have been the subject of scrutiny within the contemporary agenda for quality and safety of mental healthcare.[37,38] In Australia, multiple commissions of inquiry have investigated government and non-government institutions, and have identified serious and systematic failures of mental healthcare systems. These include the *Commission of Inquiry into the Care and Treatment of Patients in the Psychiatric Unit of the Townsville General Hospital,*[39] the *National Inquiry into the Human Rights of People with Mental Illness [Burdekin Report],*[40] and the *Report of an Inquiry Conducted by The Honourable D G Steward into Allegations of Official Misconduct at the Basil Stafford Centre [Stewart Report].*[41] Inquiries conducted in New Zealand, namely the *Royal Commission on Hospital and Related Services (1972–3)* and the *Ministerial Inquiry in respect of Certain Mental Health Services (1995–6),* arrived at similar findings.[42] The *Palmer Report*[43] uncovered systematic failures of Queensland and Commonwealth government departments when an Australian citizen, Ms Cornelia Rau, was unlawfully detained and imprisoned without adequate medical help or treatment for 10 months while experiencing acute schizophrenia. All inquiries document systemic neglect, abuse, and failure to provide safe and quality mental healthcare.

Historically, the reports *Not for Service: Experiences of Injustice and Despair in Mental Health Care in Australia* and *'Out of Hospital, Out of Mind!' A Report Detailing Mental Health Services in Australia in 2002 and Community Priorities for National Health Policy 2003–2008* table systematic failures in mental health service provision. In discussing the implementation of mental health reform in the context of community mental health service delivery, Hickie[44] asserts reports such as these reflect disorganised and dislocated health and welfare systems, and a lack of commitment to the provision of quality mental healthcare, particularly in the public sector. Moreover, Hickie argues that when any of us seeks mental healthcare we run the serious risk that our basic needs will be ignored, trivialised or neglected. Statements such as these, and others reported in the findings of the before-mentioned commissions of inquiry, document the poor quality of mental healthcare provided across Australia and New Zealand.

The multidisciplinary, community-centred and cross-jurisdictional yet fragmented nature of mental health services in Australia and New Zealand gives rise to many ethical and practical challenges for health professionals. Contributing to this has been the lack of recognition of the extent of the problem; poor diagnostics, clinician judgement and decision-making; inadequate health professional education and training; poor institutional administration and accountability; and the failure of institutions at the local, state and national level to support community-based systems of mental healthcare.[45] Barriers to providing effective mental healthcare and the treatment and management of mental illness are complex, but include a fundamental lack of recognition of the seriousness of the problem, and both its chronic and global consequences.[46]

Legislative reform for contemporary mental healthcare

Multiple reports and inquiries into the abusive care that many people have received, combined with a growing understanding of mental health, and its care and treatment, have led to changes in care and treatment and in the guiding principles that govern the management of these patients. The essence of these principles, and reflection of the flawed history of the way in which we have treated mental health patients, have been codified in law. The guiding principles of the legislation are captured well in New South Wales' *Mental Health Act 2007*. The objects of the Act (s 3) are clearly set out, and paramedics should note these and seek to work to achieve these objectives.

(a) to provide for the care and treatment and to promote the recovery of, persons who are mentally ill or mentally disordered, and

(b) to facilitate the care and treatment of those persons through community care facilities, and

(c) to facilitate the provision of hospital care for those persons on a voluntary basis where appropriate and, in a limited number of situations, on an involuntary basis, and

(d) while protecting the civil rights of those persons, to give an opportunity for those persons to have access to appropriate care and, where necessary, to provide for treatment for their own protection or the protection of others, and

(e) to facilitate the involvement of those persons, and persons caring for them, in decisions involving appropriate care and treatment.

The objects reflect the guiding principles that mental healthcare is about upholding the rights of the individual to ensure that they are involved in decision-making regarding their care and treatment, that they have get access to care, that that care be provided in the least restrictive environment possible to maintain the wellbeing of the patient and others, and that persons who fall under the provisions of the law are provided access to treatment to prevent harm to themselves or others.

The Victorian *Mental Health Act 2014* states that a person is not considered to have mental illness by reason only of any one or more of the specific conditions or states that historically were used erroneously in the past. Consideration of the elements of this list 'does not prevent the serious temporary or permanent physiological, biochemical or psychological effects of using drugs or consuming alcohol from being regarded as an indication that a person has mental illness' (Pt 1, s 4). What is not, on its own, to be considered a mental illness is that:

(a) that the person expresses or refuses or fails to express a particular political opinion or belief;

(b) that the person expresses or refuses or fails to express a particular religious opinion or belief;

(c) that the person expresses or refuses or fails to express a particular philosophy;

(d) that the person expresses or refuses or fails to express a particular sexual preference, gender identity or sexual orientation;

(e) that the person engages in or refuses or fails to engage in a particular political activity;

(f) that the person engages in or refuses or fails to engage in a particular religious activity;

(g) that the person engages in sexual promiscuity;

(h) that the person engages in immoral conduct;

(i) that the person engages in illegal conduct;

(j) that the person engages in antisocial behaviour;

(k) that the person is intellectually disabled;

(l) that the person uses drugs or consumes alcohol;

(m) that the person has a particular economic or social status or is a member of a particular cultural or racial group;

(n) that the person is or has previously been involved in family conflict;

(o) that the person has previously been treated for mental illness. (Pt 1, s 4).

New South Wales has a similar list (s 16), which reflects the broader national view that definitions and understandings of what constitutes mental illness have moved on and are more standardised than they may have been in the past.

Moreover, principles are established by which people with a mental illness or disorder should, as far as practicable, be provided with the best possible care and treatment in the least restrictive environment that enables the effective provision of that care and treatment (*Mental Health Act 2007* (NSW), s 68(a)). Other guiding principles include:

(b) people with a mental illness or mental disorder should be provided with timely and high quality treatment and care in accordance with professionally accepted standards,

(c) the provision of care and treatment should be designed to assist people with a mental illness or mental disorder, wherever possible, to live, work and participate in the community,

(d) the prescription of medicine to a person with a mental illness or mental disorder should meet the health needs of the person and should be given only for therapeutic or diagnostic needs and not as a punishment or for the convenience of others,

(e) people with a mental illness or mental disorder should be provided with appropriate information about treatment, treatment alternatives and the effects of treatment and be supported to pursue their own recovery,

(f) any restriction on the liberty of patients and other people with a mental illness or mental disorder and any interference with their rights, dignity and self-respect is to be kept to the minimum necessary in the circumstances,

(g) any special needs of people with a mental illness or mental disorder should be recognised, including needs related to age, gender, religion, culture, language, disability or sexuality,

(g1) people under the age of 18 years with a mental illness or mental disorder should receive developmentally appropriate services,

(g2) the cultural and spiritual beliefs and practices of people with a mental illness or mental disorder who are Aboriginal persons or Torres Strait Islanders should be recognised,

(h) every effort that is reasonably practicable should be made to involve persons with a mental illness or mental disorder in the development of treatment plans and recovery plans and to consider their views and expressed wishes in that development, (h1) every effort that is reasonably practicable should be made to obtain the consent of people with a mental illness or mental disorder when developing treatment plans and recovery plans for their care, to monitor their capacity to consent and to support people who lack that capacity to understand treatment plans and recovery plans,

(i) people with a mental illness or mental disorder should be informed of their legal rights and other entitlements under this Act and all reasonable efforts should be made to ensure the information is given in the language, mode of communication or terms that they are most likely to understand,

(j) the role of carers for people with a mental illness or mental disorder and their rights under this Act to be kept informed, to be involved and to have information provided by them considered, should be given effect. (*Mental Health Act 2007* (NSW), s 68)

Such provisions are fundamental to the human rights and dignity of individuals experiencing mental illness, and feature prominently and systematically in Mental Health Acts across Australia and New Zealand.

Mental health and the law in Australia and New Zealand

Mental health law is a special area of law and sits in what is called the *protective jurisdiction*, alongside other areas of law that protect vulnerable people; for example, child protection and guardianship laws. As such, you will find that the overriding principles of the law make specific reference to the need to uphold the guiding principles of the legislation which protect the vulnerable patient from harm. The key principles of the protective jurisdiction are that the human rights apply to all people, regardless of their ability to advocate for themselves. The protective jurisdiction of the law recognises that there are people within particular groups who may sometimes be unable to advocate for themselves—children and the mentally ill or disordered—and that there is therefore a need to have provisions within the law that allows someone else to act as if they were the person in that person's stead and in that person's best interest. This affords the person human worth and dignity.

In Australia and New Zealand, mental health services are provided within multidisciplinary, cross-jurisdictional arrangements. Under the Australian Constitution, states and territories are principally responsible for the delivery of health services to its citizens.[47] While the Australian federal government has no specific constitutional responsibility for health under section 51 of the Australian Constitution, it does have reserved power for responsibilities not stated in the Australian Constitution of 1901 via a doctrine of implied powers. States and territories may agree to refer constitutional authority up to the Commonwealth for matters that are the constitutional responsibility of the states/territories, such as the regulation of health professionals. Therefore, in some areas such as health, there is an overlap of federal and state/territory responsibility and authority. As New Zealand is a single entity, the New Zealand Parliament has the power to make laws on all matters under section 15 of the *Constitution Act 1986*.

Mental health is one area, however, where the responsibility and authority between the Commonwealth and each of the states and territories are sharply demarcated. In each Australian state and territory, Acts of Parliament govern and regulate the care provided to those experiencing mental illness. Mental health in Australia has been developed at a

Table 9.2 Relevant mental health legislation	
Jurisdiction	**Legislation**
Australian Capital Territory	*Mental Health (Treatment and Care) Act 1994* (ACT)
New South Wales	*Mental Health Act 2007* (NSW)
Northern Territory	*Mental and Related Services Act 2009* (NT)
Queensland	*Mental Health Act 2016* (Qld)
South Australia	*Mental Health Act 2009* (SA)
Tasmania	*Mental Health Act 2013* (Tas)
Victoria	*Mental Health Act 2014* (Vic)
Western Australia	*Mental Health Act 1996* (WA)
New Zealand	*Mental Health (Compulsory Assessment and Treatment) Act 1992*

state/territory level. That means that each state and territory has its own laws with respect to the management of mental healthcare and treatment. There are many similarities between the various jurisdictions, but it is advisable that you familiarise yourself with the particular law that applies in your state or territory to ensure that you comply with any state-specific particularities. The laws that apply in each state and territory are listed below. It is simple to search for them online. Mental health laws are prescriptive, which means that they set out in detail, step-by-step, what is required to be done to comply with the law. The relevant Acts across Australia and New Zealand are summarised in Table 9.2.

There are a variety of legal definitions for 'mental illness'. In New South Wales, the definition is:

> **mental illness** means a condition that seriously impairs, either temporarily or permanently, the mental functioning of a person and is characterised by the presence in the person of any one or more of the following symptoms:
> (a) delusions,
> (b) hallucinations,
> (c) serious disorder of thought form,
> (d) a severe disturbance of mood,
> (e) sustained or repeated irrational behaviour indicating the presence of any one or more of the symptoms referred to in paragraphs (a)–(d). (s 4, 'mental illness')

New South Wales also differentiates mental illness from mentally disordered. It defines a 'mentally disordered person' as:

> A person (whether or not the person is suffering from mental illness) is a mentally disordered person if the person's behaviour for the time being is so irrational as to justify a conclusion on reasonable grounds that temporary care, treatment or control of the person is necessary:
> (a) for the person's own protection from serious physical harm, or
> (b) for the protection of others from serious physical harm. (s 15)

This piece of law provides an opportunity for a patient who is experiencing an acute episode of illness that may risk the safety of themselves or others to be treated under the provisions of the Act without necessarily having to be diagnosed with a mental illness first, or indeed at all. In Victoria, 'mental illness' is defined as a 'medical condition that is characterised by a significant disturbance of thought, mood, perception or memory'. This is similar to Tasmania's definition, which is: 'For the purposes of this Act a person has a mental illness if the person suffers from a disturbance of thought, mood, volition, perception, orientation or memory that impairs judgment or behaviour to a significant extent' (*Mental Health Act 1996* (Tas), s 4(1)). The Northern Territory puts elements of both New South Wales and Tasmania's definition together. It says:

(1) A **mental illness** is a condition that seriously impairs, either temporarily or permanently, the mental functioning of a person in one or more of the areas of thought, mood, volition, perception, orientation or memory and is characterised:

(a) by the presence of at least one of the following symptoms:

(i) delusions;

(ii) hallucinations;

(iii) serious disorders of the stream of thought;

(iv) serious disorders of thought form;

(v) serious disturbances of mood; or

(b) by sustained or repeated irrational behaviour that may be taken to indicate the presence of at least one of the symptoms referred to in paragraph (a). (*Mental Health and Related Services Act 1998* (NT), s 6)

These and other Mental Health Acts in Australia are drafted to comply with the *National Standards for Mental Health Services*,[48] the *United Nations Principles for the Protection of Persons with Mental Illness and for the Improvement of Mental Health Care*, and a model for mental health legislation agreed to by all Australian and New Zealand jurisdictions. Similar to mental health legislation in other Commonwealth countries—such as the United Kingdom—the Acts described in Table 9.2 are intended to reflect contemporary national and international trends in mental healthcare and broad community expectations.

The Mental Health Acts of Australia and New Zealand provide for the involuntary assessment and treatment, and the protection, of persons (whether adults or minors) who have mental illnesses, while at the same time safeguarding their rights.[49] Importantly, people may opt to seek assessment and treatment voluntarily.[50] The voluntary admission of individuals for mental healthcare is not regulated formally by Acts of Parliament, but is covered by legislation relating to the function of health organisations and by common law. However, if a voluntary patient withdraws consent, the person may be admitted involuntarily if they meet the legislative criteria. An important aim of the Acts is to reduce the stigma associated with mental illness and to protect the rights of patients. Paramedics and other health professionals must be mindful of the prevailing legislative frameworks for the jurisdiction within which they work, particularly if they work across jurisdictions.

The context of paramedic practice and mental illness: roles, models and obligations

Paramedics encounter patients experiencing the broad spectrum of mental illness in pre-hospital emergency care.[51] They and other emergency service workers are also called upon to respond to and manage mental health emergencies in which an individual's mental illness presents an immediate danger to the individual or to others, often characterised by delusions, hallucinations and/or serious disorders of the thought, mood or memory. The popular culture that represents ambulance paramedics in the media, particularly more recently on television, is one of heroism,[52] routinely responding to life-and-death situations seemingly with ease.[53] However, research suggests that the majority of the patients paramedics encounter are not experiencing mental health emergencies.[54] Rather, the vast majority of paramedic work with respect to mental illness relates to patients who experience non-life-threatening conditions or disorders that are chronic and debilitating; typically, anxiety and depression. Notwithstanding, paramedics have specific obligations, skills and expertise when it comes to managing individuals with mental illness and mental health emergencies.[55,56–61]

The decentralisation of mental health services that was key to the reform of mental healthcare in Australia in the 1990s resulted in increased attendance by patients with mental health problems at emergency departments and to emergency medical services. This increase in presentations of general mental illness and mental health emergencies is well documented in Australia[62–72] and around the world.[73–75] This body of research provides considerable evidence that emergency personnel encounter patients experiencing mental health problems more frequently than before. The increasing contact emergency healthcare workers have with mental health patients has had consequences for their professional practice. Moreover, many studies of problem-solving in mental health[76–84] illustrate the complexity and difficulty faced by health professionals, such as physicians, nurses and social workers, and non-health professionals, such as police officers. Other research has documented the lack of education and training in mental illness across these health and non-health professions.[85–87] Paramedic participation in the wider mental healthcare system has been asserted in the published literature.[88–90] In some countries, such as India, paramedics are taking on new mental health counselling roles in the pre-hospital emergency care setting.[91]

The way in which paramedics manage individuals in the pre-hospital emergency care setting is prescribed by key regulatory documents, described in Table 9.2. Ambulance-specific Acts establish ambulance services, and provide paramedics with broad and far-reaching powers to protect individuals from real or potential harm or injury, which may include, but are not limited to, basic and advanced life-support procedures.

In the contemporary setting, paramedics are expected to be *protectors* and *transporters,* the origins of which are steeped in military traditions and acts of Good Samaritans.[92] From their earliest beginnings, as early as the religious crusades of the 11th century, paramedics have been expected to protect individuals from harm. This practice continued for centuries, when in the 1700s it was adapted for use in formal military conflict. In a bid to reduce the high rates of morbidity and mortality during battle, Napoleon's

Surgeon General Baron Dominique Jean Larrey introduced *stretcher-bearers* into Napoleon's armies—individuals who would retrieve injured soldiers from the battlefield and ferry them on foot to makeshift field hospitals. Their role was to protect the injured soldiers by retrieving them from the frontline and transporting them to makeshift field hospitals for definitive medical care. Their key role was *protection* by retrieval and *transport*, as it is now.[93] This emphasis on protection and transportation is illustrated by the framing of paramedic practice and ambulance services, in that they are considered an emergency service rather than a health service, largely due to the professional self-regulation.[94]

An important feature of protocols and case management guidelines in ambulance services is the expectation that paramedics' clinical judgement and decision-making of mental illness places on the transportation of patients. Paramedic practice is commonly guided by protocols and case management guidelines.[95] Bendall and Morrison report that all Australian ambulance services operate using either protocols or clinical practice guidelines, or a combination of both.[96] These guidelines typically consist of case entry script, providing information regarding diagnostic patterns and guiding principles, and a decision-tree or algorithm. Decision-trees and algorithms are intended to guide paramedics in their practice in the field. Generally speaking, decision-trees are normative and prescriptive instruments for clinical judgement and decision-making.[97] That is, they describe how the judgements and decisions should be made, and they assist in this process. Decision-trees work by breaking down problems into smaller decisions and choices, and include a comprehensive risk analysis to identify all possible risks, which are assigned a relative weight based on their probability of occurrence.[98] The decisions alluded to within the tree are based on the predictability of events using probability and statistical occurrence. Once each choice has been assigned a probability—assuming this is possible—the option with the highest utility for the decision-maker can be calculated.[99] Such models attempt to quantify the probability of the most likely and most desirable event in an attempt to assist the individual or group in making the judgement or decision.

When it comes to decision-making, the literature describes that paramedics adopt a model referred to as the *systematic approach*, a model of problem-solving whereby the assessment and analysis of data will arrive at a summary of the patient and their problems.[100] The model calls on paramedics to use a mix of knowledge, skill, experience, attitudes and intuition when managing patients. The approach has a singular aim: providing the 'best possible outcome'. However, recent research has revealed that while paramedic clinical judgement and decision-making of mental illness does follow a form of systematic approach, it is not a simple technicist activity.[101] Rather, it is a highly individualised, complex and sophisticated component of paramedic practice. Research by Shaban has revealed that conceptually, paramedic clinical judgement and decision-making of mental illness is comprised of contextual, practice and mediating elements.[102]

Fundamental to judgement practice was the *contextual element*, an amalgam of organisational and occupational factors associated with various historical, cultural, educational, political and regulatory dimensions of the Queensland pre-hospital emergency-care setting. The contextual element established the framework for the formal roles of paramedics within a hierarchy of medical treatment.

The *practice element* consisted of field actions for problem-solving and a range of individual-specific factors. The paramedics' field actions consisted of an individualised, enacted systematic approach that articulated their expectations of the protection and transportation of the patient. Actions included gathering and assessing data, describing the problem in objective detail, assessing the nature and severity of the problem, making a provisional diagnosis, and implementing actions to achieve the best possible outcome.

Coupled with field actions were *individual factors*; namely, knowledge, experience, interpersonal skills and personal traits. These individual factors augmented the paramedics' field actions for problem-solving and employing the systematic approach in differing measure, according to the individual jobs and patients they encountered.

The *mediating element* was comprised of paramedics' interactions within the scene, with the patient, and with individuals in authority. These interactions influenced the success of their clinical judgement and decision-making; in particular, their interactions with the patient, physicians, relatives, bystanders and other individuals in authority. The roles paramedics ascribed to those individuals were integral to their actual judgement practice.

Moreover, the study by Shaban[103] illustrated how paramedics' responses to the many competing priorities and demands influenced their clinical judgement and decision-making, meaning that they were not wholly governed by the formal regulatory expectations of practice that had otherwise contextualised their practice.

In 2018, Australia joined the small, yet ever-increasing pool of countries with national regulation for paramedicine.[104] In May 2018 the newly constituted Paramedicine Board of Australia and the Australian Health Practitioner Registration Authority established registration and other standards for paramedics as registered health professionals.[105] This brings with it particular obligations for paramedics with respect to their role and powers under mental health legislation.

Paramedics and mental health legislation roles and powers

Paramedics are referenced widely in Mental Health Acts in Australia. In New South Wales, paramedics are still referred to in the Act as 'ambulance officers'. 'Ambulance officer' means a member of staff of the NSW Health Service who is authorised by the Secretary to exercise the functions of an ambulance officer under the Act. It is likely that this term will be amended to 'paramedic' at some later time. Until it is amended, there is a potential for the term 'ambulance officer' to extend to any other ambulance employee of New South Wales who may be referred to as an 'ambulance officer'.

The powers of an 'ambulance officer' under the *Mental Health Act 2007* in New South Wales include the transporting of a patient to a declared mental health facility on an involuntary basis:

if the officer believes on reasonable grounds that the person appears to be mentally ill or mentally disturbed and that it would be beneficial to the person's welfare to be dealt with in accordance with this Act. (s 20)

This power is also found in Mental Health Acts in the Northern Territory (s 31), South Australia (s 56; where a paramedic is referred to as 'an authorised officer'), Tasmania (s 212) and the ACT (s 80). This piece of law places a great deal of power in the hands of paramedics, as it authorises them to detain and transport someone against their will. An individual's liberty is as prized by many as their life, so having the power to remove an individual's freedom should be taken very seriously. Remember, these patients have not broken any laws. They are not like criminals who have been tried, convicted and sentenced to jail and thus have lost their liberty as a price for committing crime. Mental health patients are the only other members of our adult society who have legal limits placed on their freedom.

Paramedics have to use a two-stage test to exercise this power. They should be sure that they have 'reasonable grounds' for making the decision. 'Reasonable grounds' requires more conviction from the paramedic than mere suspicion or 'gut instinct', but less evidence than conclusive proof (*George v Rockett* (1990) 70 CLR 104)[106] that (1) the person 'appears to be mentally ill or mentally disturbed', and (2) that it would be 'beneficial to the person's welfare to be dealt with in accordance with this Act'. This assessment is essentially subjective, but it is recommended that paramedics make this assessment in accordance with their clinical guidelines and provide supportive evidence for their assessment. In other words, this determination should not be made purely on the basis of a 'gut instinct'.

It should also be noted that the Act itself reminds paramedics of the criteria for assessing whether a patient should be transported to a mental health facility on an involuntary basis; that is, the patient has not asked to be transported. The criteria include an assessment that the patient is in fact mentally ill or mentally disordered, as defined in the Act (see above), and:

> (2) In considering whether a person is a <u>mentally ill person</u>, the continuing condition of the person, including any likely deterioration in the person's condition and the likely effects of any such deterioration, are to be taken into account. (*Mental Health Act 2007* (NSW), s 14(2))

In making this determination, paramedics can gather information:

> … personally/by audio visual link examining or observing the person, account may be taken of other matters not so ascertained where those matters:
>
> (a) arise from a previous examination of the person, or
>
> (b) are communicated by a reasonably credible informant. (*Mental Health Act 2007* (NSW), Sch 1, Note 2)

There is a further power that allows ambulance officers to request police assistance 'if they are of the opinion' that there are serious concerns about the safety of the person or other persons if they were to take the person to a mental health facility without the help of a police officer (*Mental Health Act 2007* (NSW), s 20(2)). This provision is designed to allow paramedics to seek police help when necessary, but places the decision in the hands of health professionals rather than law enforcement.

In terms of the force that may be used to exercise the powers set out in the Act, it is noted at section 81(2) that a person authorised under the Act to take a person to a mental health facility (which therefore includes paramedics as noted above), may:

(a) use reasonable force in exercising functions under this section or any other provision of this Act applying this section, and

(b) restrain the person in any way that is reasonably necessary in the circumstances.

Restraint does extend to sedation, but again this should be considered in conjunction with the paramedic's clinical guidelines. In South Australia, a paramedic may administer a drug for restraining only if they are authorised to do so under the *Controlled Substances Act 1984* (*Mental Health Act 2009* (SA), s 56(6)). The law stipulates that 'the person may be sedated … for the purpose of being taken to or from a mental health facility or other health facility under this Act if it is necessary to do so to enable the person to be taken safely to or from the facility'(*Mental Health Act 2007* (NSW) Ch 4, Pt 1). There are similar laws authorising restraint, apprehension, search and transportation in most other jurisdictions.

'Reasonable force' means force that is proportionate to the exercise of the function. It does not mean excessive force, but nor does it mean no force. In the ACT law, the limit of force that can be sued is the 'minimum amount of force necessary to apprehend the person and remove them to a mental health facility' (*Mental Health Act 2015* (ACT), s 263). This way of thinking about the force that can be used may be more useful and safer for paramedics than the term 'reasonable force'.

It should be noted that this provision of the law provides paramedics with even more power to limit a person's liberty, but authorises them to 'restrain' a person 'in any way' that is 'reasonably necessary'. Again, the key for paramedics here in terms of working inside the law is to refer to professional clinical guidelines, and exercise professional judgement about the most legal and ethical way to exercise the powers that paramedics are given to work in the best interests of the patient. The principles of the law must be kept in mind: that the patient is to be treated in the least restrictive way possible to provide them with the care and treatment they need.

A further power that the *Mental Health Act* authorises for paramedics is the power to carry out a frisk search. A 'frisk search' means:

(a) a search of a person conducted by quickly running the hands over the person's outer clothing or by passing an electronic metal detection device over or in close proximity to the person's outer clothing, or

(b) an examination of anything worn or carried by the person that is conveniently and voluntarily removed by the person, including an examination conducted by passing an electronic metal detection device over or in close proximity to that thing. (*Mental Health Act 2007* (NSW), s 81(6))

Again, this places an enormous degree of power in the hands of paramedics that can be used, and potentially abused, against vulnerable patients. The appropriate exercise of these powers requires paramedics to act at all times with the utmost professionalism. At law, an individual has a right to bodily inviolability; that is, the individual controls who can touch them, when and how. Any unauthorised touching of an individual can amount to an assault. An example of authorised touching includes when the person gives consent to be touched, but there are also examples where the person does not give consent; for example, when a person is arrested.

Paramedics are among the most trusted professionals in our society, and it is essential that paramedics maintain that trust in order for them to do their job. Paramedics are frequently required to act in the best interest of vulnerable patients, commonly when the patient is unable to give, or refuses, consent to touch. The treatment of mental health patients is a further example of the role of the paramedic to act by placing the patient's interests first and to protect the trustworthy position they have been given. The powers given to paramedics to conduct frisk searches is an example of power given to someone other than the individual to infringe on that individual's right to bodily inviolability. This responsibility should be taken extremely seriously.

This responsibility can be a concern among paramedics when they are dealing with suicidal patients. The law is clear that a person who expresses suicidal thoughts or ideation is not necessarily mentally ill (*Stuart v Kirkland-Veenstra* [2009] HCA 15; (2009) 237 CLR 215), so the expression of suicidal thoughts is not enough on its own for a paramedic to transport a patient to hospital to protect them from themselves. In order for the paramedic to be authorised under the ACT law to apprehend and transport a person involuntarily to a mental health facility, the paramedic must have formed a 'reasonable' belief that the person has a mental disorder or mental illness *and* the person has attempted or is likely to attempt suicide (*Mental Health Act 2015* (ACT), s 80(1)(a), (b)(i)).

If paramedics transport a patient directly to a mental health facility in the Australian Capital Territory, they are required to provide a written statement containing a description of the action taken under that section of the Act, and specifically include the following:

(a) the name and address (if known) of the person taken to the facility;

(b) the date and time when the person was taken to the facility;

(c) detailed reasons for taking the action;

(d) the nature and extent of the force or assistance used to enter any premises, or to apprehend the person and take the person to the facility;

(e) the nature and extent of any restraint, involuntary seclusion or forcible giving of medication used when apprehending the person or taking the person to the facility;

(f) anything else that happened when the person was being apprehended and taken to the facility that may have an effect on the person's physical or mental health. (*Mental Health Act 2015* (ACT), s 83(1))

This information should also map against clinical practice guidelines, and is an example of best practice from a legal perspective.

From time to time paramedics may be required to work across borders, and the state-by-state nature of mental health laws mean that there may be confusion about specific provisions of the respective Acts of each state/territory. The legislation of the state/territory in which you are treating the patient is the law that generally applies. However, it is likely that there will exist an agreement between the border states that addresses which law should apply. For example, there is an agreement in place between Victoria and New South Wales on the transfer of patients between states.[107]

Consent and capacity

There is a large amount of information that you should be aware of with regards to the legal understanding of consent, but for the purposes of this chapter this will be brief outline of the key elements. In short, *capacity* is the ability of a person to understand the nature, purpose and consequences of a decision. The term 'capacity' is often used interchangeably with 'competence'. For the purpose of this chapter the two terms will mean the same thing.

Patients have a right to make decisions about their medical treatment. The High Court of Australia has said that 'except in cases of emergency or necessity, all medical treatment is preceded by the patient's choice to undergo it'.[108] This right exists even if the patient has a mental illness or disorder. It is possible in the case of a patient with a mental illness or disorder that they may move in and out of capacity to consent to or refuse treatment. It is critical that paramedics undertake good clinical assessments of the patient's capacity to consent or refuse consent for treatment, which is a competent adult's right.

There is a presumption at law that anyone over the age of 18 has capacity, and it is up to the paramedics who may doubt the capacity of their patient to consent or refuse consent to treatment to assess and provide evidence to support any claim suggesting that a patient has lost capacity to make decisions for themselves. Those under the age of 18 are presumed to be not competent to consent or refuse consent for treatment. Therefore, if a paramedic makes an assessment that a person under 18 is in need of treatment and the person is refusing, the onus is on the person to demonstrate that they have the capacity to refuse. New South Wales, South Australia and the Northern Territory have laws that allow medical practitioners to provide emergency treatment to children without consent for a broad range of emergency care, but again it is likely that a person providing treatment to a person without capacity may be authorised to do so under the principle of necessity, or in the case of New South Wales and Tasmania under legislation, if that treatment is necessary to save a person's life, prevent serious damage to the patient's health or prevent the patient from suffering or continuing to suffer significant pain or distress (*Guardianship Act 1987* (NSW), s 37).

It is common for paramedics to treat patients who do not have capacity. An example is an unconscious patient. In the case of an unconscious patient, the paramedic may look to see whether there is a surrogate decision-maker authorised to make decisions on behalf of the incompetent patient. In the case *Re F*,[109] Lord Goff discussed which legal principle could apply to medical treatment given without consent. He did not find 'implied consent', which is a common misunderstanding amongst paramedics. He instead found the *principle of necessity*. The necessity principle is one that can be used to attempt to justify behaviour if the behaviour would otherwise be a breach of the law. For example, if one is speeding to get a patient to hospital urgently because of a life-threatening condition and you break the law to do so, then this may be justified on the basis of necessity: that it was necessary to break the law in order to save the person's life. This same principle is applied to almost all paramedic work where there is a patient requiring immediate lifesaving interventions and the patient cannot give consent and there is no one else who is legally able to give or refuse consent on the patient's behalf.

Often with elderly patients who may suffer from dementia that is transient—that is, it comes and goes—they may have a health guardian appointed who is authorised to made decisions on the patient's behalf when the patient is not competent to do so. The overarching principle of guardianship law is that the guardian is to act as if they were the patient. Mental health runs on the same principles, and, as stated earlier, falls into the same protective jurisdiction of the law. If the patient is not competent to make decisions for themselves, it may be that there is a guardian who is authorised to do so. If not, and the treatment is necessary to be administered in order to prevent a further harm from occurring to the patient, then paramedics may rely on the principle of necessity. This offers them a defence against any charge of assaulting the patient (i.e. touching the patient without consent). There have been no cases in Australia of a paramedic having been charged with assault for treating an incompetent patient under the principle of necessity.

Often mental health patients do not realise that they are in need of care and treatment. They may or may not be competent to make their own decisions about their care. It is therefore necessary for paramedic to carefully assess the patient's capacity to do so, and it should not be assumed that just because the patient has a mental illness or disorder that they are lacking in capacity. A good example is a patient who has bipolar disorder, a recognised mental illness, but is well managed with medication and is perfectly capable of making decisions about their own life and wellbeing.

As mentioned above, there is a presumption at law that anyone over the age of 18 is competent to consent or refuse consent for treatment. If the patient is unconscious and treatment is necessary to save further harm to the patient, then the paramedic can act without consent unless there is an advanced care directive that specifically refuses consent for treatment. Often in mental health cases where a paramedic is required to assess a mental health patient for involuntary transport to a mental health facility, it is likely that the patient either cannot consent or is refusing consent for treatment. If the paramedic suspects that the person is not competent, the onus is on the paramedic to show this.

A way to check this is to ask: Was the patient free of 'undue influence' at the time of refusing treatment? Does the refusal cover the action that is being planned? Was the person competent at the time they made the decision? In determining competence, the paramedic will establish whether the person has comprehended and retained the relevant information, believed it and weighed the information up, and communicated a decision.[110]

Safeguards within mental health legislation

There are a number of safeguards within the mental health law beyond just the list of the items at the beginning of the Act that are not mental illnesses. The ACT and Victoria are what is referred to as *human rights jurisdictions*, because, although human rights are the rights that humans have just by virtue of the fact that they are human, these two jurisdictions have chosen to explicitly consider and include references to human rights in their law-making. In section 15 of the *Mental Health Act 2014* (Vic), for example, this inclusion is reflected in the right of the patient to communicate with any person for the purpose of seeking legal advice or legal representation. Under the law, the staff of a mental health service are required to ensure that reasonable steps are taken to assist an inpatient to communicate lawfully with any person. This is because historically, for example, patients have been placed in locked mental health facilities with no way for them to make contact with those on the outside for often extensive periods of time. Another example of a protection that is provided to patients is a statement of rights which sets out a person's rights under the *Mental Health Act*. Further, as well as a written statement, there is a legal requirement that an oral explanation of this statement of rights be given as soon as the patient is capable to understanding the information (s 13).

Confidentiality and privacy

There is a legal and ethical requirement for paramedics to work to preserve the confidentiality and privacy of their patients. This does mean that paramedics should not engage in the promotion of patient information in any public forum, be it television or social media. The rule to remember is that the information you collect as a part of the privileged position of being a trusted professional paramedic is not your information to share. There are rare public health exceptions under the respective privacy laws of each state that allow for the sharing of patient information to health authorities if it is necessary to prevent harm to other persons, but this sharing of information should be considered carefully. It is critical that paramedics place the interests of their patient ahead of any other interest, including that of their employer.

Conclusion (and future challenges)

Emergency mental health has been, and will become, an increasingly important component of community and primary healthcare in the pre-hospital context.[111] In an environment where the demands for quality and safety in healthcare dominate the healthcare reform agenda, the ways in which paramedics make and account for clinical decisions take on crucial importance. The interdisciplinary integration of hospital and community services such as ambulance services is vital to the provision of quality continuity of care, as emphasised by the following comments by Chan and Noone:

> The safe and effective management of mental health emergencies is a very important component of a comprehensive system of services to individuals with mental illness and their families. Often, that is the point of entry to treatment, and frequently, it is a time of distress and turmoil. Good quality care at this point prepares a path for recovery and constitutes a critical opportunity to affect both immediate and long-term benefits.[112]

Paramedics are at the point of entry to the mental healthcare system, and are not considered peripheral health workers when it comes to mental health. Increased opportunities for paramedic participation in mental healthcare are needed.[113] Interconnected with efforts for professional regulation are standards of education, training and professional development. The fact that paramedics in Australia are now regulated health professionals brings with it increasing professional requirements and obligations. Future education and training programs must take stock of the dynamic nature of paramedic practice, and prepare paramedics to assess and manage mental illness in the field. Critical to this is the sufficiency of education and training programs and their integration with clinical guidelines, policy and legislation for ensuring quality practice.[114] At issue for paramedics' future participation as professionals in mental healthcare is the sufficiency of the prevailing legal, regulatory and processional practice frameworks for enabling high-quality and safe mental healthcare in the pre-hospital emergency-care setting.[115]

Review Questions

1 In what circumstances could a mental illness be considered a mental health emergency?

2 What is the role of the paramedic when assisting a person with a voluntary admission or when involved in an involuntary admission, and what sections of the relevant Acts apply?

3 What section of the Act in your jurisdiction defines the criteria for involuntary assessment and treatment?

4 What conditions are excluded as sole criteria for involuntary assessment and treatment in your jurisdiction? Can paramedics transport mental health patients directly to a mental health facility rather than to an emergency department for treatment? Refer to the law, policy and practice in your jurisdiction.

PRACTICE TIPS

Practice tip 1   Although the vast majority of mental illnesses do not constitute a mental health emergency, paramedics have obligations to care for all patients who are mentally ill.

Practice tip 2   Understand the distinction between mental illness, intellectual/learning disability and neurological conditions that may influence the person's presentation and ability to comprehend and respond to questions (e.g. cerebral palsy).

Practice tip 3   Critical to the paramedic's assessment and treatment of patients with mental illness is the ability to build a rapport with the patient, acknowledging the patient's concerns and problems, and understanding them and their cultural and contextual characteristics.

Practice tip 4   History-taking is essential to the comprehensive mental health assessment of the patient.

Practice tip 5   The person's conduct and language may be a function of their mental illness and beyond their control.

PRACTICE TIPS continued

Practice tip 6   Know the relevant law and policies for paramedics in your jurisdiction. Stay updated, because the law frequently changes. Thoroughly research your obligations within your professional organisation and employment setting. Seek advice and confirm your understanding with other suitably qualified individuals.

Practice tip 7   Objective, comprehensive and concise records are critical to facilitating timely, quality and safe healthcare. They are also fundamental to professional practice standards.

Practice tip 8   Managing mental illness in the pre-hospital emergency care is often challenging and stressful, and at times can be dangerous. Ensure you are appropriately supported by allied professionals, including police, physicians and other relevant personnel. Operational debriefing, peer support, and counselling services are critical to the ongoing health and wellbeing of paramedics if they are to provide optimal mental healthcare services to patients in the pre-hospital emergency care.

Endnotes

1 World Health Organization (WHO). (2010). *Mental health: strengthening our response.* [Fact sheet.] Geneva: WHO. Online. Available: https://www.who.int/news-room/fact-sheets/detail/mental-health -strengthening-our-response.

2 *Mental Health Act 2016* (Qld), s 10.

3 Shaban, R.Z. (2011) *Paramedic clinical judgement and decision-making of mental illness in the pre-hospital emergency care setting: a case study of accounts of practice.* (PhD thesis, Griffith University, Brisbane, Australia.)

4 Groom, G., Hickie, I., Davenport, T. (2003) *'Out of Hospital, Out of Mind!' A Report Detailing Mental Health Services in Australia in 2002 and Community Priorities for National Mental Health Policy for 2003–2008.* Canberra: Mental Health Council of Australia.

5 Shaban, R. (2009) *Invited Submission for Review of Western Australia Mental Health Policy and Mental Health Services.* Perth: Minister for Mental Health, Government of Western Australia.

6 Shaban, R. (2009) Paramedics and the mentally ill. In: C. Grbich and P. O'Meara (eds), *Paramedics in Australia: Contemporary Challenges of Practice* (pp. 112–133). Frenchs Forest, NSW: Pearson Education Australia.

7 Mental Health Council of Australia. (2005) *Not for Service: Experiences of Injustice and Desperation in Mental Health Care in Australia.* Canberra: Mental Health Council of Australia.

8 American Psychiatric Association. (2013) *Diagnostic and Statistical Manual of Mental Disorders*, 5th ed. Text Revision (DSM-V-TR). New York: American Psychiatric Association.

9 World Health Organization (WHO). (2018). *Fact Sheet 220—Mental Disorders.* Geneva: WHO.

10 Vigo, D., Thornicroft, G. and Atun, R. (2016) Estimating the true global burden of mental illness. *The Lancet Psychiatry* 3(2), 171–178.

11 WHO, *Fact Sheet 220—Mental Disorders*.

12 World Health Organization (WHO). (2001) *The World Health Report 2001—Mental Health: New Understanding, New Hope*. Geneva: WHO. Available: https://www.who.int/whr/2001/en/whr01_en .pdf?ua=1.

13 World Health Organization (WHO). (2018) *Suicide*. [Fact sheet.] Geneva: WHO. Online. Available: https://www.who.int/news-room/fact-sheets/detail/suicide.

14 Australian Institute for Health and Welfare (AIHW). (2018). In brief. *Australia's Health 2018*: Cat. No. AUS222. Canberra: AIHW. Available: https://www.aihw.gov.au/getmedia/fe037cf1-0cd0-4663-a8c0-67cd09b1f30c/aihw-aus-222.pdf.aspx?inline=true.

15 Ibid.

16 Australian Health Ministers' Advisory Council. (2006) *Council of Australian Governments National Action Plan on Mental Health 2006–2011*. Canberra: Australian Government.

17 Groom et al., *'Out of Hospital, Out of Mind!'*; Shaban, *Invited Submission for Review of Western Australia Mental Health Policy and Mental Health Services*; Shaban, Paramedics and the mentally ill; Mental Health Council of Australia, *Not for Service*.

18 Australian Institute for Health and Welfare (AIHW). (2010) In brief. *Australia's Health 2010*. Cat. No. 122. Canberra: AIHW.

19 World Health Organization (WHO). (2001) *Mental Health Problems: The Underdefined and Hidden Burden*. Fact sheet No. 218. Geneva: WHO. Online. Available: https://www.who.int/mediacentre/factsheets/fs218/en/.

20 Ibid.

21 Shaban, *Paramedic clinical judgement and decision-making of mental illness in the pre-hospital emergency care setting*.

22 American Psychiatric Association, *DSM-V-TR*.

23 World Health Organization (WHO). (2018) *International Statisical Classification of Diseases and Related Health Problems*, 11th ed. (ICD-11.) Geneva: WHO.

24 American Psychiatric Association, *DSM-V-TR*.

25 Office of the United Nations High Commissioner for Human Rights. (1991) *United Nations Principles for the Protection of Persons with Mental Illness and for the Improvement of Mental Health Care*. New York: United Nations General Assembly.

26 Ibid.

27 WHO, *Mental Health*; Groom et al., *'Out of Hospital, Out of Mind!'*; Mental Health Council of Australia, *Not for Service*.

28 Commonwealth Department of Health and Aged Care. (2000) *The National Mental Health Report 2000: Changes in Australia's Mental Health Services under the First National Mental Health Plan of the National Mental Health Strategy 1993–1998*. Canberra: Australian Government.

29 Palmer, M.J. (2005) *Inquiry into the Circumstances of the Immigration Detention of Cornelia Rau*. Canberra: Department of Immigration and Multicultural and Indigenous Affairs.

30 Commonwealth Ombudsman. (2006) *Report into Referred Immigration Cases: Mental Health and Incapacity*. Report No. 07–2006. Canberra: Department of Immigration and Multicultural Affairs, at p. 27.

31 Department of Parliamentary Services. (2005) *The Detention of Cornelia Rau: Legal Issues*. Canberra: Parliament of Australia.

32 Doessel, D., Scheurer, R., Chant, D. et al. (2005) Australia's mental health strategy and deinstitutionalisation: some empirical results. *Australian and New Zealand Journal of Psychiatry* 39(11–12), 989–994.

33 Wand, T. and Happell, B. (2001) The mental health nurse: contributing to improved outcomes for patients in the emergency department. *Accident and Emergency Nursing* 9(3), 166–176.

34 Sharrock, J. and Happell, B. (2000) The role of the psychiatric consultation-liaison nurse in the general hospital. *Australian Journal of Advanced Nursing* 18(1), 34–39.

35 Salkovkis, P.M., Storer, D., Atha, C. et al. (1990) Psychiatric morbidity in an accident and emergency department: characteristics of patients at presentation and one month follow-up. *British Journal of Psychiatry* 156, 483–487.

36 Fontaine, K.L. and Fletcher, J.S. (1999) *Mental Health Nursing*, 4th ed. Sydney: Addison Wesley.

37 Mental Health Council of Australia, *Not for Service*.

38 Whiteford, H.A. and Buckingham, W.J. (2005) Ten years of mental health service reform in Australia: are we getting it right? *Medical Journal of Australia* 182(8), 396–400.

39 Carter, W.J. (1991) *Report of the Commission of Inquiry into the Care and Treatment of Patients in the Psychiatric Unit of the Townsville General Hospital between 2nd March 1975 and 20th February 1988.* Brisbane: Queensland Government.

40 Human Rights and Equal Opportunity Commission. (1993) *Burdekin Report: Report of the National Inquiry into the Human Rights of People with Mental Illness.* Canberra: Human Rights and Equal Opportunity Commission.

41 Criminal Justice Commission. (1995) *Report of an Inquiry Conducted by the Honourable D G Steward into Allegations of Official Misconduct at the Basil Stafford Centre.* Brisbane: Queensland Government.

42 Brunton, W. (2005) The place of public inquiries in shaping New Zealand's national mental health policy 1858–1996. *Australia and New Zealand Heath Policy* 10(2), 24.

43 Palmer, *Inquiry into the Circumstances of the Immigration Detention of Cornelia Rau.*

44 Mental Health Council of Australia, *Not for Service*.

45 Brunton, The place of public inquiries in shaping New Zealand's national mental health policy 1858–1996.

46 WHO, *Fact Sheet 220—Mental Disorders*.

47 Forrester, K. and Griffiths, D. (2010) *Essentials of Law for Health Professionals*, 3rd ed. Sydney: Elsevier.

48 Commonwealth Department of Health and Aged Care. (1997) *National Mental Health Strategy: National Standards for Mental Health Services.* Canberra: Commonwealth Department of Health and Aged Care.

49 *Mental Health Act 2016* (Qld).

50 Ibid.

51 Shaban, *Paramedic clinical judgement and decision-making of mental illness in the pre-hospital emergency care setting*.

52 Reynolds, L. (2009) Contextualising paramedic culture. In: P. O'Meara and C. Grbich (eds), *Paramedics in Australia: Contemporary Challenges* (pp. 28–43). Frenchs Forest, NSW: Pearson Education Australia.

53 Shaban, *Paramedic clinical judgement and decision-making of mental illness in the pre-hospital emergency care setting*.

54 Ibid.

55 Ibid.

56 Chan, A. and Noone, J.A. (eds). (2006) *Emergency Mental Health Educational Manual.* Vancouver, BC: Mental Health Evaluation and Community Consultation Unit, University of British Columbia.

57 Shaban R. (2004) Mental health and mental illness in paramedic practice: a warrant for research and inquiry into accounts of paramedic clinical judgment and decision-making. *Journal of Emergency Primary Health Care* 2(3), 3–4.

58 Roberts, L. (2007) *The implications of mental health call outs on paramedic practice*. Adelaide: Department of Paramedic and Social Health Sciences, Flinders University; 2007.

59 Roberts, L. and Henderson, J. (2009) Paramedic perceptions of their role, education, training and working relationships when attending cases of mental illness. *Journal of Emergency Primary Health Care* 7(3), 1–6.

60 Townsend, R. and Luck, M. (2009) Protective jurisdiction, patient autonomy and paramedics: the challenges of applying the NSW *Mental Health Act*. *Journal of Emergency Primary Health Care* 7(4), http://dx.doi.org/10.33151/ajp.7.4.185.

61 Shaban R. (2008) Mental illness in the emergency care setting: a global challenge—emergency mental health: where are we now? *Australasian Emergency Nursing Journal* 11(2), 67–69.

62 Sharrock and Happell, *The role of the psychiatric consultation-liaison nurse in the general hospital;* Townsend and Luck, Protective jurisdiction, patient autonomy and paramedics.

63 Kalucy, R., Thomas, L., Lia. B. et al. (2004) Managing increased demand for mental health services in a public hospital emergency department: a trial of 'hospital-in-the-home' for mental health consumers. *International Journal of Mental Health Nursing* 13(4), 275–281.

64 Kalucy, R., Thomas, L. and King, D. (2005) Changing demand for mental health services in the emergency department of a public hospital. *Australian and New Zealand Journal of Psychiatry* 39(1–2), 74–80.

65 Brunero, S., Fairbrother, G., Lee, S. et al. (2007) Clinical characteristics of people with mental health problems who frequently attend an Australian emergency department. *Australian Health Review* 31(3), 462–470.

66 Fry, M. and Brunero, S. (2004) The characteristics and outcomes of mental health patients presenting to an emergency department over a twelve month period. *Australian Emergency Nursing Journal* 7(2), 21–25.

67 Wooden, M.D., Air, T.M., Schroder, G.D. et al. (2009) Frequent attenders with mental disorders at a general hospital emergency department. *Emergency Medicine Australasia* 21(3), 191–195.

68 Broadbent, M., Creaton, A., Moxham, L. et al. (2010) Review of triage reform: the case for national consensus on a single triage scale for clients with a mental illness in Australian emergency departments. *Journal of Clinical Nursing* 19(5–6), 712–715.

69 Wand, T. and White, K. (2007) Examining models of mental health service delivery in the emergency department. *Australian and New Zealand Journal of Psychiatry* 41(10), 784–791.

70 Knott, J., Pleban, A., Taylor, D. et al. (2007) Management of mental health patients attending Victorian emergency departments. *Australian and New Zealand Journal of Psychiatry* 41(9), 759–767.

71 Lowthian, J., Curtis, A.J., Cameron, P. et al. (2010) Systematic review of trends in emergency departments attendances: an Australian perspective. *Emergency Medicine Journal* 28(5), 373–377.

72 Dent, A.W., Phillips, G.A., Chenhall, A.J. et al. (2003) The heaviest users of an inner city emergency department are not general practice patients. *Emergency Medicine* 15(4), 322–329.

73 Salkovkis et al., Psychiatric morbidity in an accident and emergency department.

74 Saliou, V., Fichelle, A., McLoughlin M. et al. (2005) Psychiatric disorders among patients admitted to a French medical emergency services. *General Hospital Psychiatry* 27(4), 263–268.

75 Dent, A., Hunter, G. and Webster, A.P. (2010) The impact of frequent attenders on a UK emergency department. *European Journal of Emergency Medicine* 17(6), 332–336.

76 Broadbent et al., Review of triage reform.

77 Schmidt, T.A., Atcheson, R., Federiuk, C. et al. (2001) Hospital follow-up of patient categorized as not needing an ambulance using a set of emergency medical technicians protocols. *Prehospital Emergency Care* 5(4), 366–370.

78 Spooren, D., Buylaert, W., van Heeringen C. et al. (1998) Police involvement in psychiatric emergency referrals to an urban general hospital. *Pre-hospital Immediate Care* 2, 10–13.

79 Spooren, D., Buylaert, W., Jannes, C et al. (1996) Patients with psychiatric emergencies transported by an ambulance in an urban region. *European Journal of Emergency Medicine* 3(1), 14–18.

80 Pajonk, F.G., Bartels, H.H., Biberthaler, P. et al. (2001) Psychiatric emergencies in preclinical emergency service: incidence, treatment and evaluation by emergency physicians and staff. *Der Nervenarzt* 72(9),685–692.

81 Doyle, T.J. and Vissers, R.J. (1999) An EMS approach to psychiatric emergencies. *Emergency Medical Services* 28(6), 87, 90–93.

82 Torrey, E.F. (1971) Emergency psychiatric ambulance services in the USSR. *American Journal of Psychiatry* 128(2), 153–157.

83 Nordberg, M. (1999) Paramedics provide care to mentally ill. *EMS Magazine* p. 8.

84 Green, G. (1999) Emergency psychiatric assessments: do outcomes match priorities? *International Journal of Health Quality Assurance* 12(7), 309–313.

85 Ibid.; Wand and Happell, The mental health nurse; Sharrock and Happell, The role of the psychiatric consultation-liaison nurse in the general hospital; Salkovkis et al., Psychiatric morbidity in an accident and emergency department.

86 Bell, G., Hindley, N., Rajiyah, G. et al. (1990) Screening for psychiatric morbidity in an accident and emergency department. *Archives of Emergency Medicine* 7(3), 155–162.

87 Anstee, B.H. (1972) Psychiatry in the casualty department. *British Journal of Psychiatry* 120, 625–629.

88 Shaban, *Paramedic clinical judgement and decision-making of mental illness in the pre-hospital emergency care setting*.

89 Naved, R.T., Rimi, N.A., Jahan, S. et al. (2009) Paramedic-conducted mental health counselling for abused women in rural Bangladesh: an evaluation from the perspective of participants. *Journal of Health, Population and Nutrition* 27(4), 477–491.

90 Saddichha, S. and Vibha, P. (2011) Behavioural emergencies in India: would psychiatric emergency services help? *Prehospital and Disaster Medicine* 26(1), 65–70.

91 Ibid.

92 Shaban, *Paramedic clinical judgement and decision-making of mental illness in the pre-hospital emergency care setting*.

93 Ibid.

94 Ibid.

95 Ibid.

96 Bendall J. and Morrison, A. (2009) Clinical judgement. In: P. O'Meara and C. Grbich (eds), *Paramedics in Australia: Contemporary Challenges of Practice* (pp. 96–111). Frenchs Forest, NSW: Pearson Education Australia

97 Shaban, *Paramedic clinical judgement and decision-making of mental illness in the pre-hospital emergency care setting*.

98 Thompson, C. and Dowding, D. (2001) *Clinical Decision Making and Judgement in Nursing*. London: Churchill Livingstone.

99 Ibid.

100 Shaban, *Paramedic clinical judgement and decision-making of mental illness in the pre-hospital emergency care setting*.

101 Ibid.

102 Ibid.

103 Ibid.

104 Townsend, R. (2017) *The role of law in the professionalisation of paramedics in Australia.* (PhD thesis, Canberra, Australian National University.)

105 Paramedicine Board of Australia. (2018) *Registration Standards.* Melbourne: Australian Health Practitioner Regulation Agency.

106 *George v Rockett* (1990) 170 CLR 104.

107 Eburn, M. (2018, 25 October) Mental health services by paramedics across the NSW/Victoria border. *Australian Emergency Law.* Online. Available: https://emergencylaw.wordpress.com/2018/10/25/mental -health-services-by-paramedics-across-the-nsw-victoria-border/.

108 *Rogers v Whitaker* (1992) 175 CLR 479, at [14].

109 *Re F (Mental Patient: Sterilisation)* [1990] 2 AC 1.

110 *Re C (Adult: Refusal of Medical Treatment)* [1994] 1 WLR 290.

111 Lowthian et al., Systematic review of trends in emergency departments attendances

112 Chan and Noone (eds), *Emergency Mental Health Educational Manual.*

113 Shaban, *Paramedic clinical judgement and decision-making of mental illness in the pre-hospital emergency care setting.*

114 Ibid.

115 Ibid.

Chapter 10
Paramedics, privacy and confidentiality

Bruce Baer Arnold

Learning objectives

After reading this chapter, you should be able to:

- understand privacy and confidentiality as concepts, and areas of disagreement
- understand international and national legal frameworks regarding privacy and confidentiality
- understand the interaction of law, practitioner codes and ethics regarding privacy and confidentiality
- understand the operation of privacy and confidentiality in paramedicine.

Definitions

Confidentiality A duty not to inappropriately disclose or misuse sensitive corporate or personal information, protected under confidentiality law.

Privacy A human right involving a freedom from inappropriate physical interference or observation, conceptualised in different ways and protected under a range of law.

Introductory cases

Privacy and confidentiality cases

Paramedics, institutions and the people with whom they deal navigate an often turbulent sea of personal and corporate information. Consider some of the following instances where there is likely to be disagreement about social expectations, technologies, practitioner codes, ethics and law.

Continued

> ## Introductory cases continued
>
> A paramedic places images of a comatose female celebrity on Instagram and Facebook. Another tweets pictures of the celebrity's distressed children as mummy is stretchered out of her Gold Coast apartment. An ambulance service demands that all employees undergo weekly blood tests after a tabloid headline about the theft of painkillers. A trainee paramedic chooses to opt out of the national My Health Record scheme after reading that the risks outweigh the benefits. A senior colleague calls for a mandatory e-health card that would contain unencrypted personal medical data to assist in accidents. A journalist reveals that the state emergency services' network was hacked 2 years ago without detection: personnel files are now for sale on the dark web, going cheap. A manager shares technical specifications with his sister-in-law, who wants an edge in bidding for a big equipment supply tender. A technician hides a digital camera in the showers so he can record female employees unawares. Inter-state, another paramedic is distressed to find that a senior colleague has been sharing intimate snaps made in her bedroom before their relationship fell apart.
>
> *All of the above scenarios pose questions about privacy and confidentiality, which are increasingly salient matters in a world of social media, digital networks, and conflicts between professional ethics and personal benefit. This chapter offers both a research perspective and guidance in navigating cases such as these.*

Introduction

Privacy and confidentiality are of increasing community and professional concern in a world of social media, networked databases, litigation and practitioner discipline.[1]

Those concerns encompass respect for people who are assisted by paramedics, and, importantly but often unrecognised, respect for the paramedics themselves. The concerns also encompass the behaviour of institutions, such as ambulance services, that have responsibilities for users of paramedicine, paramedicine professionals and the broader community.

This chapter deals with the Australian and New Zealand privacy and confidentiality regimes in relation to paramedicine. The literature on the privacy aspects of new technologies and new social practices—such as 'revenge porn' and 'sexting', or the hacking of networked medical devices—is expanding rapidly. Yet it is often confusing, for specialists and non-specialists alike, in part because legal frameworks and their associated practice codes vary widely from one jurisdiction to another.

Surprisingly, although there is substantial case law and scholarship on privacy problems involving law enforcement—for example, police officers improperly accessing official networks to aid an associate or harass a colleague—and much research on health data access/integrity in hospitals, alongside a rich body of scholarship about confidentiality as a fundamental for the clinician–patient relationship, there is little literature on the privacy aspects of paramedicine in the Australian and New Zealand jurisdictions.

One conclusion is that the absence of extensive published research reflects both the under-recognition of paramedicine as an important profession,[2] and delays in the establishment of coherent practitioner codes at the national rather than state/institutional levels.[3]

This chapter begins by discussing privacy and confidentiality in principle, before mapping the varying frameworks for those fields of law in Australia and New Zealand. The frameworks are challenging for paramedicine practitioners, legal practitioners and researchers alike, because they are notably inconsistent. The chapter highlights salient statute and case law. It next analyses the practitioner code and guidelines, both in the abstract and in relation to their interpretation by particular institutions. It notes the significance of the *Health Practitioner Regulation National Law Act* in Australia as providing paramedics with authority to reinforce the profession's expectations regarding ethics if there is conflict with ministerial policy in a specific jurisdiction. It contextualises issues and practices, such as those highlighted above, that are likely to be increasingly contentious in the emerging data-rich health services environment.[4]

That analysis draws on both scholarly literature and an examination of recent Australian and New Zealand case law regarding privacy and confidentiality in relation to paramedicine.

Making sense of privacy and confidentiality

An effort to understand privacy and confidentiality should start with a recognition that, although both are important for paramedicine, they are not identical.

Privacy is an aspect of human dignity[5] that is discernible in law over many centuries,[6] and is often respected (e.g. through trespass, crime and data protection law, rather than merely through a discrete 'Privacy Act') in widely different ways.[7] In essence, privacy relates to people rather than to private-sector corporations and government agencies. It is concerned with the private or personal sphere; in particular, personal information about individuals.[8] It involves a balance between collective and purely personal goods, with courts recurrently construing the 'public interest' in terms of social benefit rather than public curiosity.[9] It is important but not an absolute; enactments accordingly generally feature major exclusions or exceptions in order to balance the competing rights, responsibilities and objectives.[10]

Confidentiality has a broader scope.[11] It encompasses sensitive personal information; for example, information provided to a lawyer or a clinician that was imparted in circumstances that meant the recipient had a duty not to improperly misuse or disclose that information. Importantly, it also encompasses non-personal information, such as trade secrets (e.g. technical specifications and test data) and business plans or proposals that are not in the public domain.[12] Confidentiality typically arises as a consequence of a specific relationship; for example, an employee's duty of loyalty to the employer, or a clinician's duty to safeguard disclosures made by a patient. In some circumstances it may provide stronger protection than specific privacy enactments; for example, through the scope for large-scale compensation payments to deter disregarding of confidentiality. It is not an absolute, and will be lawfully disregarded in some circumstances.[13]

Paramedicine professionals and the entities for which they work are subject to a patchwork of privacy law and confidentiality law. Those legal frameworks, as noted above, cover the dealings that professionals have with people who use paramedicine services, and the families or associates of those people. The frameworks also cover paramedics themselves, both in terms of their duty to employers and as individuals who should be protected from inappropriate surveillance by their employers and peers.

It is unlikely that we will see a fundamental simplification of those frameworks in the immediate future, although New Zealand's human rights regime hints at a way forward.[14] Several Australian jurisdictions have discrete human rights enactments that, consistent with international agreements such as the *International Covenant on Civil and Political Rights*, refer to privacy, but in practice they are aspirational rather than providing substantive remedies in instances where an individual's privacy has been disregarded.[15]

Privacy as freedom from inappropriate interference

Privacy as a matter of principle and practice in paramedicine is challenging, because there is disagreement about what it means, why it is important and how it is to be given effect. Some people claim, whether disingenuously or naïvely, that privacy is unachievable, or unnecessary or simply so outdated as to be meaningless. However, while the slogans 'It has gone, so get over it' and 'If you have done nothing wrong, you have nothing to hide' provide nice sound-bites for high-school debating teams or proponents of tougher law and order, they are at odds with the realities of most people's lives.[16] Few readers, for example, would be comfortable with some of the incidents noted at the beginning of this chapter, such as video being taken of themselves or loved ones in intimate situations, or the undisclosed (and thus typically unauthorised) sharing of personal information. A succession of surveys has demonstrated that most Australians do care about privacy, and that their disquiet about the disregarding of privacy is increasing, in part because there is a growing awareness of the implications and frequency of that disregard.[17]

Theorists have sought to *systematise* our understanding, and enable the development of effective law and administrative protocols by characterising privacy in different ways.[18] One approach, of particular relevance for paramedicine professionals and policymakers, is a multi-faceted notion of 'health privacy': a sectoral characterisation that would sit alongside a narrower 'financial privacy' and 'information privacy'.

Another approach is to refer to *characterisations* such as locational or geospatial privacy (increasingly important, for example, in tracking employees across a precinct, city or region), physical privacy (extending from not being observed in a bathroom through to restrictions on cavity or other searches or the coerced provision of blood samples), intellectual privacy (important for young people in exploring heterodox ideas without the chill attributable to being monitored by 'Big Sister' and 'Big Brother') and information privacy (for some people a matter of not being comprehensively profiled on public/private databases, and thereby being treated as a set of identifiers rather than as a person).

A third approach, drawing on an understanding of privacy as a matter of information collection and distribution, is to address it under a *rubric of data protection*.[19] That rubric is salient for professionals in Australia and New Zealand, because we increasingly benchmark our privacy regimes against those in Europe, where much of the language emphasises privacy as an inalienable human right rather than a commodity, but often refers to data protection; for example, the *General Data Protection Regulation (GDPR)* in place from mid-2018.[20] The GDPR is an EU-wide law that affects Australian and New Zealand businesses dealing with consumers in Europe. However, it does not cover all aspects of privacy in that region.[21]

A persuasive and succinct characterisation of privacy comes from the United States over 120 years ago, with privacy being summarised by Warren and Brandeis as a freedom from inappropriate interference, a freedom for all people rather than merely for the rich and powerful.[22] It is a freedom that may be more important to individuals and groups at particular times in their life or in particular circumstances. This characterisation is valuable for two reasons.

The first is that, in referring to 'inappropriate', the characterisation recognises that privacy is a matter of balance rather than an absolute. That balance will be encountered by paramedics in their professional practice and in their daily lives.

It is appropriate, for instance, for parents/guardians to observe toddlers, and thereby provide them with the safety and healthcare to which all children are entitled as humans. Australian law formally allows disclosure of contact details, such as 'silent numbers' in emergencies, where that disclosure will assist in saving a person's life.[23] It allows the use of data on Medicare and other cards as part of the delivery of publicly-funded health/welfare services.[24] It is, however, not appropriate for disgruntled ex-partners to share intimate images of the person with whom they shared a bed. It is not appropriate for a professional to engage in the unauthorised dissemination of images of people encountered in the course of duty as a paramedic; for example, by selling photographs of the live/dead victims of a car crash, or of a celebrity in an ambulance after an overdose.[25]

Expectations regarding privacy/confidentiality may be over-ridden by mandatory reporting requirements, which are specifically provided for in the *Health Practitioner Regulation National Law Act* in Australia.[26] Professionals can expect those requirements to become more comprehensive and more stringent in the coming decade.[27] Note that such reporting is not 'to the world at large'. Note, also, that protection for whistleblowers—otherwise known as public interest disclosure—is highly contentious.[28]

Inappropriateness may be signalled by the law, by practitioner codes and—more subtly—by practitioners asking 'Is there a justification for this?' and 'Would you like it done to you?' Professionals recognise that just because something is technologically feasible or administratively convenient does not mean it should be done. The notion of 'inappropriate' encompasses a rejection of arbitrariness—in other words, a rejection of decision-making that is outside formal guidelines that cannot be justified in principle, is idiosyncratic, or is determined by the benefit to the decision-maker rather than to the community at large.

The second reason that the characterisation of privacy as freedom from inappropriate *interference* is valuable is because it is not technology-specific or sector-specific, in contrast to many enactments of Australian parliaments that are solely concerned with privacy in terms of an audio device, or a video device or an identifier such as the ubiquitous Tax File Number.[29] Reference to 'interference' is sufficiently broad as to cover a range of environments, with an emphasis on the protection of people in situations where they reasonably have an expectation of being left alone and thereby respected. Interference accordingly encompasses the bedroom and bathroom, the individual's personal finances and demographical data collected by taxation and census agencies, and matters such as what a person is reading, where the person is travelling and with whom the person associates.

Australian and New Zealand courts, informed by privacy theorists, are increasingly construing the appropriateness of an activity that reduces privacy by asking whether that action is *proportionate*. Can an agreed public policy objective, for example, be reached in ways that are not unduly invasive? A health department or ambulance service with a legitimate objective of protecting paramedicine professionals and the general public by identifying and addressing the consumption of behaviour-modifying substances might demand weekly blood tests of all employees. A more proportionate mechanism might be the random provision by employees of hair samples and buccal swabs, which are less invasive than a blood test. Disagreements about privacy are often attributable to administrators assuming that if they have a hammer then every problem must be treated as a nail (a disproportionate response that erodes trust), or that any news is good news.[30]

The notion of interference recognises that in Australia and New Zealand, alongside other liberal democratic states, people typically have the freedom to make choices. This freedom is often manifested in contracts. Some of those choices relate to personal information or other aspects of the individual's private life. In thinking about privacy, readers of this chapter should recognise that some people will on occasion engage in 'over-sharing' or make errors of judgement about whom they trust. Some disclosure by individuals about themselves and associates, in particular about their children and friends, may be uninformed. An area of growing contention in law is whether the agreements used by many private-sector entities involve genuine consent. Both Australia and New Zealand will eventually emulate the practice in the European Union regarding properly informed consent as the basis of data collection, data analysis and data sharing.[31]

Professionals should be wary of the claim that because most people using social media share images and other personal information means that they do not care about privacy, or that any harms are trivial. Apart from a wide range of survey results that demonstrate the falseness of the claim, remember that using Facebook to share pictures of the person's birthday party is not the same as a paramedicine professional arbitrarily tweeting images from a crash scene or an employer selling health records to an insurer.

Confidentiality as respect for relationships

Confidentiality co-exists with, and is broader than, privacy law. As noted above, it encompasses both personal information (and thus potentially serves as a strong mechanism for the protection of health and other data) and trade secrets or other information that has nothing to do with interference with the personal sphere. It can best be understood as a matter of respect for relationships, rather than in terms of specific types of data or their format. Salient court judgements regarding confidentiality have accordingly included disputes about medical records, marital 'pillow talk',[32] celebrity weddings[33] and mundane devices such as carpet fasteners and hole punches.[34]

In essence, confidentiality seeks to legally recognise and thereby reinforce relationships in the health sector and other areas of life. Many of those relationships have a strongly commercial basis. A salient example is the relationship between the employee and the employer—what used to be dubbed the 'master–servant relationship'—in which employees have a legally enforceable duty to put the employer's interests ahead of their own, and accordingly, for example, must safeguard information that is sensitive, and to which they gained privileged access in the course of employment.[35] Paramedics will owe that duty to ambulance services, health departments and other employers. That duty is typically reinforced by the employment contract, and further reinforced through parliamentary enactments that are specific to the health sector.[36] Professionals will also be aware of the relationship between clinicians and patients, with an understanding that non-disclosure of data acquired in the course of diagnosis and treatment is essential to the trust that is the foundation of both public health and the legitimacy of the health professions.

As with privacy, confidentiality is not an absolute. Not every exchange of information between a clinician and a patient, a lawyer and a client, an employer and an employee is confidential. 'Will it rain this afternoon?' is, for example, qualitatively different from 'I haven't told my wife I'm sleeping with other men.' Patient expectations can be validly breached in exceptional circumstances—for example, to prevent harm to the patient, to the practitioner or to a third party. It is also axiomatic that samples will often be shared with pathology labs, and that information gained by a general practitioner in the course of a consultation will be shared with a specialist. That sharing cannot, however, be to the world at large.

As with privacy, it is important to note that neither administrative convenience nor public curiosity is a justification for the disclosure of confidential health data beyond what would be reasonably considered by a court to be necessary for diagnosis and treatment.

Law and practice frameworks

What does that mean for paramedicine practitioners and administrators? We can contextualise both confidentiality and privacy by recognising that privacy ecosystems are dynamic, diverse and, unfortunately, often misunderstood.

Australian and New Zealand privacy law is a patchwork

Much public discussion and media reporting about confidentiality assumes that it is identical to privacy, and indeed that privacy is solely a matter of information (e.g. about the sharing of medical records or the hacking of credit-card databases). Much discussion involves reference to rights, typically to a transcendent 'right to privacy', and without much sense of responsibilities. That discussion is problematical, because in Australia there is no comprehensive right to privacy.

Privacy and confidentiality do not feature in the national constitution, so (unlike Europe) it thus cannot be invoked to invalidate a national, state or territory enactment that removes privacy. The range of national enactments regarding privacy, surveillance and data protection typically co-exist with rather than override state/territory law. Australian courts have chosen not to recognise a comprehensive privacy right; instead, they have— sometimes idiosyncratically—sought to protect the personal sphere on an instance-by-instance basis through contract law, criminal law (e.g. stalking and trespass), confidentiality law, and remedies under a diverse range of the privacy-specific enactments of the different legislatures.

One result is that paramedicine practitioners need to be conscious of a patchwork of law, rather than assuming that a coherent framework is established by a single privacy enactment and thence given effect through a single, readily-understood practitioner code. The situation in New Zealand is somewhat simpler, because that nation does not have a federal system of law.

This chapter highlights the significance of the courts, because law, from a pragmatic perspective (i.e. what actually happens rather than what theorists want to happen), is ultimately what courts decide in applying enactments and principles. There are clear references to privacy in numerous global human rights agreements, such as the 1948 *Universal Declaration of Human Rights*, but those agreements have no effect, apart from potentially influencing public opinion, unless they are reflected in enactments and positively interpreted by the relevant Australian and New Zealand courts.

The absence of a comprehensive agreement about privacy alongside the lack of a Commonwealth power to impose an enactment that extends from trespass to cavity searches, the handling of medical records and vetting of future practitioners means that there is no overarching national health enactment, health privacy enactment or general privacy enactment. Consistent with the above comment regarding a dynamic ecosystem, practitioners are instead likely to encounter a range of law regarding privacy in the course of their careers and private lives, with substantial variation across Australia and across the Tasman.

Privacy law predates paramedicine

As noted above, much privacy is a function of traditional law that is not specific to paramedicine. All of the jurisdictions criminalise unauthorised entry to residential and other premises apart from in exceptional circumstances, consistent with the rubric that an Englishperson's home is their castle and that they protect the private sphere by shutting the door and pulling the curtains.[37] Theft of items that contain private or confidential information—including diaries, photo albums and laptops—is similarly criminalised. Unauthorised access to, and dissemination of, information from a computer network is also criminalised, but specialists note that the penalties may be of little consolation if personal or corporate data has been illicitly shared with the world at large. Law also criminalises unauthorised searching or other contact with an individual. Much of that criminal law is accompanied by a scope for action under tort law—in other words, civil litigation for physical injury or distress.

New technologies and practice

The environment becomes more challenging when we consider devices that capture still/moving images (including the smartphones that are carried by most adults), audio or other data formats. Law regarding the invasive use of such devices is inconsistent, with some jurisdictions, for example, lagging behind by specifically criminalising the unauthorised use of listening devices (often conceptualised as the wire-taps that feature in old crime dramas), but not covering the use of video. That inconsistency is partially offset by law that prohibits the unauthorised recording in particular locations or of particular activities, notably the undisclosed use of a video device in a changing room for the purposes of sexual gratification. Closed-circuit television cameras (CCTV) have proliferated in streets, retail malls, hospitals, airports and educational institutions over the past decade. That surveillance is permissible on the basis that it does not extend to locations in which people have a reasonable expectation of privacy (e.g. in a toilet), that the surveillance is not covert, and that there is no arbitrary sharing of recorded images.

Employers, employees and privacy

We encounter similar inconsistencies in considering the privacy aspects of employment law. The Australian jurisdictions have adopted different stances regarding the use of tracking devices to monitor the movement of ambulances and other corporate vehicles. Those devices will become ubiquitous. The position in Australian law is broadly that their use is permissible if employees are alerted that tracking does or might occur. Employees are deemed to have consented to be tracked by entering into the employment relationship, whether specifically through an individual contract or through a workplace agreement that is not specific to the particular individual.

What about privacy in relation to corporate networks, including employer-issued phones rather than merely desktop devices? The longstanding position in law is that if you use the network you are bound by the employer's terms and conditions, which typically include 'use' provisions that allow the employer to monitor what the employee might consider to be private email and web-surfing via that network. That surveillance is reflected in a growing number of instances in which employers have been found to have lawfully dismissed or disciplined a staff member or contractor.

Preceding paragraphs have referred to tests for substances that are perceived as likely to affect an employee's performance, in particular alcohol and cocaine. That testing is sometimes contentious, with critics for example arguing that neither employers nor society at large have any right to interfere with what employees do outside the workplace. A conventional rejoinder is that comprehensive testing, which does not single out a specific individual, is appropriate because of potential harms and may be proportionate. Requirement for the provision of a urine sample would, for example, be less invasive than a blood sample, with a buccal swab potentially providing both accurate results and being less intrusive than the supervised collection of a waste product.

Contracts may also specifically reinforce duties of non-disclosure or other misuse of confidential information other than personal information, strengthening the protection of confidentiality under the master–servant relationship noted above.

What is 'information privacy'?

Most people in Australia and New Zealand now have some sense of 'privacy law' as a matter of an information privacy enactment; in particular, the collection and handling of personal information in print and electronic databases. One reason that the privacy ecosystem is challenging is that there is a range of such enactments. Some jurisdictions, for example Western Australia and South Australia, have no Privacy Act. In contrast, the Australian Capital Territory has a discrete *Information Privacy Act* (covering the territory government), a *Workplace Privacy Act* (covering public and private employers) and a *Health*

Records (Privacy and Access) Act (covering public and private health records).[38] Across the border in New South Wales, that state's Health Records Act deals with public hospital/clinic records but not the private health sector.[39]

The state/territory enactments co-exist with a range of national enactments, of which the best-known but often misunderstood are the *Privacy Act 1988* (Cth) and the controversial *My Health Records Act 2012*. They are not the only the national enactments dealing with privacy; there are discrete privacy provisions in over 212 national enactments; for example, law regarding the taxation system, the population census and Medicare.

The 1993 New Zealand *Privacy Act* covers how public- and private-sector entities—including businesses, hospitals, schools and government agencies—collect, use, disclose, store and give access to personal information (i.e. about identifiable living people). It provides the basis for several more detailed codes regarding specific industries, activities and types of personal information. A salient example is the *Health Information Privacy Code*.

The 1988 Australian *Privacy Act* is another information privacy enactment, made by Australia's national government. It was initially restricted to the operation of most national government agencies (with important exclusions regarding, for example, national security agencies and law enforcement activity). Since then, it has been extended to cover many businesses, including entities in the health sector. Importantly, it does not cover state/territory government agencies, which are instead covered by state/territory enactments in those jurisdictions where the government has enacted an information privacy statute. The process of extension and modification over the past 30 years means that the enactment is cumbersome and often confusing, resulting in a growing number of disputes in the Federal Court.

The Act centres on 13 *Australian Privacy Principles (APPs)*; in essence, broad statements that are interpreted with the assistance of detailed guidelines issued by the Office of the Australian Information Commissioner (OAIC).

The Australian Privacy Principles

The APPs are structured in five parts, which need to be read together rather than in isolation. Part 1 articulates principles that require APP entities (public and private) to consider the privacy of 'personal information', including management of that information in an open and transparent way. Part 2 articulates principles dealing with the collection of that information, including unsolicited personal information. Part 3 articulates principles about how APP entities deal with personal information and government-related identifiers, such as Tax File Numbers. Part 4 provides principles about the integrity (e.g. security and quality) of personal information. Part 5 articulates complementary principles regarding requests for access to and correction of personal information.

As noted above, the APPs feature substantial exceptions—for example, regarding public/private health ('permitted health situations'), law enforcement, defence and the location of missing persons ('permitted general situations'). Importantly, the APPs expressly refer to 'reasonable belief' and 'reasonable action', which as interpreted by the OAIC foster a lowest common denominator approach in contrast to practice in Europe under the GDPR.

In summary, *APP1* provides for 'open and transparent management of personal information'. That means that the entity must take reasonable steps in the circumstances to implement 'practices, procedures and systems' to ensure compliance with the APPs and any registered APP code. In particular, the public/private entity must have a clear and accessible privacy policy statement regarding its management of personal information.

APP2 relates to 'anonymity and pseudonymity', and is multi-faceted. It specifies that an individual must have the option of not identifying themselves (or of using a pseudonym) except where there is a requirement under law for identification (e.g. opening a bank account or a mobile phone account), or where it is impracticable for the entity to deal with anonymous or pseudonymous people. Businesses and government agencies may lawfully require you to provide identification.

APP3 deals with the 'collection of solicited personal information', which covers both non-sensitive solicited personal information (collection of which is prohibited 'unless the information is reasonably necessary for, or directly related to, one or more of the entity's functions or activities') and sensitive information (collection of which is prohibited unless the individual consents to the collection, and the information is reasonably necessary for one or more of the entity's functions or activities). The consent requirement is disregarded in several circumstances; for example, when collection is required by law or by a court order, or where there is a 'permitted health situation', or a government agency 'reasonably believes' that collection is 'reasonably necessary for, or directly related to' one of its functions or activities.

APP4 relates to 'dealing with unsolicited personal information'. If an entity receives unsolicited personal information it must, within a reasonable period, determine whether collection was possible under APP3. If not, it must as soon as practicable (if it is lawful and reasonable to do so) de-identify or destroy the information.

APP5 deals with 'notification of the collection of personal information'. The expectation is that individuals who are properly notified may choose not to provide information, and will have scope for action if information has been misused.

APP 6 deals with the 'use or disclosure of personal information', again a focus of complaints. There must be no use or disclosure of the information for any other 'secondary' purpose unless there was consent or the individual would reasonably expect the entity to use/disclose it for the secondary purpose, there is requirement under law, a 'permitted general situation' or 'permitted health situation', or the entity 'reasonably believes' that use/disclosure is 'reasonably necessary' for enforcement-related activities.

APP7 deals specifically with 'direct marketing'. The APP provides that an entity holding personal information must not use/disclose that information for the purpose of direct marketing. There are, however, significant exceptions, in use/disclosure for direct marketing with the person's consent. Note that the APP sits alongside the electronic non-interference enactments.[40]

APP8 deals with 'cross-border disclosure of personal information', a special provision regarding the movement and processing offshore of personal information, given that Australian law does not extend to other jurisdictions. An entity must take reasonable steps to ensure that an overseas recipient does not breach the APPs. Exceptions include provision for express consent by individuals, disclosure being required by law or under an international agreement regarding information-sharing (e.g. national security), or reasonable belief that disclosure is 'reasonably necessary' for enforcement-related activities.

APP9 deals with the 'adoption, use or disclosure of government related identifiers'; in essence, non-government entities are prohibited from using a government-related identifier (e.g. the Medicare Number) for its own identification of a person unless that is required by law.

APP10 deals with the 'quality of personal information', with the APP entity taking reasonable steps to ensure that personal information is 'accurate, up-to-date, complete and relevant'. The 'relevant' is significant.

APP11 deals with the 'security of personal information': entities are required to take 'reasonable steps' to protect any information they hold from misuse, interference, loss, unauthorised access, modification or disclosure, and to destroy or de-identify the information.[41] Readers should note increasing concerns within the privacy and information technology communities regarding the ineffectiveness of both the destruction and the de-identification of health, financial and other sensitive data.[42]

APP12 deals with 'access to personal information'. An entity must, on request, give an individual access on a timely basis to any personal information about that person which is held by the entity. Exceptions provide for restrictions, including refusal of access on the basis of a reasonable belief that it would pose a serious threat to an individual's life, health or safety, or to public health and safety. Any charges for access must not be 'excessive'.

APP13 deals with the 'correction of personal information'. An APP entity must take reasonable steps to ensure that the information is accurate, up-to-date, complete, relevant and not misleading. Individuals may seek to require a statement be associated with their personal information—in essence, a note or flag—indicating that they consider the information to be inaccurate, out-of-date, incomplete, irrelevant or misleading.

Protection for paramedicine practitioners

Paramedicine practitioners have some protection in their lives outside the workplace under the national *Privacy Act*. While they have duties to their employers as employees, they are also potentially protected from privacy abuses as employees, and more generally as individuals, who have a reasonable expectation that a peer or a stranger will not intrude into a private space, such as the bedroom, share a recording of an intimate moment or make a recording without their knowledge. The people with whom they deal as paramedicine professionals similarly have an expectation that the paramedics will not inappropriately disregard the privacy of accident victims, other people in need, or bystanders. Simply put, practitioners will behave professionally.

That respectful behaviour is required by two groups of law specific to practitioners.

The first is the enactment/s in each jurisdiction that establishes and regulates paramedicine services, such as the *Ambulance Services Act* and the *Health Care Act* in Victoria and South Australia, respectively.[43] The second is the *Health Practitioner Regulation National Law Act* (known as 'the National Law'), consistent enactments by the different jurisdictions to provide a uniform regime covering health practitioners, including paramedicine practitioners.

The *Health Practitioner Regulation National Law Act*

In terms of both privacy and confidentiality, the National Law is significant for three reasons.

The first is that it recognises paramedicine as a profession, as distinct from a trade or other occupation. That recognition embodies expectations regarding accreditation (in the first instance relating to both training and fitness to practice, through, for example, satisfaction of character tests), behaviour (ethical practice guided by practice codes, as discussed below) and competence. It also acknowledges a substantial degree of self-regulation by the profession, which is deemed to be capable of articulating and administering standards. One consequence of the National Law is that in dealing with privacy relating to practice, paramedicine professionals will be held to a higher standard than people who are not professionals. As noted above, privacy is a matter of responsibilities rather than merely rights; both practitioners and paramedicine administrators are expected to be conscious of privacy and confidentiality issues.

The second reason is that the National Law provides the basis for a uniform paramedicine regime across Australia, bringing together the different state/territory governments in a desirable manner that allows for consistent administration, the mobility of practitioners in search of employment, and the identification of practitioners whose performance means that they are likely to seek to subvert regulation by moving from one jurisdiction to another. As with character tests—where peers and administrators alike expect comprehensive disclosure by candidates and the checking of criminal record databases to prevent entry to the profession of people who cannot be trusted—while the sharing of information about disciplined or de-registered practitioners may be considered by those people as contrary to their privacy, in principle it is both necessary and proportionate.

The third reason is the most direct. The National Law gives authority for the national Australian Health Practitioner Regulation Agency (AHPRA), which oversees the national boards for 14 regulated health professions, as well as, saliently, the Paramedicine Board of Australia. The National Law establishes adjudication bodies (e.g. the state Health Ombudsman in Queensland) and dispute resolution bodies (e.g. the Queensland Civil and Administrative Tribunal), with further disputes being addressed by the courts. In giving effect to overarching regulation of the various health professions, the National Law also gives authority to practitioner codes and interpretative guidelines that deal with matters such as the use of social media, and which are backed by sanctions such as de-registration and termination of employment.[44]

Practitioner code and guidelines

The National Law does not seek to provide exhaustive day-by-day instructions regarding privacy and confidentiality. The existence of other privacy-specific and privacy-related law is taken as a given; co-existing rather than being superseded. Consequently, the paramedicine code and guidelines are more detailed than the National Law from which they draw their authority. They deal with the behaviour of paramedicine practitioners in general. They also specifically refer to both privacy and confidentiality. They will accordingly be referred to tribunals and courts in instances, for example, where there are disputes about discipline and de-registration.[45]

The introduction to the *Interim Code of Conduct* (June 2018) thus states:

Practitioners have ethical and legal obligations to protect the privacy of people requiring and receiving care. Patients or clients have a right to expect that practitioners and their staff will hold information about them in confidence, unless information is required to be released by law or public interest considerations. Practitioners need to obtain informed consent for the care that they provide to their patients or clients. [46]

Part 1 goes on to note that the Code is not a charter of rights, and that it:

... does not address in detail the range of general legal obligations that apply to practitioners, such as those under privacy, child protection and anti-discrimination legislation; responsibilities to employees and other individuals present at a practice under workplace health and safety legislation; and vicarious liability for employees under the general law. Practitioners should ensure that they are aware of their legal obligations and act in accordance with them.[47]

Part 3.2, on the relationship between practitioners and the person in care, refers to a 'high standard' of personal conduct, including:

... protecting the privacy and right to confidentiality of patients or clients, unless release of information is required by law or by public interest considerations, and communicating appropriately with and providing relevant information to other stakeholders, including other treating practitioners, in accordance with applicable privacy requirements. [48]

Part 3.4 provides more specific guidance, stating:

Practitioners have ethical and legal obligations to protect the privacy of people requiring and receiving care. Patients or clients have a right to expect that practitioners and their staff will hold information about them in confidence, unless release of information is required by law or public interest considerations. Good practice involves:

a) treating information about patients or clients as confidential and applying appropriate security to electronic and hard copy information

b) seeking consent from patients or clients before disclosing information, where practicable

c) being aware of the requirements of the privacy and/or health records legislation that operates in relevant states and territories and applying these requirements to information held in all formats, including electronic information

d) sharing information appropriately about patients or clients for their healthcare while remaining consistent with privacy legislation and professional guidelines about confidentiality

e) where relevant, being aware that there are complex issues relating to genetic information and seeking appropriate advice about disclosure of such information

f) providing appropriate surroundings to enable private and confidential consultations and discussions to take place

g) ensuring that all staff are aware of the need to respect the confidentiality and privacy of patients or clients and refrain from discussing patients or clients in a non-professional context

h) complying with relevant legislation, policies and procedures relating to consent

i) using consent processes, including formal documentation if required, for the release and exchange of health and medical information, and

j) ensuring that use of social media and e-health is consistent with the practitioner's ethical and legal obligations to protect privacy. [49]

Part 3.16 of the code notes that good practice involves:

> ... facilitating arrangements for the continuing care of all current patients, which may include the transfer or appropriate management of all patient records while following the law governing privacy and health records in the jurisdiction. [50]

Part 11.2 notes the privacy aspect of research ethics, an area discussed by Wendy Bonython in Chapter 15 ('Paramedic research') in this book.

The National Law code for paramedicine practitioners reflects the Australia and New Zealand College of Paramedicine (ANZCP) *Code of Conduct*, which, for example, states:

> ANZCP Members will hold in confidence any information obtained in a professional capacity, using professional judgment only where there is a clear need to share information for the therapeutic benefit and safety of a person. This includes the injudicious use of any form of social media to breach patient confidentiality. Members will understand and apply the principles of informed consent. [51]

For the sake of both consistency and economy, there is currently some sharing of guidelines across the professions under the National Law. Therefore, they should be consulted by paramedicine practitioners in interpreting the code. One example is the interim mandatory notification guideline. Another is the (thinner) interim social media policy document (June 2018), which practitioners can expect to be substantially expanded in coming years.

Institutional requirements

Consistent with the above characterisation of privacy as an ecosystem—in which the performance of individual practitioners is shaped in varying ways and determined by different bodies such as the ANZCP and AHPRA—both the National Law and the code recognise that employers have a role to play in articulating and enforcing privacy and confidentiality.

While there is no uniform policy document and detailed standards, employers instead deal with expectations regarding privacy and confidentiality through policy statements, operational manuals and tools such as warnings when accessing a corporate network. This means that the material and its implementation through training and supervision vary. Practitioners should therefore familiarise themselves with the material in place within their organisations, and on occasion may contribute to the enhancement of that material, given the recognition in the National Law of paramedicine as a profession.

One example of a privacy and confidentiality philosophy is provided by the Ambulance Service of New South Wales, which states:

> All staff will ensure that they keep all information they may obtain or have access to, in the course of their work, private and confidential. The trust of our patients and clients is paramount. [52]

Accordingly:

I will never:

- Use official information without proper authority or for purposes that breach privacy law
- Use or disclose official information acquired in the course of my employment outside of my workplace or professional relationships (eg Professional Colleges) unless required by law or given proper authority to do this
- Misuse information gained while undertaking my work role for personal gain.

I will always comply with the Privacy and Personal Information Protection Act 1998, Health Records and Information Privacy Act 2002 and PD2005 362 (Privacy Manual) with regard to personal information held by the Ambulance Service.

In doing this I will:

- Follow privacy and security procedures in relation to any personal information accessed in the course of my duties
- Preserve the confidentiality of this information
- Inform the appropriate person immediately if a breach of privacy or security relating to information occurs
- Only access personal information that is essential for my duties. This includes accessing any records relating to other staff
- Ensure that any personal information is used solely for the purposes for which it was gathered
- Only divulge personal information to authorised staff of the Ambulance Service who need this information to carry out their duties. …

I will:

- Ensure that unauthorised parties cannot readily access confidential and/or sensitive official information held by me, in any form whether documents, emails, computer files etc
- Maintain the security of confidential and/or sensitive official information overnight and at all other times when my place of work is unattended
- Only discuss confidential and/or sensitive official information with authorised people, either within or outside the Ambulance Service. [53]

Conclusion

Although new technologies and new social practices will continue to raise challenges for practitioners in their professional and private lives, the principles underlying privacy and confidentiality law will remain stable and relevant. In an era where privacy is being abused by governments and businesses, such as Cambridge Analytica, those principles are more relevant than ever.

Nevertheless, both practitioners and institutions are fallible. Mistakes will occur; sometimes there will be conflicts. Professional ethics and guidance by practitioner bodies therefore remain important; although some failures will be addressed through litigation.

Finally, principles are often abstractions that are given effect through detailed guidelines and operational protocols. The profession, under the National Law, has agreement about the significance of privacy and confidentiality as foundations of the trust that is fundamental to the delivery of services, and to the social contract between the profession and the people who receive care. The specifics of what those principles mean in practice will be influenced in coming years by institutional agendas and the evolving of more detailed guidance under the code.

Review Questions

1 What law applies to your tweeting of images from a crash scene?

2 Are there ethical rather than legal restrictions on such tweeting?

3 You are aware that a colleague's substance misuse problem raises questions about her performance. She says that you cannot alert a supervisor or another agency because it would breach her privacy. Is she correct?

4 The corporate wifi network in your agency is insecure: its password is 'password'. What can you do about potential exposure of personnel and incident records?

5 Your union is considering agreement to mandatory urine and blood tests of all employees in return for a small salary increase and increased job security. Should you agree?

Endnotes

1   Solove, D. (2011) *Nothing to Hide: The False Tradeoff Between Privacy and Security*. New Haven: Yale University Press; Bonython, W. and Arnold, B.B. (2015) Privacy, personhood, and property in the age of genomics. *Laws* 4(3), 377–412; Bygrave, L. (2002) *Data Protection Law: Approaching its Rationale, Logic and Limits*. The Hague: Kluwer Law; Rosen, J. (2004) *The Naked Crowd: Reclaiming Security and Freedom in an Anxious Age*. New York: Random House; Nasheri, H. (2005) *Economic Espionage and Industrial Spying*. Cambridge: Cambridge University Press.

2   Joyce, C.M., Wainer, J., Piterman, L. et al. (2009) Trends in the paramedic workforce: a profession in transition. *Australian Health Review*, 33(4), 533–540; Williams, B., Onsman, A. and Brown, T. (2009) From stretcher-bearer to paramedic: the Australian paramedics' move towards professionalisation. *Australasian Journal of Paramedicine*, 7(4). Available: https://ajp.paramedics.org/index.php/ajp/article/view/191

3   Wardle, J.L., Sibbritt, D., Broom, A. et al. (2016) Is health practitioner regulation keeping pace with the changing practitioner and health-care landscape? An Australian perspective. *Frontiers in Public Health* 4, 91–97.

4   Solove, D. (2004) *The Digital Person: Technology and Privacy in the Information Age*. New York: New York University Press.

5   Kateb, G. (2011) *Human Dignity*. Cambridge, Mass: Harvard University Press; Nussbaum, M. (2006) *Frontiers of Justice: Disability, Nationality, Species Membership*. Cambridge, Mass: Harvard University Press.

6   See, for example, Igo, S. (2018) *The Known Citizen: A History of Privacy in Modern America*. Cambridge, Mass: Harvard University Press.

7   Solove, D. (2002) Conceptualizing privacy. *California Law Review* 90(4), 1087–1156; Sofsky, W. (2009) *Privacy: A Manifesto*. Princeton: Princeton University Press; Wacks, R. (1993) *Personal Information: Privacy and the Law*. Oxford: Oxford University Press.

8   Regan, P. (2002) Privacy as a common good in the digital world. *Information, Communication and Society* 5(3), 382–405; Cohen, J. (2013) What privacy is for. *Harvard Law Review* 126, 1904–1933; Inness, J. (1992) *Privacy, Intimacy and Isolation*. Oxford: Oxford University Press.

9   *Attorney General (NT) v Heinemann Publishers Pty Ltd* (1987) 10 SLWLR 86, at 91; *Commonwealth of Australia v John Fairfax and Sons Ltd* (1981) ALJR 45, at 49; *Director of Public Prosecutions v Smith* [1991] 1 VR 63, at 75.

10   Delany, H. and Carolan, E. (2008) *The Right to Privacy*. Dublin: Thomson Round Hall; Warby, M., Moreham, N. and Christie, I. (2011) *Tugendhat and Christie: The Law of Privacy and the Media*. Oxford: Oxford University Press; Paterson, M. (2015) *Freedom of Information and Privacy in Australia: Information Access 2.0*. Chatswood: LexisNexis Butterworths.

11   Aplin, T., Bently, L., Johnson, P. and Malynicz, S. (2012) *Gurry on Breach of Confidence: The Protection of Confidential Information*. Oxford: Oxford University Press; Pattenden, R. and Sheehan, D. (2016) *The Law of Professional–client Confidentiality*. Oxford: Oxford University Press.

12   *Coco v AN Clark (Engineers)* [1969] RPC 1; *Saltman Engineering v Campbell Engineering* (1948) 65 RPC 20; *Seager v Copydex* [1967] 2 All ER 415; *Moorgate Tobacco v Philip Morris (No 2)* (1984) 156 CLR 414.

13   *X v Y* (1987) 13 IPR 202, [1988] 2 All ER 648; *R (Axon) v Secretary of State for Health* [2006] EWHC 37 (Admin); *W v Edgell* [1990] 1 Ch 35.

14   Rishworth, P., Huscroft, G., Optican, S. et al. (2003) *The New Zealand Bill of Rights*. Melbourne: Oxford University Press; Australian Law Reform Commission (ALRC). (2014) *Serious Invasions of Privacy in the Digital Era*. ALRC Report 123. Sydney: ALRC. See also *Armfield v Naughton* [2014] NZHRRT 48 and *Holmes v Housing New Zealand Corporation* [2014] NZHRRT 54.

15   Joseph, S, Schultz, J. and Castan, M. (2004) *The International Covenant on Civil and Political Rights: Cases, Materials and Commentary*, 2nd ed. Oxford: Oxford University Press. See *Human Rights Act 2004* (ACT), s 12, and *Charter of Human Rights and Responsibilities Act 2006* (Vic), s 13.

16   Sprenger, P. (2009) Sun on privacy: 'Get over it'. *Wired* 7(1), 34–35; Bagaric, M. (2007, 22 April) Privacy is the last thing we need. *The Age*, p. 15.

17   See, for example, Office of the Australian Information Commissioner (OAIC). (2017) *Australian Community Attitudes to Privacy Survey 2017*. Sydney: OAIC. Online. Available: https://www.oaic.gov.au/engage-with-us/community-attitudes/australian-community-attitudes-to-privacy-survey-2017; King, T., Brankovic, L. and Gillard, P. (2012) Perspectives of Australian adults about protecting the privacy of their health information in statistical databases. *International Journal of Medical Informatics*, 81(4), 279–289.

18   Nissenbaum, H. (2004) Privacy as contextual integrity. *Washington Law Review* 79(1), 119–158; Solove, Conceptualizing privacy.

19   Jay, R. (2012) *Data Protection Law and Practice*. London: Sweet and Maxwell; Kuner, C. (2007) *European Data Protection Law, Corporate Compliance and Regulation*. Oxford: Oxford University Press; Kuner, C. (2013) *Transborder Data Flows and Data Privacy Law*. Oxford: Oxford University Press.

20   Voigt, P. and Von dem Bussche, A. (2017) *The EU General Data Protection Regulation (GDPR)*. Berlin: Springer.

21   Albrecht, J.P. (2016) How the GDPR will change the world. *European Data Protection Law Review* 2, 287–289; Bennett, S. (2018) GDPR: Change to European privacy laws and its impact on Australian businesses. *Governance Directions* 70(2), 85–89.

22   Warren, S. and Brandeis, L. (1890) The Right to Privacy. *Harvard Law Review* IV(5), 193–220.

23   *Telecommunications Act 1997* (Cth), ss 276(1)(a)(iv), 277(1)(a)(ii), 285(1)(a) and 285(2).

24   *Healthcare Identifiers Act 2010* (Cth), ss 25A and 26.

25 Loughlin, P., McDonald, P. and Van Krieken, R. (2010) *Celebrity and the Law*. Leichhardt: Federation Press.

26 *Health Practitioner Regulation National Law Act 2009* (Qld), Sch, Pt 8, s 140; Pt 10, s 237. Note the mandatory reporting by education providers under Pt 8, s 143.

27 Wolf, G. (2017) Compelling safety: reforming Australian treating doctors' mandatory reporting obligations. *Sydney Law Review* 39(2), 199–232.

28 Pascoe, J. and Welsh, M. (2011) Whistleblowing, ethics and corporate culture: theory and practice in Australia. *Common Law World Review* 40(2), 144–173; Ryan, H. (2014) The half-hearted protection of journalists' sources: judicial interpretation of Australia's shield laws. *Media and Arts Law Review* 19, 325–357.

29 *Data-Matching Program (Assistance and Tax) Act 1990* (Cth).

30 *TV Works and The Order of St John* [2009] NZBSA 5.

31 Kosta, E. (2013) *Consent in European Data Protection Law*. Leiden: Martinus Nijhof.

32 *Argyll v Argyll* [1967] Ch 302.

33 *Douglas v Hello!* [2001] 2 ALL ER 289.

34 *Saltman v Campbell* (1948) 65 RPC 203; *Seager v Copydex* [1967] 2 All ER 415; *Woolworths Ltd v Olsen* (2004) 63 IPR 258.

35 Irving, M. (2012) *The Contract of Employment*. Chatswood: LexisNexis Butterworths.

36 See, for example, *Ambulance Services Act 1986* (Vic); *Emergencies Act 2004* (ACT); *Ambulance Service Act 1982* (Tas); and *Health Services Act 1997* (NSW).

37 *Semayne's case* [1572] EngR 333 and *Bostock v Saunders* (1773) 2 Wm Bl 912, endorsed in *Monis v The Queen* [2013] HCA 4.

38 *Information Privacy Act 2014* (ACT); *Workplace Privacy Act 2010* (ACT); and *Health Records (Privacy and Access) Act 1997* (ACT).

39 *Health Records and Information Privacy Act 2002* (NSW).

40 *Do Not Call Register Act 2006* (Cth); *Spam Act 2003* (Cth).

41 It is reinforced through the data breach reporting scheme introduced under the *Privacy Amendment (Notifiable Data Breaches) Act 2017* (Cth).

42 El Emam, K. (2013) *Guide to the De-Identification of Personal Health Information*. Boca Raton: CRC Press.

43 *Ambulance Services Act 1986* (Vic); *Health Care Act 2008* (SA).

44 *Health Practitioner Regulation National Law*, Sch, Pt 5, ss 39 and 41.

45 *ER 24 Pty Ltd t/a ER 24 v Ms Jennifer May Elliot* [2017] FWC 391.

46 Paramedicine Board of Australia. (2018) *Interim Code of Conduct for Registered Health Practitioners*. Melbourne: Australian Health Practitioner Regulation Agency, at p. 5. Online. Available: https://www.paramedicineboard.gov.au/professional-standards/codes-guidelines-and-policies/code-of-conduct.aspx (accessed 3 December 2018).

47 Ibid., at p. 6.

48 Ibid., at p. 10.

49 Ibid., at p. 11.

50 Ibid., at p. 15.

51 Australian and New Zealand College of Paramedicine (ANZCP). *Code of Conduct*. Leichhardt, NSW: ANZCP. Online. Available: https://www.anzcp.org.au/anzcp-website-subscriber-terms-and-conditions (accessed 27 February 2019).

52 Ambulance Service of New South Wales. (2007) *Code of Conduct*. Sydney: Ambulance Service of New South Wales, at 1.4.1.

53 Ibid., at 1.4.1s.

Chapter 11

Record-keeping and the patient healthcare record

Peter Lang

Learning objectives

After completing this chapter, you will be able to:

- describe the purpose of a patient healthcare record and its uses
- outline the type of information that should be included in the record
- describe the method for correcting errors in a record
- identify what right a patient has to gain access to their record
- list the circumstances under which a patient or other person can be allowed access to paramedic records.

Definitions

Patient healthcare record (PHCR) A document containing personal, sensitive and healthcare information, including a patient's medical history and the healthcare provided by health professionals to facilitate the ongoing safe care and treatment of a patient. The PHCR does not just relate to a traditional ambulance 'case sheet', but may also include referral letters, plans, forms, 'schedule' or 'section' documents, and transfer-of-care records, and may be on paper, be electronic or be a combination of both (hybrid).

VACIS system A computerised patient healthcare record system designed by Ambulance Victoria that is now used by a number of Australian ambulance services. ('VACIS' is an acronym for 'Victorian Ambulance Clinical Information System'.)[1]

An introductory case

Paramedic witness

It is 06:00 h, and you are a single on-call paramedic who has been called to a person who is unconscious with 'cardiac problems'. On arrival you assess the scene, and all is quiet. A calm, elderly male meets you in the street and leads you to a supine body under a blanket on a mattress on the grass in a backyard of a residential home. On your way across the driveway you ask the bystander what has happened. You are told a jumbled story about the patient collapsing because his heart gave out. Your questions are evaded with other rambling, confused responses. Things look quiet and nothing looks suspicious, so you continue in. As you approach the patient, you see that he is in his late 20s, and you start to realise something is not right. You are told that 'It wasn't me, it was him—Max did it', as you kneel down and pull the blanket off the patient. As you ask 'Where's Max? What did he do?', you notice that the patient has a bullet hole in the centre of his chest. He is almost as pale as you have suddenly become; he is not breathing and has no pulse. You nervously look at the bystander, as he says, 'Max did it, Max killed him—then he took off in my car.' Shortly afterwards, the police enter the scene and take control. You hear the police ask the bystander for an account of what happened, and you hear the bystander say that he just found the patient lying there and that he has no idea what happened.

This chapter will explain the importance of correct, contemporaneous and complete documentation, and what aspects of paramedic practice this can impact on. In cases such as this one, a paramedic's notes and what a paramedic hears and sees are often used and relied on, not only in the clinical context, but as evidence in a number of different environments. In this case, a statement made to the paramedic by the bystander differs from accounts given later to police. Statements made to the paramedic, things the paramedic witnesses, and written documentation made by the paramedic about a case will at times become part of the evidence, and may be significant for police, the coroner and the courts. In this case, the reference to 'Max' by the bystander may be significant in giving the police a lead as to the possible suspect, and, unless the bystander gives this information to police, the paramedic may be the only one who can provide police with the information.

Introduction

Healthcare professionals, including paramedics, must document details of their assessment of, management of, and interaction with every patient. This important information is recorded on a document(s) commonly known as the *patient healthcare record (PHCR)*. The record must be compiled at the time of the interaction or incident, and finalised shortly afterwards. This is commonly known as *writing contemporaneously*, and is more likely to ensure that an accurate record is made. In the Australian and New Zealand environment, the traditional central ambulance patient record is commonly either handwritten on a carbonised printed form (usually in triplicate) or typed electronically into a computer program designed for this purpose.

This central document is increasingly being supplemented or augmented by referral and transfer-of-care letters, pro-forma documents, care plans, and other documentation associated with legislative activity (i.e. sections and schedules of mental health legislation). These records, however obtained and recorded, become confidential PHCRs, and are an essential component of the patient's healthcare journey. The record becomes a form of reference to be used by clinicians to assist in the understanding of, and the ongoing delivery of, healthcare to the patient. It is also used as a resource for a number of secondary and future purposes.

In some situations, the PHCR may also be given to the patient or another healthcare professional at the conclusion of the paramedic interaction, particularly if the matter is non-urgent and the patient will be referred on, left in their own care or left in the care of others to later present to their chosen healthcare professional. This record may also at times be called on by a court or investigator as evidence, providing support to, or acting as, primary evidence of names, dates, times and places, and providing details of what the paramedic saw, heard, was told or did in a particular situation. In other situations, the documentation may give effect to a legislative function, such as limiting freedom or liberty under a section or schedule of, for example, mental health legislation.

Effective, clear and concise documentation of objective, relevant and first-hand information is essential to capturing the requisite detail onto the document, so that it is not only credible, but is useful in providing a record that contributes to the holistic care of the patient. The correction of errors must be performed in an appropriate way to ensure that the integrity of the record is not compromised, or its reliability rendered invalid.

Importantly, a PHCR is a private and confidential document about the patient with whom a paramedic interacts. Maintaining the privacy of those records is not only an ethical responsibility for paramedics, it is also a legal one. In every jurisdiction in which a paramedic works, the government has legislation protecting an individual's rights to privacy with respect to the collection, storage and use of their medical records. This legislative requirement therefore impacts on the way in which paramedics and paramedic services collect, store and use that information appropriately. Privacy is an important responsibility of all healthcare workers.

This chapter will explore:

- the nature of a patient healthcare record
- electronic records
- record ownership
- confidentiality and privacy
- record access
- what a record should contain
- correction of errors in the record.

What is a 'patient healthcare record'?

A *patient healthcare record (PHCR)* is a record that is created by a clinician, usually immediately after an interaction with a patient. It generally contains details to identify the individual the record pertains to, as well as an account of the patient's health information and any information that is linked with the patient's episode of care. (See Appendix 11.1 for an example.) This may include their medical history of previous illnesses, injuries and treatments, and medications the patient is currently taking and has been previously prescribed. It may also contain results of any assessments, blood tests, scans, X-rays, details of any sensitivities or allergies, and any other relevant information related to the patient's health, such as social details, family history, disabilities and details of any health professionals who have been involved with the patient. A paramedic's record, case sheet, slip, electronic record, transfer form, referral letter or any other document that is used by a paramedic to record details of an incident or personal health information is considered a PHCR.

The PHCR is predominantly used as a confidential source of information given by paramedics to other authorised healthcare professionals who take responsibility for that patient. Documentation supports the verbal handover report given as the patient is physically transferred, and provides a point of reference for the receiving clinicians to understand the events leading up to the patient's current condition(s), observations made, including signs and symptoms, their previous medical history, allergies and sensitivities, their current medications, any treatments and procedures performed by the paramedic, and any outstanding or unresolved issues. This information informs and supports the continuation of treatment as the patient continues their journey through the healthcare system.

In the paramedic context, a PHCR may also contain other non-medical information, such as private health insurance details, government support systems' entitlement status and details, employment status, workplace or institution billing details, patient's address and telephone number(s), relatives' contact details, equipment used to treat the patient, and various forms of demographic information. This information is often collected to enable the paramedic service to obtain funding, substantiate a claim for cost recovery, provide demographic details of work performed, and establish a data set to improve service delivery or to provide contact information for patients or their relatives for further use.

In some organisations and jurisdictions, certain data from the record are also used in a number of other contexts, including in the gathering of statistical information and research data, both medical and organisational, for a number of purposes, including organisational performance, clinical research, motor vehicle crash data analysis, crime statistics, population demographics and clinical outcomes. These data are normally de-identified, and extracted for analysis as required. The record can also be used in clinical auditing for individual paramedic or service performance, and the monitoring of medication administration and equipment usage at a number of organisational levels.

Electronic records

For many years, health records have been collected in paper form. Data may have been collected from these forms, or may have been scanned into electronic form. Doing this was not only labour-intensive, but the data collected were subject to interpretation at the point of transfer, or errors may have been made in the transcription process. With the advent of modern technology, records are increasingly made in electronic form at the patient's side. In 2005, Ambulance Victoria established the *Victorian Ambulance Clinical Information System (VACIS)*, a standardised 'episode'-based electronic patient care record designed for paramedics to enter patient healthcare information and data at the point of care using a portable tablet-style computer.[2] The record (and data) entered by the paramedic is uploaded to a centralised secure data centre for storage and further analysis. The functionality of the system potentially allows for electronic transfer of selected parts of the patient's record to the health facility taking over care of the patient, or for the printing of the report in the ambulance for traditional paper-based record transfer.[3]

A number of state ambulance services in Australia joined to form the *VACIS collaboration*, a non-profit entity enabling the member state services to 'work(ing) together collaboratively to develop, implement and enhance VACIS throughout Australia'. These member services included ACT Ambulance Service, Ambulance Service of New South Wales, Ambulance Tasmania, Ambulance Victoria and Queensland Ambulance Service. Drawing data from these large ambulance services provides a powerful database for research, analysis and service delivery improvement.

An example of one such collaboration is the *Australian Resuscitation Outcomes Consortium (Aus-ROC)*, which 'aims to increase research capacity in the area of out-of-hospital cardiac arrest, with a specific focus on improving rates of survival and outcomes for survivors'.[4] This consortium uses data from a total of eight ambulance services currently, with two more soon to join. Currently Ambulance Victoria, SA Ambulance Service, St John Ambulance Western Australia, St John Ambulance Northern Territory, Queensland Ambulance Service, St John Ambulance New Zealand, Wellington Free Ambulance and Ambulance Tasmania contribute data, with the NSW and ACT ambulance services to join in the near future.[5]

As with all technology, data can be lost or transferred outside secure areas if safety and security systems are not put in place. Governments have been working to keep up with technology by legislating to ensure that safety systems and data security are requirements of any electronic record system. Systems are designed and required to protect privacy and limit access to information.

Systems like the *VACIS electronic medical record (eMR)* (see Fig. 11.1) are kept on secure networks, with password-enabled access and multi-level security clearances preventing unauthorised access. The Australian government is rolling out *My Health Record*, a centralised electronic health records system for all Australians. This system will hold a range of medical records, including allergies, test results and discharge summaries for future use, and provides unique security challenges for the Australian Digital Health Agency, which is the systems operator of My Health Record.[6] The linkages between paramedics and My Health Record are yet to be developed.

Record ownership

The custodial ownership of medical records generally lies with the organisation, individual or facility that collects the information.[7] In most cases of paramedics' practice, the custodian of the records is the body for whom the healthcare professional works, and on whose behalf they collect the records. Paramedics who work for an organisation do not

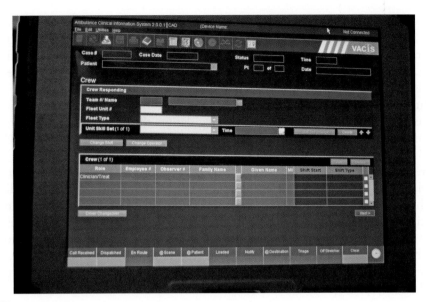

Figure 11.1
VACIS electronic medical record Source: VACIS(R) ©2007

automatically have a right to use the information for their own personal use or for research purposes, despite having collected it on the organisation's behalf. While standards of record storage and security in all jurisdictions are generally similar in intent, the laws that apply depend on where the organisation sits or for which organisation the paramedics practise. Those services provided by the state/territory or by state/territory contractors are required to comply with state/territory legislation. Importantly for paramedics, records should be stored in authorised facilities in accordance with the organisation's record-keeping procedures, which should comply with the relevant jurisdiction's laws.

Confidentiality and privacy

Medical records contain personal, sensitive and private details. As such, society wants to ensure that this information remains private and is protected by laws to prevent it from being misused or disclosed to persons who have no right to it.

In Australia, there are a number of pieces of legislation that aim to maintain privacy for individuals. See Chapter 10 for further discussion on this legislation. Stemming from the legislation are the *Australian Privacy Principles (APPs)*, of which 11 relate to health and hospitals. Many Australian states and territories have enacted their own complementary legislation, which is very similar to, or mirrors, the concepts of the Commonwealth Information Privacy Principles, and have also enacted legislation and policies to protect personal information and provide secure mechanisms for patients and others to access information. Each government department and any health organisation, in turn, must develop policies and practices that support these principles.

In New Zealand, the *Privacy Act 1993*, which contains 12 generic privacy principles, and the *Health Information Privacy Code 1994* aim to maintain privacy for individuals. However, the New Zealand government is currently in the process of making changes to the *Privacy Act*. The proposed changes look to enhancing the powers of the Privacy Commissioner, and introduce mandatory reporting of all privacy breaches.[8] (See Chapter 10 for further discussion on privacy.)

In Australia, there are various pieces of legislation that relate to healthcare records, depending on which jurisdiction the particular organisation operates in and what type of organisation it is. For example, a private paramedic service operating in Western Australia is required to abide by the *Privacy Act 1998* (Cth)[9] and the *Privacy Amendment (Private Sector) Act 2000* (Cth),[10] whereas a public service operating in Western Australia comes under the jurisdiction of the *State Health Act 1911* (WA).[11] This multiple legislative complexity derives from the way in which the Commonwealth of Australia was created and how it operates under the Australian Constitution, with states and the Commonwealth having the ability to create legislation in their respective jurisdictions. However, most of the pieces of legislation are similar, in that they usually mirror or comply with generally accepted privacy principles.

Access to medical records

Access to medical records is an essential aspect of privacy that paramedics should be aware of. In the section 'Patient access to their own records', we explore a patient's ability to gain access to their own healthcare records; and in the section 'Who else can gain access to records?', we look at others who are able to access records and for what purpose. Paramedics are occasionally requested to provide information, and it is necessary for the paramedic as custodian of confidential information to know who they can release information to, and when, and also how to advise a patient should they ask the paramedic for access to their own records. A paramedic should be aware of their institution's policies and processes on record access, and know where applications for such information should be directed.

Patient access to their own records

Case 11.1 illustrates a common occurrence a paramedic may be faced with when interacting with the public. What right does Mr Wilson have to access his records? What advice would you give him on how he might go about obtaining them? We explore this scenario and discuss the answers to these questions in the following text.

Case 11.1 A patient's right to access their PHCR

Mr Wilson knocks on the ambulance station door, wishing to thank the paramedics who assisted him when he fell over in the supermarket last month. He shows off the cast covering his fractured left arm. Mr Wilson also requests a copy of the paramedic's record so he can use it to sue the supermarket for causing his pain and suffering.

The healthcare record is about the patient and their current medical situation, and it could be assumed that, as the record is about the patient, the patient should be entitled to access its content. Generally, the patient is entitled to access any information held about them within the public sector. Applications to obtain personal healthcare records can often be made directly to the organisation where the records are held, and, if this is not possible, through the Australian state or Commonwealth commissioners[12] or via the provisions of the freedom of information Acts in each jurisdiction.

However, access to records in the private sector has not always been possible. In 1995, Ms Breen brought a case against her surgeon, Dr Williams, in the Supreme Court of New South Wales to get access to her records. Although Dr Williams had records pertaining to her, the access was refused, based on the argument that the doctor had not made the notes with the intent of her copying and reading them. Ms Breen subsequently lost her appeal to the New South Wales Court of Appeal, and to the High Court of Australia, on the basis that a doctor can provide information to the patient from their notes without disclosing the entire notes, and therefore should not be compelled to do so.[13]

Following this case, a number of changes were made to improve the ability of patients to access information held by private practitioners, including the establishment of the information privacy principles (specifically APP 6) under the *Privacy Act 1988* (Cth), as well as the enactment of the *Privacy Amendment (Private Sector) Act 2000* (Cth) and the establishment of the Commonwealth Privacy Commissioner,[14] who is now known as the Australian Information Commissioner.

In New Zealand, applications for access to records can be made through the record-holder, and can be refused only in exceptional circumstances, as described in the *Privacy Act 1993*. Private organisations can charge reasonable fees for copies of X-rays and other images; however, if the fees will be over $30, the cost details must be provided to the applicant prior to them incurring the costs. Access to records in New Zealand is governed under the *Health Information Privacy Code 1994*, which has the force of law. Any complaints, lack of action or over-charging for records can be referred to the New Zealand Privacy Commissioner, who can investigate and rule on the complaint.[15]

Generally, paramedics' records may be accessed by patients,[16] and so paramedics should be aware that at some point their documentation will not only be read by other clinicians, but may also be read by the patient. Patients wishing to gain access to their records should be directed to the appropriate office for access. It is impractical and unreasonable for paramedics to be expected to supply a copy of a record to a patient on the spot, so paramedic service providers should have up-to-date policies on how to deal with applications from patients wishing to access their records. These policies should comply with the relevant laws in the jurisdiction in which the organisation operates. Paramedics should be aware of, and familiarise themselves with, these policies, so that they are able to inform and direct patients to the correct office or person when approached.

Who else can gain access to records?

Paramedics routinely hand over a copy of their completed PHCR when they hand responsibility of a patient to another health professional at a hospital. In Case 11.2, we

Case 11.2 To share or not?

You attend to and treat Mr Jones, a 73-year-old man who has open leg wounds after his leg collided with a table corner as he was walking around in his home. In taking a history, you discover that he also has chronic circulation problems as a result of his type 2 diabetes mellitus. You dress his wounds, but you are concerned about his healing capacity given his co-existing conditions. However, the patient decides he does not wish to be transported to hospital, and will instead attend his local general practitioner at the local medical clinic.

examine a situation where a paramedic might consider divulging health information to another person outside of the typical situation, and in the following text we explore the legal context of that information transfer.

In this case, you are unsure about what you are legally permitted to share with the patient's general practitioner. We explore the legal context of this situation in the following text.

The record can sometimes contain pertinent information that can be relied on to substantiate claims, refute accusations, justify actions or provide details that lead to a conclusion. Courts often call on paramedics and their records to assist in court proceedings, particularly where the paramedic attended a person who is now subject to court proceedings. Police, the coroner and the courts can gain access to a person's records by subpoena. Often, when making insurance claims, a claimant is required to sign a release to permit the insurance provider access to health record information prior to a claim being reviewed.[17] On occasions, the details of a record can be scrutinised closely and may be pivotal in deciding a claim or case.

Under the national privacy principles in both Australia and New Zealand, and in legislation in most jurisdictions, any health information collected must not be used or disclosed without consent for a secondary purpose, unless it is directly related to the primary purpose for which it was collected,[18] or unless releasing it is necessary for the prevention of serious threat to life. In the case study of Mr Jones, the information was collected to deliver health services to Mr Jones, and the release of information by the paramedics to Mr Jones's general practitioner or to another health professional involved in the continuation of his treatment and healthcare for the same conditions would be permitted under this principle.

Content of a record

Case 11.3 illustrates the importance of being objective in documenting your observations. Paramedics often see things that conflict with what they have been told, so it is important to identify and clearly document what has been witnessed first-hand, and what has been said to have occurred. In this case, the paramedic observes that Mrs Peterson is no longer

Case 11.3 Dealing with inconsistencies

A paramedic has responded to a motor vehicle crash involving two cars. On arrival he finds an elderly female, who identifies herself as Mrs Peterson, sitting in the gutter near a car. She tells the paramedic that she was in the sedan with front-end damage. Her car has both passenger- and driver-side doors open. The other car, which has been hit side-on, contains a deceased male. The paramedic commences assessment of Mrs Peterson, and during his secondary survey he notices that, among other injuries, she has a visible seatbelt haematoma mark crossing from her left shoulder to her right hip. The paramedic asks where she was sitting in the car at the time of the crash and whether anyone else was with her, and she reports that she was the only occupant and that she was driving.

in the car, both front doors of the car are open, and she has a seatbelt haematoma consistent with someone who had been sitting on the passenger side of the vehicle. Mrs Peterson informs the paramedic that she was the only occupant and that she was driving. Is it possible she was the driver? Is it possible she was the passenger and the driver has absconded from the scene? What would you do if you were the paramedic, and how should this case be documented?

The most appropriate way to deal with this is to clarify the information with Mrs Peterson, including having a discussion about the seatbelt marks, and in doing so you would express your concern for anyone else who may have been in the vehicle who may have serious injuries. There may be a valid explanation for these inconsistencies; however, you need to explore them in case a third person is injured somewhere. Document the facts, including the direction of the seatbelt haematoma, clearly state that you found the patient out of the vehicle on your arrival, and note that the patient informed you that she was driving. It will also be necessary to inform the police of your suspicions and why, as the information you have will not otherwise be available to them, and it will assist them in making inquiries about the possibility of another occupant in the vehicle. The records you keep of this incident could be called on by the police, the courts, the hospital or even Mrs Peterson's doctor, so it is vitally important you record the information properly.

Record formatting and the content of the health information collected vary greatly from jurisdiction to jurisdiction, as there is no one model to follow. Traditionally, each ambulance service designed its own paper-based (usually A3-format) triplicate form to record an event or patient interaction, the medical details, the billing details and any other relevant information. (But increasingly they are now also being used to collect data for later analysis.) Each jurisdiction developed its own format, and, while based on similar health information, generally these formats were structured around each organisation's needs and did not necessarily collect the same information. Many organisations progressed from handwritten notes to a combination of free text and tick boxes and coloured-in fields to enable scanning and data collection.

In Australia in particular, with the state ambulance authorities forming the Convention of Ambulance Authorities, a standardised data collection set was agreed on,[19] and the mandatory fields have subsequently helped to focus documentation on particular sets of data. As we have already discussed in this chapter, in recent years standardised eMR systems have been, or are being, introduced into state/territory ambulance services. Many of the services are using the same eMR system, thus standardising data collection and the general format of the central medical record.

Additional specific paper-based documents have been implemented in some jurisdictions to use to hand over a patient to non-traditional (i.e. not an emergency department) healthcare practitioners, particularly where the traditional PHCR is not practical or requires augmentation. Examples include a paper referral letter to a general practitioner where a patient is being referred away from the traditional emergency department pathway to their general practitioner, or where a tool or pro-forma is used to support the handing over of specific information to specialist health providers (or departments), such as when formally enacting a section of mental health legislation, providing specific transfer-of-care information associated with a detailed assessment (e.g. acute myocardial infarction, stroke) or to highlight a particular risk (e.g. increased risk of falls). All of these tools are designed to support and augment the handover of clinical information to provide an ongoing continuum of care.

The importance of how a medical record is written is highlighted in Case 11.4. Ultimately, this was a case that more relevantly revealed the court's view of paramedics, and its understanding and valuing of paramedics' work. From the lawyers representing the plaintiff, through the state courts and up to the High Court, the sentiment was the same. At no time was a paramedic called to explain the meaning of the notes, nor to allow the court to determine whether the notes were expert opinion or, indeed, simply a lay opinion based on the things the paramedic writing the notes had heard and seen for himself. Case notes are recognised at law as 'business records', and as such they can be admitted to the court and used as evidence of what has or has not happened, without the court necessarily having to rely on a direct account from the person who wrote them. However, given the dispute over, first, the importance or not of the question mark and, secondly, the discussion about 'opinion' evidence, and, more specifically, the opinion of the paramedics, one would have thought the paramedics themselves would have been called to offer an explanation to the court.

Indeed, the court demonstrated a lack of understanding as to why the paramedics would make such a notation at all. Paramedics understand that the mechanism of a patient's injury can assist in diagnosis and treatment. The court seemed to think that the opinion was recorded for possible future investigations as to the cause of the injury (e.g. coronial inquiry) or because they are required to do so as a matter of 'training'. They supposed that the question mark was placed in the statement because it was 'merely something that would be consistent with training, that is to say, not to be adamant but to put forward one's best opinion taking into account all the circumstances'.[20] In fact, the High Court

Case 11.4 The importance of punctuation

In the early hours of the morning, an ambulance was called to a man in a drain in a park in Lithgow, New South Wales. The man, Mr Jackson, was found at the foot of a 1.5-m high drain wall. He had multiple injuries, including a serious head injury that rendered him unconscious. The paramedic case notes recorded the history as '? Fall from 1.5 metres onto concrete'. The paramedics treated the man, and he was taken to hospital. The man later sued the council for negligence for failing to erect a fence that would have prevented him suffering his multiple injuries.

There was a dispute as to how the man's injuries had been caused, because there were a number of different ways by which he could have arrived at the bottom of the drain. If Mr Jackson could prove, on the balance of probabilities, that he had suffered the injury as a result of falling off the 'high', unprotected side of the drain, he would be eligible for compensation for his injuries. He relied on the ambulance notes to prove his case.

The court was presented with the case notes without the '?' included. It had been cut off in the photocopying of the documents. The court thought that the statement 'Fall from 1.5 metres onto concrete' was the opinion of the treating paramedic, and thus it added weight to Mr Jackson's case. The case came before another court; however, once it was discovered that the '?' had been missing from the material tendered to the original court, the second court had to consider whether the missing question mark made a difference to Mr Jackson's case. To resolve this matter the case went all the way to the High Court. The High Court said that the paramedic statement '? Fall from 1.5 metres' was so 'ambiguous as to be irrelevant', and that, as such, the question mark did not matter. In addition, the court found that it was 'not possible positively to find that [the paramedic notes] stated an opinion' as to the cause of Mr Jackson's injuries. The case was dismissed.[21]

did not think that the paramedics were expressing an opinion about the cause of the injury at all, and as such the notes were inadmissible.

The following sets of information are generally accepted as required in any PHCR:

- patient identification
- critical information (such as allergies)
- important and relevant information (such as mechanism of injury)
- presenting problem, conditions, provisional diagnosis
- history and assessment findings (including pertinent negatives)
- current medications and other conditions
- treatment given and medications administered.

In the following sections, we shall outline each of these types of information.

Patient identification

The patient must be identified, or the record must be clearly identifiable as pertaining to this particular patient as part of the record, and each page should clearly contain the same identification information. First name, surname, date of birth, age, address, medical record number or healthcare card number are all examples of identifying information that is specific to a patient and is used for their identification.[22] This is essential to ensure that the documentation and subsequent information contained within pertains to the correct patient. Errors of identification are common, and incorrect identification can have dire consequences, such as the incorrect administration of medication, which in some cases has caused the death of a patient.

Critical information

Information of a critical nature, such as allergies, medication reactions, blood disorders, immune deficiencies and other critical information must be recorded clearly and obviously on each page, so other clinicians can clearly see and check for these alerts prior to administration of medications.[23] Not knowing this information can result in medications being given that will cause serious harm to the patient.

Important and relevant information

Paramedics often exclusively gain insight and gather other information from the patient, the scene of an incident and bystanders, which can be essential in the assessment, management and ongoing care of a patient further along the timeline. If this information is not recorded, it is often lost, and lack of this knowledge may impact on the accuracy and time taken to diagnose and manage a patient. The mechanism of injury in trauma patients is often helpful in understanding possible injuries, particularly where a patient has suffered a range of major injuries and pinpointing a specific internal injury is proving problematic. This includes, but is not limited to, the angle of impact, the estimated speed, distance of fall, type and amount of damage to vehicle, airbag deployment, location of patient, ejection from or presence in vehicle, length of knife (in stabbings), type and calibre of weapon, accelerant type in burns, or type of medication, chemical or poison ingested. This information may be important at a later stage, and should be included if possibly linked to the patient's condition.

Presenting problem, conditions, provisional diagnosis

In paramedic practice the presenting problem is a standard piece of information that is provided to ensure that others reading the documentation are clear on what the patient's main reason for calling or chief complaint was. Generally the patient is seeking assistance in relieving the chief complaint. Depending on the paramedic's level of training and experience, and on the organisational procedures, a provisional diagnosis may also be provided and documented on the record. A provisional diagnosis is made when a paramedic uses experience, understanding and knowledge to evaluate the patient's condition, using clinical signs and symptoms, information gained through assessment and exploration of the patient's history and other possible causes, to establish a working hypothesis of what the most likely underlying problem or cause is, so as to implement a treatment regimen.

History and assessment findings

The history of the patient's current condition and/or pre-existing conditions, and any clinical findings identified by primary and secondary assessments, must be documented to provide other clinicians with a clear record of what information the paramedic found and based their provisional diagnosis and treatments on. Any injuries, illness, events leading up to the situation, medications taken, actions, signs, symptoms, observations and history should all be documented as they relate to the patient's current condition.[24] It is important to also provide a negative finding or pertinent negative to a specific test or assessment, particularly if it is best practice for that assessment to be carried out in that circumstance. For example, if a diabetic patient was feeling unwell, it would be best practice to assess whether the patient's blood glucose level is within normal ranges. The details of that assessment should be documented, regardless of its result, to demonstrate that it was undertaken.

Current medications and other conditions

Noting current medications and co-existing conditions is essential in providing the overall medical condition of the patient, and will inform and impact on the continuance of care for the patient. For example, a diabetic will require additional consideration due to the effects of the condition on micro-circulation. Additionally, monitoring of blood glucose levels and dietary considerations must be made if the patient requires admission into a health facility or if extended pre-hospital care is required.

Treatment given and medications administered

Details of any advice given, treatment applied or medications administered should also be detailed in the health record, including the time of administration, the amounts in weight and volume, the route of administration and the authority for the administration.[25] If not already obvious (i.e. in some private practices where a number of loose sheets may be in use for one patient), the identity of the individual must be clearly documented on each individual page. This provides a clear record of what was provided to the patient for future reference.

Other considerations

In addition, paramedics must ensure that their documentation is objective, presented fairly, completely factual, and without influence from emotional or personal prejudices. It should be accurate, where due care has been applied to record all of the relevant facts based on what was observed, with no doubt, speculation, assumption or hearsay included in the record. Records must be concise, authentic and timely, made at the time of the incident or event, and must contain only accurate and real timelines. Records must be legible and easily read by those who need to read them, so no misunderstandings or incorrect assumptions can be made based on poorly written or constructed records. A record should only contain recognised symbols, abbreviations and shorthand.[26] Misinterpretation and errors may occur as a result of using poor or not universally recognised abbreviations.

National regulation: Paramedicine Board of Australia and the National Law

In the Australian context, from late 2018, as paramedics become registered with the Paramedicine Board of Australia they are required to meet national standards and other associated guidelines and codes set and enforced by the board. In relation to documentation, there are two documents that make particular reference to health records and keeping records. One is the *Interim Code of Conduct*, which was developed under section 39 of the *Health Practitioner Regulation National Law Act* 2009 (Qld)—also known in the abbreviated form as 'the National Law'—and describes a range of behaviours that are expected in the practice of paramedicine. Section 8.4 of the interim code outlines the following:[27]

Section 8.4 Health records

… Good practice involves:

a. keeping accurate, up-to-date, factual, objective and legible records that report relevant details of clinical history, clinical findings, investigations, information given to patients or clients, medication and other management in a form that can be understood by other health practitioners

b. ensuring that records are held securely and are not subject to unauthorised access, regardless of whether they are held electronically and/or in hard copy

c. ensuring that records show respect for patients or clients and do not include demeaning or derogatory remarks

d. ensuring that records are sufficient to facilitate continuity of care

e. making records at the time of events or as soon as possible afterwards

f. recognising the right of patients or clients to access information contained in their health records and facilitating that access, and

g. promptly facilitating the transfer of health information when requested by patients or clients.

In addition to the code of conduct, the Paramedicine Board of Australia has (under section 38 of the National Law) adopted interim *Professional Capabilities for Registered Paramedics*. This document provides guidance on how paramedics should perform. In relation to records and documentation, a subsection of 'Domain 4: Safety, risk management and quality assurance' outlines the following expectations:[28]

---

4. Maintains records appropriately

Record information systematically in an accessible and retrievable form

keep accurate, comprehensive, logical, legible and concise records

use only accepted terminology in completing patient care records, and

---

review, communicate, record and manage patient/service user information accurately, consistent with protocols, procedures and legislative requirements for maintaining patient/service user records.

Patient/service user information management must comply with confidentiality and privacy. The registered paramedic must demonstrate awareness of the legislative requirements about ownership, storage, retention and destruction of patient/service user records and other practice documentation.

Correction of errors

Case 11.5 is an example of a not-so-common but plausible mistake that a paramedic may encounter in their documentation. We explore the correct way to deal with this type of error, and the rationale for this action. Should Barry go back and scribble out the error? How should the paramedic deal with the issue? How should it be corrected? We will explore the correct manner of dealing with this type of error and others in the following text.

In documentation, there are a number of errors that commonly occur, and these are easily dealt with if a few basic principles are applied. It is important to note that mistakes happen and that everyone makes them, so being clear and open about the mistake is best practice. Hiding errors (or scribbling them out or using corrective fluid to change them) only adds complexity to a simple problem, as well as introducing doubt as to what was written underneath, and opens speculation as to what is being covered up. Clarity and open corrections are easier to explain.

In the event of writing an incorrect word, figure or statement while making notes, the best form of correcting the mistake is to put a line through the error—do not delete, obliterate, obscure or completely block out or use correction fluid or tape. Providing an explanation, or notation 'written in error' or similar, in the notes, and signing, dating

Case 11.5 When terminology matters

Paramedic Barry Smith completes a healthcare record following a case. The case involved a semi-conscious patient who had suffered a traumatic head injury, and was experiencing a difficult airway. After off-loading the patient, Barry is replenishing the medications kit at the station at the end of the shift and notices an error, where the medication 'morphine' has been written instead of 'metoclopramide'. Barry has already lodged the PHCR as part of the hospital's records. It appears from the written record that paramedic Smith administered 10 mg morphine IV to a patient, when in practice he actually administered metoclopramide.

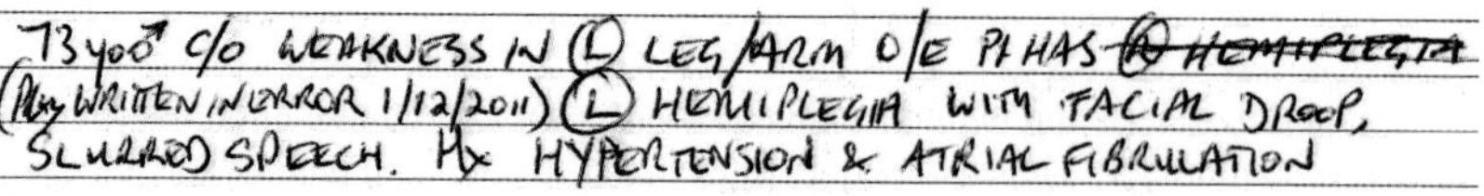

Figure 11.2 Correcting documentation

and noting the time on the record before continuing on with the correct information is the best and most transparent way of correcting an error (see Fig. 11.2).[29] This method identifies that the crossed-out section is deliberately crossed out, and provides details of why it was crossed out, the identity of who corrected it, and when it was corrected.

If the correction is brought into question at a later time, the document is easily analysed, and what was written in error can be identified, removing any doubt or speculation that what was changed was anything other than a genuine mistake. In the case of carbonised handwritten paramedic records, the corrections will be transferred to all copies by the carbonated paper, so copies left at the health facility at handover will corroborate the original documents held by the paramedic service, further validating that the corrections were made at the time of the incident. With electronic paramedic notes, corrections made during the creation of the document will of course be made in the text, up until the record is printed or electronically transferred to the receiving facility at the handover of the patient.

In the event of an error being identified much later, such as in the case of Barry mentioned in Case 11.5, the most appropriate action is to make an addendum to the record by whatever method is possible without changing the original record.[30] Changing the original document after it was written would diminish its value as a contemporaneous note. As most records are copied or shared with the receiving health facility, any changes to only one copy would also seriously compromise the reliability of the document as a form of evidence. An element of doubt would be introduced as to the validity of the document as a true record of events, and anything on it would then be brought into question. The creation of an addendum or subsequent record provides two clear records, with both individual records standing alone without being tampered with—one that was made at the time, and a second that was made when the new information came to light. The new record requires cross-referencing information to the older one, with dates, times, signatures and reasons for changes to ensure that it is linked appropriately. Depending on the systems of record-keeping in use at the paramedic service, and the method of storage, this may be as hard copy or in electronic form.

In Case 11.5, Barry's first action is to clarify the correct information verbally with the receiving facility. This correction of the account would be recorded by the facility in their healthcare records. A correct record must also be lodged within the record system of the paramedic service, and, depending on the type of system used, this may be on a subsequent record, in an electronic system or some other method of recording, and should be clearly cross-referenced to allow someone reading either record to be made aware of the other.

Conclusion

Patient healthcare records are an important part of the patient care continuum. They are used to record all aspects of a patient's healthcare, and are also used as a tool to transfer important information from one provider to another. In the case of paramedics, the PHCR is used to collect, collate and record all aspects of the patient interaction for further use by receiving clinicians. The information is also sometimes used for other statistical, medical and administrative purposes. The record is an important record of fact, and the information recorded must be objective, concise and detailed. Any errors made must be dealt with appropriately, so as not to reduce the integrity of the document. The document must be stored and dealt with appropriately to maintain the privacy of the individual. Only authorised persons may access the record, and its information can only be used for the purpose for which it was collected.

Review Questions

1. What is a 'healthcare record', and what are the key characteristics of a good healthcare record?
2. Who owns your healthcare record, and under what circumstances can other people access your record?
3. What are the correct ways to deal with mistakes and errors on a written healthcare record, and why?
4. What jurisdiction do you currently work in (or, if you are a student, imagine you are working in your local service), and what legislation does a healthcare record completed by you need to comply with?
5. Does your organisation have a policy or procedure on how to deal with a patient or other person asking for a copy of the record you have just completed? Investigate and consider what you would advise and where you would direct them if you were asked for a copy.
6. What does the code of conduct say about record-keeping?

Appendix 11.1 A patient healthcare record (with kind permission from the Ambulance Service of New South Wales)

Endnotes

1   Ambulance Service of NSW. *Latest news*. Online. Available: http://www.ambulance.nsw.gov.au/Media
    -And-Publications/Latest-News/Ambulance-moving-forward-with-digital-recording-innovation.html
    (accessed 12 February 2019).

2   Ibid.

3   Ibid.

4   Australian Resuscitation Outcomes Consortium (Aus-ROC). [Home page.] Online. Available: https://
    www.ausroc.org.au (accessed 1 October 2018).

5   Australian Resuscitation Outcomes Consortium (Aus-ROC). *Collaborating organisations*. Online. Available:
    https://www.ausroc.org.au/epistry/collaborating-organisations/ (accessed 1 October 2018).

6   Australian Digital Health Agency. *My Health Record: Frequently asked questions*. Online. Available: https://
    www.myhealthrecord.gov.au/for-you-your-family/howtos/frequently-asked-questions (accessed 1 October
    2018).

7   Office of the Australian Information Commissioner. *Who owns the records?* Online. Available: https://
    www.oaic.gov.au/individuals/privacy-fact-sheets/health-and-digital-health/privacy-fact-sheet-49 (accessed 12
    February 2019).

8   Health Information Strategy Steering Committee. (2005) *Health Information Strategy for New Zealand*.
    Wellington: Ministry of Health. Available: https://www.health.govt.nz/system/files/documents/
    publications/health-information-strategy_0.pdf (accessed 5 February 2019).

9   Office of the Australian Information Commissioner. *Information Privacy Principles*. The Privacy Act 1988
    (Cth) Schedule 3 (private), Section 14 (public). Online. Available: https://www.oaic.gov.au/privacy-law/
    privacy-act/ (accessed 28 November 2018).

10 Office of the Australian Information Commissioner. (2001) *Guidelines on Privacy in the Private Health
    Sector*. Online. Available: https://gp2u.com.au/static/documents/Guidelines-on-Privacy-in-the-Private
    -Health-Sector-2001.pdf (accessed 28 November 2018).

11 Staunton, P. and Chiarella, M. (2013) *Nursing and the Law*, 7th ed. Sydney: Elsevier, at p. 247.

12 *Privacy Act 1988* (Cth), Pt 3, APP6, s 6.1. Online. Available: https://www.oaic.gov.au/individuals/
    privacy-fact-sheets/general/privacy-fact-sheet-17-australian-privacy-principles#australian-privacy-principle
    -6-use-or-disclosure-of-personal-information (accessed 12 February 2019).

13 Staunton and Chiarella, *Nursing and the Law*, at p. 245.

14 Ibid, at pp. 246–247.

15 Morris, K.A. (2017) *Cole's Medical Practice in New Zealand*, 13th ed. Wellington: Medical Council of New
    Zealand, at p. 429. Available: https://www.mcnz.org.nz/news-and-publications/cole-s-medical-practice-in
    -new-zealand/ (accessed 28 November 2018).

16 *Privacy Act 1988* (Cth), Pt 3, APP 6, s 6.1. Online. Available: https://www.oaic.gov.au/individuals/
    privacy-fact-sheets/general/privacy-fact-sheet-17-australian-privacy-principles#australian-privacy-principle
    -6-use-or-disclosure-of-personal-information (accessed 12 February 2019).

17 Ibid.

18 Ibid.

19 Australian Resuscitation Outcomes Consortium (Aus-ROC). *Variables*. Online. Available: https://
    www.ausroc.org.au/epistry/variables/ (accessed 12 February 2019).

20 *Lithgow City Council v Jackson* [2009] HCATrans 184.

21 Ibid.

22 Council of Standards Australia. (1999) *AS 2828:1999—Paper-based health care records*. Sydney: Standards
    Australia International Ltd.

23   Ibid.

24   Ibid.

25   Ibid.

26   Ibid.

27   Paramedicine Board of Australia. (2018) *Interim Code of Conduct for Registered Health Practitioners.* Melbourne: Australian Health Practitioner Regulation Agency. Online. Available: https://www. paramedicineboard.gov.au/professional-standards/codes-guidelines-and-policies/code-of-conduct.aspx (accessed 5 October 2018).

28   Paramedicine Board of Australia. (updated 13 December 2013) *Professional Capabilities for Registered Paramedics.* Online. Available: https://www.paramedicineboard.gov.au/Professional-standards/Professional -capabilities-for-registered-paramedics.aspx (accessed 5 October 2018).

29   Council of Standards Australia. *AS 2828:1999—Paper-based health care records.*

30   Ibid.

Chapter 12
The use of drugs in pre-hospital care

Ruth Townsend and Alisha Hensby

Learning objectives

After completing this chapter, you will:

- have been introduced to the laws that govern the use of drugs in Australia, and why they exist
- have an understanding of drug schedules, and how they apply to paramedic practice
- know how and why drugs should be stored and recorded
- know how paramedics are authorised to administer drugs, and which drugs they are authorised to administer
- have a broader understanding of the key issues affecting paramedics and drugs, including self-prescribing and medication administration errors.

Definitions

Drug substitution Where a drug is replaced by a non-authentic replacement, most commonly with restricted drugs. For example, fentanyl is replaced with water.

Poisons Standard A Commonwealth instrument that is designed to promote the uniform scheduling of substances, and uniform labelling and packaging requirements throughout Australia.

Prescription The authorisation, by an authorised person, to another to be supplied a restricted drug.

Restricted drugs Schedule 4 and schedule 8 drugs as defined by the Poisons Standard. These are sometimes referred to as 'controlled drugs' because they are addictive.

An introductory case

Multiple patient overdose

A paramedic is called to the scene of a New Year's Eve party where a multiple patient overdose is suspected to have taken place. On arriving at the scene, the paramedic discovers four people with altered levels of consciousness, varying from extreme agitation to unresponsive. All patients had self-presented to the medical tent, where their condition deteriorated, at which time the ambulance was called. The paramedics are informed that all of the patients were known to have ingested tablets of unknown origin and makeup. Because it is New Year's Eve, emergency services are stretched and back-up may not arrive in time.

After an initial examination, the patients are found to be hyperthermic, tachycardic and hypertensive. Due to the patients' agitation, the paramedics may administer midazolam or ketamine along with fluid administration to address this clinical presentation.

There are a number of issues to be concerned about and be aware of with regard to paramedic practice and the regulation of drugs. This chapter will introduce you to the main areas of the law that are required to be known and understood. This will assist paramedics to provide safe care to their patients, to avoid legal liability with regard to the administration of drugs that may harm a patient, and to comply with the stringent laws that apply to drug storage, recording and administration.

Introduction

All paramedics administer, or at least come into contact with, medication as an inherent part of their role. Whether transporting a patient from home to hospital or back again, part of the role of the paramedic is to ensure that there is a continuity of care with respect to the medications that have been prescribed for, and/or administered to, the patient. In the pre-hospital care setting this information can contribute to the paramedic forming a holistic view of what might be going on with the patient, and certainly assists with collecting a medical history about the patient. Further to this, it assists paramedics to make informed decisions about the administration of drugs, and what the likely impact of drug administration may be on the patient.

In addition, there are tight legislative controls around medicines in all states and territories, and concerning the ways in which they are used. Only certain professionals are legally allowed to prescribe drugs, and distributing medications without legal justification is a criminal offence. This chapter will allow paramedics to understand the rules regarding the storage, recording, carrying and administration of medication in paramedic practice.

Regarding the nomenclature used in this chapter, many ambulance services refer to the drugs they administer as 'medicines', whereas the term 'drugs' commonly refers to street drugs. For the purposes of this chapter, medicines will be referred to as 'drugs' to remain consistent with the legislation. Where this chapter refers to 'ambulance officers', this is because the relevant legislation still refers to paramedics as 'ambulance officers'. The terms should be used interchangeably.

The governance of drugs

There are laws regarding the supply and use of medications at state/territory and Commonwealth levels in Australia. It is the responsibility of each individual health practitioner to know, understand and comply with these laws. The use of drugs is governed by a national classification scheme. Drugs are classified according to the *Standard for the Uniform Scheduling of Medicines and Poisons* (SUSMP), which is published by the National Drugs and Poisons Schedule Committee, established under the *Therapeutic Goods Act 1989* (Cth). The Poisons Standard is a Commonwealth instrument that is designed to promote the uniform scheduling of substances, and uniform labelling and packaging requirements throughout Australia.

What are the 'schedules' of drugs?

Poisons are classified according to the schedules in which they are included. Table 12.1 provides a general description of the schedules. For the legal definitions, however, it is necessary to check with each relevant state or territory authority.

The scheduled drugs that paramedics most commonly encounter are: schedule 2 or 3, over-the-counter medications (e.g. paracetamol or ibuprofen); schedule 4, prescription-only medications (e.g. midazolam); schedule 8, controlled drugs (e.g. morphine); and schedule 7, some farm chemicals (e.g. organophosphates).

Who may possess and supply certain drugs?

The term 'supply' in the context of drugs has a specific meaning in law. It effectively means that a person who is licensed to do so may legally make a drug available to another person. The licensing of a person to supply obviously imposes restrictions on the availability of drugs, and that includes restrictions on the amount of a drug that may be available to supply. In turn, there are restrictions on who may possess drugs. In legal terms, 'possess' means the physical or manual control of a drug. For example, under the *Poisons Regulations 2018* (Tas):

> (d) an ambulance officer, paramedic or interstate ambulance officer—
>
> may possess and use any narcotic substances for the purposes of his or her profession or employment. (reg 14)

In New South Wales, the *Poisons and Therapeutic Goods Regulation 2008* authorises a person:

> (i) who is employed in the Ambulance Service of NSW as an ambulance officer or as an air ambulance flight nurse, and
>
> (ii) who is approved for the time being by the Director-General for the purposes of this clause.
>
> … to have possession of, and to supply, drugs of addiction. (reg 101)

Table 12.1 General description of the poisons schedules	
Schedule 1	There are no longer any schedule 1 poisons.
Schedule 2	**Pharmacy medicine**—Substances the safe use of which may require advice from a pharmacist, and which should be available from a pharmacy or, where a pharmacy service is not available, from a licensed person.
Schedule 3	**Pharmacist-only medicine**—Substances the safe use of which requires professional advice, but which should be available to the public from a pharmacist without a prescription.
Schedule 4	**Prescription-only medicine** or **Prescription animal remedy**—Substances the use or supply of which should be by or on the order of persons permitted by state or territory legislation to prescribe, and should be available from a pharmacist on prescription.
Schedule 5	**Caution**—Substances with a low potential for causing harm, the extent of which can be reduced through the use of appropriate packaging with simple warnings and safety directions on the label.
Schedule 6	**Poison**—Substances with a moderate potential for causing harm, the extent of which can be reduced through the use of distinctive packaging with strong warnings and safety directions on the label.
Schedule 7	**Dangerous poison**—Substances with a high potential for causing harm at low exposure, and which require special precautions during manufacture, handling or use. These poisons should be available only to specialised or authorised users who have the skills necessary to handle them safely. Special regulations restricting their availability, possession, storage or use may apply.
Schedule 8	**Controlled drug**—Substances which should be available for use, but require restriction of manufacture, supply, distribution, possession and use to reduce abuse, misuse and physical or psychological dependence.
Schedule 9	**Prohibited substance**—Substances which may be abused or misused, the manufacture, possession, sale or use of which should be prohibited by law except when required for medical or scientific research, or for analytical, teaching or training purposes with the approval of Commonwealth and/or state or territory health authorities.[1]

In Victoria, an operational staff member within the meaning of the *Ambulance Services Act 1986* is authorised to use those schedule 4 poisons or schedule 8 poisons listed in the health services permit held by that ambulance service. In South Australia, the penalties for the unauthorised prescribing or administering of a drug are heavy, with a fine of $10,000 or a custodial sentence of 2 years. In Western Australia, a person is authorised to possess schedule 4 and schedule 8 drugs with the permission of the chief executive officer of the Health Service.

Regulation 174 of the *Health (Drugs and Poisons) Regulation 1996* (Qld) prescribes in detail the legal requirements for staff employed by the Queensland Ambulance Service to obtain, possess or administer restricted drugs like benztropine, frusemide, haloperidol, hydrocortisone, metoclopramide, promethazine and the others listed in a clinical protocol approved by the Queensland Ambulance Service (QAS) and listed in the appendix to the regulation.

These requirements include that the paramedic be working in an ECP (extended care program) area, acting on a doctor's instruction, have undergone certain training, be acting under a clinical protocol of the QAS and other details (see the regulation). What this detail demonstrates is that obtaining, possessing, administering and/or supplying medication in healthcare is very strongly regulated and an important area for paramedics to understand.

In addition to obtaining, possessing and supplying drugs, there are laws regarding the storage and recording of restricted drugs.

Storage and recording of drugs

There are strict regulations regarding the way in which some drugs must be stored, in particular schedule 8 drugs like ketamine and morphine, which are sometimes referred to as 'controlled' drugs (e.g. *Health (Drugs and Poisons) Regulation 1996* (Qld), Sch 982A, App 2A) or 'drugs of addiction'(NSW Health).

Schedule 8 drugs are generally required to be kept in a locked place that disallows access by those unapproved to access; namely, the public. However, approval can be given by the appropriate state or territory authority for schedule 8 drugs to be kept in first-aid kits or paramedic kits.

All drugs used by an organisation should be accounted for; however, there are specific legislative requirements for the recording of some drugs on a register.[2] For example, drugs of addiction are required under regulation 111 of the *Poisons and Therapeutic Goods Regulation 2008* (NSW) to be kept in a register:

111 Drug registers to be kept

(1) A person who has possession of drugs of addiction at any place must keep a separate register (a **drug register**) at that place.

(2) A drug register is to be in the form of a book:

(a) that contains consecutively numbered pages, and

(b) that is so bound that the pages cannot be removed or replaced without trace, and

(c) that contains provision on each page for the inclusion of the particulars required to be entered in the book.

(3) Separate pages of the register must be used for each drug of addiction, and for each form and strength of the drug.

(4) The Director-General may from time to time approve the keeping of a drug register in any other form.

Registers are audited and any discrepancies must be accounted for. Those that remain unaccounted for are reportable by law under the *Poisons and Therapeutic Goods Regulation 2008* (NSW).

Case 12.1 The drug substitute

You commence work at a new ambulance station and notice the station is lax with its drug security procedures. You hear a couple of officers talking about 'drug substitution'. You ask what that means, and they explain that some medications, like the pain reliever fentanyl, are tampered with and 'substituted with other fluids'.

What are the issues to consider with 'drug substitution'?

There are some aspects of drug registration that are more difficult to manage in the pre-hospital care environment than the hospital. However, some jurisdictions legislate for these circumstances, and all service procedures have protocols outlining that the administration of restricted drugs to patients *must be witnessed* by a person other than the person administering the drug. This is sometimes difficult for paramedics if administration is required en route and the second officer is driving and unable to witness administration. It is also difficult in regional or remote areas where the paramedic may be working alone.

There is also the issue of substitution where the prescribed drug is substituted with another fluid. For example, a narcotic is substituted for saline. Consider Case 12.1.

It is a criminal offence to substitute a drug. The offence constitutes theft, and if a restricted or controlled drug is the substituted drug, then the paramedic may be guilty of unauthorised possession and, if used, administration of a restricted substance. In addition, there is a risk to the public that they do not get the pain relief they require, that they may be at risk of contamination and harm from a potentially hazardous unknown substance, and that they may be treated by a paramedic who is under the influence of drugs while administering care.[3]

What happens if not all of the schedule 8 drug is used?

If only part of an ampoule of the drug is used—for example, if pethidine comes in 100 mg ampoules but the patient only requires 75 mg—the remaining 25 mg must be discarded and recorded in the register as having been discarded. The recording of this data is necessary so that there is a mechanism available for checking that drugs are being administered in accordance with legislative intentions. For example, in New South Wales, where there may be an excess amount of a drug like morphine drawn up, the discarded amount would be documented on the electronic medical record (EMR) and disposed of at the receiving facility by the administering paramedic. This would be witnessed by their paramedic partner. Both paramedics would then sign the EMR.

What happens a discrepancy is noticed?

If a drug of addiction is lost in some way—for example, has been misplaced or incorrectly drawn up—a record must be made of this loss. In New South Wales, there is a statutory requirement that the Director General of Health be notified immediately if a drug of addiction is stolen or lost.[4] This requirement to notify police and the health department should be set out in each respective ambulance service's procedures manual. All drug inventory is subject to auditing, and this is why it is necessary to keep accurate records of drug use. There have been some instances where the use of, and access to, drugs has been examined by external authorities. For example, in New South Wales there was an investigation undertaken by police with regard to allegations of theft of drugs from the Ambulance Service of New South Wales by paramedic employees.[5]

What if the patient is drug-dependent?

It is not infrequent for an ambulance to be called to a patient who is suffering from a drug addiction and is seeking easy access to a restricted drug. The paramedic should perform a full patient assessment, and never dismiss the complaint of a patient merely by virtue of the fact that the patient has an addiction. However, there are laws that prohibit the administration, prescription, selling or supplying of restricted drugs to people *purely* for the purposes of supporting their drug dependency.

Prescribing

The 'prescription' of a drug is the authorisation, by an authorised person, to another to be supplied a restricted drug. Schedule 4 and schedule 8 drugs require a prescription, and are consequently referred to as 'restricted drugs'. In no state or territory are paramedics authorised to prescribe medications. There are specific prohibitions against the prescription of schedule 8 drugs by anyone other than a doctor, nurse practitioner, veterinarian or dentist in some jurisdictions. For example, section 16 of the Victorian *Drugs, Poisons and Controlled Substances Regulation 2006* says:

> **Persons authorised to write prescriptions**
>
> ...
>
> (2) A person other than a registered medical practitioner, veterinary practitioner, dentist, nurse practitioner or authorised midwife must not write a prescription for a Schedule 8 poison.

However, paramedics are not required to prescribe drugs, but to administer them.

Medication errors

There is a large body of literature on the ways to manage, and the reason for managing, the adverse events that arise as a result of human error in the delivery of healthcare. Medication errors by health practitioners contribute a significant percentage to those mistakes that result in harm to the patient.[6] A medication error is defined as:

> ... any preventable event that may cause or lead to inappropriate medication use or patient harm while the medication is in the control of the healthcare professional, patient, or consumer. Such events may be related to professional practice, health care products, procedures, and systems, including prescribing; order communication; product labeling, packaging, and nomenclature; compounding; dispensing; distribution; administration; education; monitoring; and use.[7]

A study conducted by Vilke et al. found that 9% of paramedic respondents admitted to making a medication error in the preceding 12 months.[8] Knowledge of adverse events in healthcare has led to a redesign of the healthcare system to allow for fewer mistakes to be made, but also to encourage practitioners to report errors. The self-reporting of errors is important, not only so that patients can be made aware of the potential harms that may have been caused as a result of the error and seek to have those addressed, but also because it allows for the identification of systems failures. This, in turn, allows for a redesign of the system in which policies, training, the environment and even the equipment may be altered to ensure staff are working in a system that makes it more difficult for them to make mistakes. Lucian Leape[9] and others argue that a number of factors contribute to errors being made, including: working in environments with poor lighting that makes it difficult to see the medications that are being administered; poor protocols that do not reflect best practice (e.g. adrenaline treatment for anaphylaxis is best administered via an intramuscular injection rather than intravenously);[10] poor equipment (e.g. an inappropriately sized syringe for the drawing up and administration of insulin); poor training that does not provide paramedics with sufficient information to make good clinical decisions (e.g. poor medication calculation skills).[11] Leape also argues that another mechanism for limiting medication error is to involve the patient in the process wherever possible.[12] This is discussed in more detail later on in this chapter.

Safety and medication administration

To maximise patient safety and minimise drug administration errors, there are a number of elements that must be addressed *prior* to the administering of a drug. These include gaining the patient's consent for the drug administration (see the section 'Consent' in Chapter 5, 'Consent and refusal of treatment'). There are many occasions where consent is not able to be gained because the patient is unable to give it, and treatment is required urgently to prevent further harm or to save the patient's life. In the case of an emergency where the patient is not competent to consent and there is no guardian, the drug may be administered. However, where the patient is competent or there is a guardian present, consent must be sought. This also involves educating and informing the patient about the proposed course of treatment, and about the associated benefits and risks of undertaking that treatment. This requires the paramedic to have a firm knowledge of the range of drugs that they are authorised to administer, and the necessary skills to impart this information to the patient so that the patient understands it. This process satisfies the legal and ethical component of autonomy and informed consent, but it also importantly acts as an additional layer of safety for the patient and the practitioner. For example, consider Case 12.2.

The five rights of drug administration

Further to involving the patient in a discussion about treatment, you should also consider the five rights of drug administration, how you will assess, evaluate and document the effects of the drug, and how you would respond were you to give a drug in error or the administration of the drug resulted in an adverse effect.

Case 12.2 The safe paramedic

You are called to a patient with chest pain. On arrival, you find the patient unconscious. After an initial primary survey and 12-lead ECG, you identify that the patient is suffering from a STEMI infarction. You are aware that the medications to treat this normally require consent from the patient, due to the known adverse effects, including uncontrolled haemorrhage and death. However, in this circumstance you are unable to get patient consent and there is no substitute decision-maker to seek consent from. You are therefore relying on the doctrine of necessity to justify your treatment of the patient, along with your professional requirement to act in the best interests of your patient. In order to ensure that you are doing so in the safest possible way, and in accordance with best practice, law and ethics, you consult with your partner, and, after developing an appropriate treatment, and in accordance with your guidelines, you make the clinical decision to administer thrombolytic medications.

- Check that you are giving:
  – the right *patient*,
  – the right *medication*, in
  – the right *dose*, at
  – the right *time*, via
  – the right *route*.
- Check that the patient has no allergies to the drug to be administered.
- Consider what an adverse effect of this drug might result in, so that you are prepared for it; for example, an overdose of a narcotic will require the quick resuscitation of the patient with naloxone and respiratory support.[13]

Medication errors are common, and may lead to serious consequences for the patient. Most occur in older people due to polypharmacy. Communication between staff and patients is essential to help reduce errors.[14] Each ambulance service will have its own protocols with regard to the safe administration of medication to a patient, and should incorporate risk management suggestions to assist staff to avoid making errors. For example, NSW Health provides a list of precautions (see Table 12.2). It also identifies the work health and safety issues that should be considered to ensure that staff also remain safe during medication administration.

Assessment and documentation of drug administration

Always ensure documentation of administration, including the drug given, the dose, the route, the time given and the patient response, including any adverse drug reactions. Always ensure that you have assessed and evaluated the effectiveness of medication administration, particularly medicines that affect respiratory rate, heart rate, blood pressure, level of consciousness or blood glucose. The patient's underlying pathophysiology and

Table 12.2 Precautions and work health and safety issues[15]	
Precautions	Name the medication you are about to give, and ask the patient whether they have had it previously, and whether they have had any reactions.
	Ensure that aseptic technique is used at all times.
	Swab sites, vials and bungs prior to administration.
	Use an ampoule opener with all glass ampoules.
	Draw up medication with a filtered drawing-up needle.
	Apply an approved syringe cap to cover the syringe hub between doses to maintain asepsis.
Work health and safety issues	Wear approved appropriate personal protective equipment during the procedure.
	Do not re-sheath needles.
	Dispose of sharps into approved sharps containers immediately.
	Ensure compliance to infection control procedures.
	Ensure compliance to relevant work health and safety and manual handling techniques.

Case 12.3 The adverse event

A paramedic is called to a patient suffering from an anaphylactic reaction. He administers adrenaline as per his protocol. The protocol states that the adrenaline can be given in incremental doses. There is no requirement to check the patient's blood pressure in between doses. The patient's blood pressure rises rapidly and results in the patient suffering an intracerebral bleed that results in severe disability.

health status should always be considered, as this may affect the metabolism and overall effectiveness of the drug. The importance of such checks can be illustrated by Case 12.3.

In this case, a failure to evaluate the effectiveness of the drug in between doses has led to harm to the patient. The paramedic followed the protocol and could, therefore, not be found negligent in their treatment of the patient. However, it could be argued that a foreseeable harm was suffered by the patient, because adrenaline is known to cause a rapid rise in blood pressure. If the paramedic had assessed the effectiveness of the dose by taking blood pressure measurements in between doses, the paramedic may have been alerted to the problem prior to it causing significant damage.

What happens if a drug is given in error?

If a medication administration error occurs, the paramedic should at least undertake the following:

- Immediately discontinue the medication.
- Assess for any adverse drug reaction (ADR) to the medication, including changes in level of consciousness, or allergic reaction.

- Treat the symptoms of the ADR as per protocol.
- Ascertain whether the patient has any known allergy to the medication given in error.
- Notify the doctor of the medication error, along with any ADR to the medication, during clinical handover.
- Apologise to the patient.
- Document the reaction and response.

Conclusion

A knowledge and understanding of the law with respect to the area of medications is necessary for the paramedic to ensure that they abide by the rules. The reason for abiding by the rules with regard to drug possession, supply, storage, recording and administration goes beyond ensuring that practitioners themselves are safe from legal action. The reason for abiding by the rules is to ensure that the patient remains safe. The high rates of harm caused to patients as a result of medication administration errors emphasise the need to consider the ethical maxim *do no harm*, and how it applies in this area.

Review Questions

1 What are the most common schedule 4 and schedule 8 drugs used by paramedics?
2 What are the rules regarding the recording of restricted drugs?
3 Why are the possession and supply of drugs regulated?
4 What is a 'medication error'?
5 What are the elements that should be considered prior to administering a drug to the patient? (This goes beyond the five rights.)
6 What should you do if you realise that a medication error has been made?
7 What does the code of conduct say about minimising risk of errors?

Endnotes

1 *Poisons Standard 2019* (Cth) Online. Available: https://www.legislation.gov.au/Details/F2019L00032 (accessed February 2019).

2 See also *Medicines, Poisons and Therapeutic Goods Regulation 2008* (ACT); *Medicine, Poisons and Therapeutic Goods Act 2018* (NT); *Health (Drugs and Poisons) Regulation 1996* (Qld); *Controlled Substances (Poisons) Regulations 2011* (SA); *Poisons Regulations 2018* (Tas); *Drugs, Poisons and Controlled Substances Regulations 2017* (Vic); *Medicines and Poisons Regulations 2016* (WA).

3 Wallace, N. (2009, 12 October) Ambos accused of stealing drugs. *The Sydney Morning Herald*; Wallace, N. (2010, 23 January) Ambos slammed over drugs. *The Sydney Morning Herald*.

4 *Poisons and Therapeutic Goods Regulation 2008* (NSW), reg 124.

5 Wallace, Ambos accused of stealing drugs; Wallace, Ambos slammed over drugs.

6   Roughead, E.E. and Semple, S.J. (2009) Medication safety in acute care in Australia: where are we now? Part 1: a review of the extent and causes of medication problems 2002–2008. *Australia and New Zealand Health Policy* 6, 18.

7   National Coordinating Council for Medication Error Reporting and Prevention (NCC MERP) (US) *Consumer information for safe medication use*. Online. Available: https://www.nccmerp.org/consumer-information.

8   Vilke, G.M., Tornabene, S.V., Stepanski, B. et al. (2006) Paramedic self-reported medication errors. *Prehospital Emergency Care* 10(4), 457–462.

9   Leape, L.L., Brennan, T.A., Laird, N. et al. (1991) The nature of adverse events in hospitalized patients: results of the Harvard Medical Practice Study II. *New England Journal of Medicine* 324(6), 377–384. See also Leape, L.L. and Berwick, D.M. (2005) Five years after 'To Err Is Human': what have we learned? *Journal of the American Medical Association* 293(19), 2384–2390.

10 Simon, G.A., Brown, R., Mullins, J. et al. (2006) Anaphylaxis diagnosis and treatment. *Medical Journal of Australia* 185(5), 283–289; Pumphrey, R.S. (2000) Lessons for management of anaphylaxis from a study of fatal reactions. *Clinical and Experimental Allergy* 30(8), 1144–1150.

11 See also Crossman, M. (2009) Technical and environmental impact on medication error in paramedic practice: a review of causes, consequences and strategies for prevention. *Journal of Emergency Primary Health Care* 7(3), 990374.

12 Leape et al., The nature of adverse events in hospitalized patients.

13 Myers, E (2006) *Nurse's Clinical Guide*, 2nd ed. Philadelphia: FA Davis Company.

14 Hilmer, S.N. (2016) Strategies to reduce medication errors. *Medicine Today* 17(7), 44–50. Available: https://respiratorymedicinetoday.com.au/sites/default/files/cpd/MT2016-07-044-HILMER.pdf

15 NSW Health. (2013; updated 14 March 2017) *Medication handling in NSW public health facilities*. Online. Available: https://www1.health.nsw.gov.au/pds/ActivePDSDocuments/PD2013_043.pdf (accessed February 2019).

Chapter 13
Employment law

Philip Groves and Erin Hillson

Learning outcomes

After reading this chapter, you should be able to:
- understand the key requirements of the *Fair Work Act*, and its application to paramedic practice
- articulate the key requirements of an employment contract
- navigate the Ambulance and Patient Transport Industry Award 2010, and know how to locate any updates to this award
- understand the differences between direct employment and independent contracting
- know the rights and responsibilities of employment, including termination, leave and employment conditions
- articulate the requirements for workplace health and safety and workers' compensation applicable to paramedic practice
- understand workplace wellness, including equal opportunity, workplace bullying, discrimination, and mental and physical health at work.

Definitions

Bullying According to the *Fair Work Act 2009* (Cth), a worker is bullied at work when 'an individual or group of individuals repeatedly behaves unreasonably towards the worker, or a group of workers of which the worker is a member, and that behaviour creates a risk to health and safety' (s 789FD).

Discrimination When a person, or a group of people, is treated less favourably than another person or group because of their background or certain personal characteristics. This is known as *direct discrimination*. It is also discrimination when an unreasonable rule or policy applies to everyone but has the effect of disadvantaging some people because of a personal characteristic they share. This is known as *indirect discrimination*.[1]

Continued

Employee A person directly engaged by a business or undertaking, paid as an individual.

Employment contract A formal contract between two parties, outlining the terms and conditions of employment. Contracts may take various forms, but require key elements, which are discussed throughout the chapter.

Independent contractor A person who works for a business or undertaking, but who is engaged and remunerated as a company, partnership, sole trader, or other business structure.

Sexual harassment An unwelcome sexual advance, unwelcome request for sexual favours or other unwelcome conduct of a sexual nature which makes a person feel offended, humiliated and/or intimidated, where a reasonable person would anticipate that reaction in the circumstances.[2]

Worker Changes to harmonise the work health and safety (WHS) legislation in 2011 introduced the term 'worker' to describe anyone involved in a workplace. Workers, in this context, include paid employees, contractors, volunteers, students, visitors, and even members of the public.

Introductory case

A cheeky injury

Amanda is a paramedic, who is engaged by an ambulance service as a contractor. She decided to become an independent contractor because it gives her more freedom to work on the weekends, and to enjoy the tax advantages of purchasing a car through her private business. While responding to an emergency, Amanda trips and fractures her jaw and cheekbone. She is unable to work for 6 months due to the complications of surgery and infection.

This chapter will provide you with some context in which to consider and reflect on this case.

Introduction

As a paramedic, you will inevitably be introduced to a range of legal contexts. One of the most important for you will involve employment law, and its related fields of safety and workers' compensation law (see Table 13.1, which indicates the legislation that governs the area of workers' compensation). These areas of law govern your day-to-day working life as a paramedic, and so it is critical that you understand the basic applications of these legal frameworks.

The requirement for the regulation of health practitioners in Australia has changed the way in which paramedics may work. They are no longer only able to be direct employees

Table 13.1 Workers' compensation legislation	
Jurisdiction	**Legislation**
Australia Capital Territory	*Workers Compensation Act 1951*
New South Wales	*Workers Compensation Act 1987*
	Workplace Injury Management and Workers Compensation Act 1998
Northern Territory	*Workers Rehabilitation and Compensation Act 1986*
Queensland	*Workers' Compensation and Rehabilitation Act 2003*
South Australia	*Workers Rehabilitation and Compensation Act 1986*
Tasmania	*Workers Rehabilitation and Compensation Act 1988*
Victoria	*Accident Compensation Act 1985*
Western Australia	*Workers' Compensation and Injury Management Act 1981*
New Zealand	*Accident Compensation Act 2001*
	Injury Prevention, Rehabilitation and Compensation Act 2001

within a state, as the current context allows subcontracting, private enterprise, and inter-state mobility. This means you will be faced with decisions regarding your employment status. Should you aim to be a direct employee or a contractor?

This chapter will not be able to provide the answer for you, because your decision may be based on a variety of factors, including personal circumstance, taxation implications, and work opportunities. What this chapter does attempt to do, however, is offer an overview of the general key issues, so you are better able to make informed judgements as you progress in your chosen career.

The chapter is divided into three sections. The first provides an overview of employment law and the employment context. The second looks at compliance requirements, such as work health and safety (WHS), insurance, and workers' compensation. The third discusses the growing area of workplace wellness, and the critical importance of psychological and physical health at work, an area which is subject to increased regulation and legal oversight.

Endnotes suggest further reading, which is encouraged, as this chapter is only able to provide a helicopter view of the topic.

Employment law

General context

Work is a constant in modern society, and it is no surprise that work is governed by a significant depth of laws and regulations. It is important to acknowledge the history of work and law. Legal intervention in the workplace has a long history, and typically involves the tempestuous relationship between employee and employer, often mediated through interest groups such as unions.

Much of the relationship between employer and employee has been characterised by a 'power imbalance', which had its roots in very real exploitation. Karl Marx,[3] for example, documented this 'exploitation' of workers, whereby the rich prosper through ownership of business and the 'means of work', while the poor remain subservient and dependent on wages.

In Australia, workplace law has enjoyed a complex development, heavily influenced by political motivations. Early case law involved the analysis of worker status. Who was a worker? What rights did workers have? Typically, and importantly, most case law surrounded responsibility for workplace experiences such as work injury and pay entitlements.

What developed from this legal wrangling was a focus on two critical areas of work: employment conditions (rates of pay, leave, overtime, termination) and workplace 'control' (who is responsible for a workplace?).

Both concepts are critical to our topic, as they define the experience of employment for paramedic professionals, and establish the duties and responsibilities placed on all workers, contractors and employers.

Laws in place

The current legal framework for employment law in Australia is governed by the *Fair Work Act 2009* (Cth) (the '*Fair Work Act*'). As a Commonwealth Act, it applies to all states and territories. It defines *minimum standards*, and provides a framework for interpreting the next part of the legal framework: modern awards. *Modern awards* establish the specific details of remuneration and conditions of employment. They are industry-specific, and the one applicable to our purpose is the Ambulance and Patient Transport Industry Award 2010. We will discuss this award in detail below. (See Appendix 13.1 for a full list of the industrial laws that apply in Australia and New Zealand.)

The third tier is *enterprise agreements*. These are effectively negotiated employment terms, which must acknowledge any relevant award as a baseline, and must also comply with the National Employment Standards (the baseline requirements outlined in the *Fair Work Act*), but allow flexibility for employment arrangements. They are typically used in the private sector or where awards do not apply (e.g. managers, etc.).

The employment contract

Regardless of the application of the National Employment Standards (NES), awards or other agreements, the employment contract remains the cornerstone of the employment relationship. An employment contract is a formal agreement between two parties. It is typically written, but it can be verbal.

Key elements of an employment contract, according to Stewart, include:
- There must be a clear offer of employment, and it must be accepted by the employee.
- The terms of the agreement must be certain (e.g. an offer to start this job, on this date, for this amount of money).
- There must be valuable consideration (e.g. I give up my time to work for you, in return for money).
- Employer and employee must be legally able to enter the contract (e.g. not a child).
- The contract must also be for a legal purpose (e.g. not intended to defraud anyone).[4]

Enterprise bargaining

The option exists, particularly supported by unions, to negotiate enterprise agreements. These must maintain the basic requirements of the NES,[5] as outlined below, and the basic elements of contract law. These agreements can be complex, and so it is important to investigate further if they apply to you. As they must follow the minimum standards, they are likely to be beneficial, at least in some ways. One key thing to note is that the paramedic profession's service is considered part of the 'public interest', and thus strike/industrial action may be considered unlawful.[6] This is where matters can become subjective. What is harsh or unreasonable? The first step is to check your employer's human resource guidelines or policies, the award and the NES. Case law has confirmed that employers cannot overwork their employees (e.g. putting them on-call for excessive periods of time),[7] but, at the same time, there is an acceptance that there is a standard of reasonableness in terms of hours and expectations.[8]

Who is an employee?

For an individual to be an *employee*, an employer must exercise control over the individual in a workplace. This may be broadly interpreted, and can include a common purpose to achieve an outcome, a direct transfer of money for service, and a variety of other factors, including who takes charge of organising work activities. See *Stevens v Brodribb Sawmilling Co Pty Ltd*[9] for a detailed analysis of these aspects. For paramedics, control and organisation is relatively clear. Instructions may be generated by radio or computer, allocating work tasks; rosters may outline work times and requirements—this would fall under the ambit of control. Supplying a uniform may also be considered a clear indication of 'employment'.[10]

Case law has dealt predominantly with contested employment cases. Was the person employed? Such cases arise when economic factors come into play, especially after a death or serious injury. Was the person an employee to whom I owed a duty of care? The elements are important to understand, particularly when we look at the subcontractual relationship.

National Employment Standards

Moving now to the specific terms of employment, the *Fair Work Act 2009* outlines 10 minimum standards that no award, contract or enterprise agreement may avoid. These are described as the *National Employment Standards (NES)*. It is important to understand their basic purpose. The account of them below is a simple summary. Should you require further explanation or detail, please consult them directly. They are easy to follow, and elucidate various aspects under the general discussion points below. The NES include:

- hours of work
- flexible working arrangements
- parental leave
- annual leave
- personal/carer's leave
- community service leave

- long-service leave
- public holidays
- termination and redundancy
- fair work statements.

Hours of work

Employees are only required to work a maximum of 38 hours per week. Employees may refuse to work more hours on reasonable grounds. What are reasonable grounds? They may include family circumstances, health and safety implications, the work context, the availability of overtime, pay expectations (e.g. if the role is paid at a higher rate on the expectation that more hours will be worked).[11] Paramedics, with available overtime and often demanding work expectations, may expect to work longer than 38 hours per week.

Flexible working arrangements

Requests for flexible working arrangements may be made by an employee under certain circumstances. The circumstances may include being a parent, being a carer, living with a disability, being over the age of 55, or experiencing family violence.[12] Specific requirements are noted, including being eligible after 12 months of full-time employment, or 'long-term' casual employment. Reasonable business grounds are an excuse for rejecting a request. Reasonable business grounds may include the request being too costly or being impractical to implement, which would result in lost productivity or reduced customer service.

Parental leave

Parental leave is available to employees (other than casuals) after 12 months of service, and long-term casual employees under certain circumstances. Leave is available for birth and adoption. Twelve months of unpaid leave is also available.[13]

Annual leave

Permanent employees are entitled to 4 weeks of annual leave per year of employment, or 5 weeks of annual leave if employees are 'shift-workers'. Leave accumulates year by year, progressively according to service (e.g. a proportion accrues in each pay period).[14]

Personal/carer's leave

For each year of employment, employees are entitled to 10 days carer's/personal leave (otherwise known as 'sick leave'). Leave accrues, year to year. Compassionate leave is also outlined; 2 days per 'event', which can include the death or serious injury of a family member. The employee must give notice of the leave being taken as soon as possible, which can be after the leave has started (e.g. if you are in hospital it may not be practical to tell your employer you are commencing sick leave).[15]

Community service leave

This includes jury duty and supporting natural disaster response (e.g. serving in the Rural Fire Service or State Emergency Services). Employees must be paid for the first 10 days of jury service. Casual workers are not included in this provision.[16]

Long-service leave

Long-service leave is calculated based on award provisions, or any employment agreement pre-dating the *Fair Work Act 2009*.[17]

Public holidays

Employees are not required to work on public holidays, unless requested to do so, and the request is reasonable. What is reasonable? This depends on the nature of the work, the personal circumstances of the employee (family, etc.), the availability of overtime, etc.[18] Paramedics are expected to work on public holidays, as allowances and overtime rates are outlined in the relevant modern award, as outlined below.

Termination and redundancy

Employers must give you written notice or payment in lieu if your employment is terminated. Minimum notice periods apply. For example, for those who have completed less than 1 year of service there is 1 week of notice, while more than 5 years of service requires 4 weeks (see section 117 of the *Fair Work Act 2009* for specific periods). Employers must add 2 weeks to the period for an employee over the age of 45 who has worked for at least 2 years with the employer.[19]

Redundancy pay is required if termination occurs because the role is no longer required, or the employer becomes bankrupt. Specific pay requirements are set out.[20]

None of the above apply to an employee terminated due to serious misconduct. This can be a particularly complex area of employment law, and so you are encouraged to seek professional advice if you face termination or redundancy.

Fair Work Information Statement

Prepared by the Fair Work Ombudsman, this is a statement that all employers must give to workers when they start, or as soon as is 'practicable'.[21] We will encounter 'practicable' in the section on workplace safety below. It is a legal term implying that business needs and economic necessity are to be considered when determining a course of action.

Ambulance and Patient Transport Industry Award 2010

The employment of paramedic professionals is covered by the Ambulance and Patient Transportation Award 2010 (the award). This award, like all modern awards, is given authority through the *Fair Work Act*, and outlines the specific terms of engagement for paramedic professionals. The following analysis provides an overview of the key elements of the award. You are encouraged to download and read the award in detail, as you should ensure you are aware of your rights and obligations as an employee. It is also important if you establish a business as a contractor, and then engage employees. This overview is only designed to familiarise you with the layout and general intentions of the award.

Variations

The award makes it possible for an employer and employee to agree to modify the terms of the award, if it meets 'genuine needs'.[22] This might include paying at a higher rate or exchanging one benefit for another. This is a potentially complicated area, and professional employment law advice should be sought for each specific context.

Change and consultation

If a change occurs, or is about to occur, in the workplace (including the introduction of new technology which will significantly affect the working life of employees), an employer must consult with employees. This requires notification, opportunity for comment, and the resolution of issues.[23]

Dispute resolution

This section is very important, as it outlines what has to happen when something goes wrong. This applies to the NES and the award. First, an attempt should be made by the employer and employee to try to resolve the issue. If that fails, the matter should be escalated through the management levels of the employer.[24] It is not discussed here, but the *Fair Work Act*[25] outlines further dispute resolutions requirements, which are mediation, conciliation and arbitration.[26] Note the whistleblower legislation outlined in Table 13.2. There is legislative protection for identifying issues in particular circumstances. Seeking relevant legal advice is recommended if you find yourself in such a position.

Types of employment

Three options for employment are outlined. Full-time (averaging 38 hours per week), part-time (averaging less than 38 hours a week, but having a regular work pattern), and casual irregular, with casual loadings specified of 25% on weekdays, 75% on weekends, and 100% on public holidays, to offset the absence of annual leave, etc.[27]

Termination

In addition to the NES, notice is required from the employee if the employee resigns. If the notice period is not worked, pay may be withheld. Also, when employment is terminated by the employer, a paid job-searching day is available.[28]

Table 13.2 Whistleblowing and public interest	
Jurisdiction	**Legislation**
Commonwealth	*Public Service Act 1999*, s 16
	Corporations Act 2001, Pt 9.4AAA, s 1317AC
	Fair Work (Registered Organisations) Act 2009, s 337A
Australian Capital Territory	*Public Interest Disclosures Act 1994*, s 26
New South Wales	*Public Interest Disclosures Act 1994*, Pt 3
Northern Territory	*Public Interest Disclosures Act 2008*, s 14
Queensland	*Public Interest Disclosure Act 2010*, s 36
South Australia	*Whistleblowers Protection Act 1993*, s 5
Tasmania	*Public Interest Disclosures Act 2002*, s 19
Victoria	*Whistleblowers Protection Act 2001*, Pt 3
Western Australia	*Public Interest Disclosures Act 2003*, Pt 3

Wages and hours

Minimum wages are detailed for all operational classifications. It is important to check and review these carefully, to make sure you know your base rate of pay. This will also have implications if you are injured at work and require time off under workers' compensation insurance. Your pay may be calculated by your base rate.[29] Allowances are detailed in section 15, with payment of wages[30] and work hours detailed.[31] There is an option to work 40 hours per week, and to take an additional 12 days of annual leave, or a rostered day off every 4 weeks.

As a paramedic, having to work repeated shifts may be an important issue. Under the award, no employee will be required to work more than 10 consecutive shifts without 24 hours off-duty. However, if you do work more than '12 consecutive shifts without 24 hours off duty, you will be paid for the 13th shift and any further consecutive shift worked, at the rate of treble time until 24 hours off duty is provided'.[32]

Note that there is a disclaimer: the provision does not apply if you exceed your normal shift time by up to an hour while completing a case. You are expected to complete your cases, despite the hour calculation requirements. This may be an important consideration, and is an inherent component of the paramedic profession. Thus, any disputes resulting from any related issue will be considered by the commissioner within the context of paramedic industry practice.

Shift allowances and rostering and penalty rates

The award details shift allowance, which is based on start and finish times.[33] Rosters are required to be placed a month (28 days) in advance, with rotating rosters where possible.[34] Overtime penalty rates are complex, and are based on hours worked and days worked; for example, double time for overtime on Saturday and Sunday. The award should be consulted for specific provisions.[35] Rest time is required after overtime,[36] or else the employee is to be paid double time until rest is made available. Rest is described as a continuous 8 hours off-duty. Employees may request time off in lieu of payment for overtime.[37] On-call allowances may also apply,[38] as do recall allowances (when recalled to duty after a rostered shift has finished),[39] control-call allowances (if required to attend to radio/telephone calls),[40] and stand-by (when requested to stand by outside ordinary work hours.[41]

It is important to understand these types of allowances, so you can be aware of them and the different work statuses you may experience.

Other

The remainder of the award deals with issues and definitions that may be important, and should therefore be consulted as and when required. For example, payments and requirements when a worker is seconded to higher duties,[42] and how excessive annual leave is measured (8 weeks for a permanent employee—or 10 if a shift-worker).[43] Finally, public holiday pay calculations are detailed.[44]

Unlawful dismissal

Your employment may be terminated for a number of reasons. Misconduct is a key reason, as is changing organisational needs (you are no longer needed). In many instances, you will have no legal redress other than to claim your outstanding leave entitlements and notice period. Some termination, however, is unlawful, including termination that is harsh, unjustified or unreasonable.[45]

To contract or not to contract

The preceding sections have discussed the employment context, including key terms, requirements and basic legal frameworks. This section now focuses on the differences between being an employee and being a contractor. The *Health Practitioner Regulation Amendment Act 2017* (NSW) and the requirement to achieve registration have consequences, with the most significant for paramedic practice being the option for paramedics to either remain as direct employees of a state ambulance service, or to establish themselves as independent contractors.

Being an employee

You may not have a choice. Your desired role may require you to be an employee, or the engaging body may require you to contract to them. The decision, in these circumstances, is simple. Regardless, here are a few discussion points to identify the key differences between being an employee and a contractor.

Employees have more rights?

Yes, they do. In terms of employment law, contractors are not covered by the *Fair Work Act 2009* and the provisions discussed above. If you have issues or grievances to raise, you will have to do that through alternative avenues, as provided for in your contract.

Contractors have more liability?

Yes, they do. If an employee makes a mistake, their employers will typically support them through any legal process, and personal liability is unlikely to attach to the individual worker. This is due to the doctrine of *vicarious liability*,[46] whereby a test of 'relative closeness'[47] applies to liability. For example, if an employee paramedic injures a patient by making a mistake, the paramedic's employer is likely to be held liable due to the inherent requirement to train and assess competency expected of employers, all part of the 'relative closeness' between the worker, the task and the patient. However, if you are a contractor you must take out relevant insurance, because you may be considered liable for a mistake or negligent action. You also have greater liability under work health and safety (WHS) legislation, as will be discussed below.

Is there any value in being a contractor?

Yes, there is, but it will depend on your financial situation, and family and other considerations. You will earn more money (generally) as a contractor, because the engaging organisation will typically not have to pay your workers' compensation insurance, professional indemnity insurance (if required), superannuation, etc. You will have to organise these things yourself. Depending on your business structure, you may be able to arrange your affairs to benefit you. It is a balance, and there is no right or wrong path—it is all about what will work for you and will give you employment/engagement!

Compliance requirements

This section focuses on what a contractor must do, but it also gives an insight into employees' duties, especially those attaching to WHS legislation.

Work health and safety (WHS)

The harmonised legislation in 2011 brought a semi-standardised approach to *occupational health and safety* (see Table 13.3 for the main sources of legislation in Australia and New Zealand relevant to occupational health and safety). While some states have not followed the harmonised legislation (Victoria and Western Australia), and others have amended the original Act (Queensland), the basic concepts of WHS remain consistent across all Australian states and territories. With minor exceptions, the purpose and scope of WHS legislation is consistent.

The first step is to identify the jurisdiction applicable to you. This may be complicated if you run a national or international organisation. Typically, your workers are governed by the safety laws in the state or territory where they do work. This can include their home office, if they work from home.

The legal hierarchy of safety (for WHS)

WHS law fits within a general legal hierarchy, and the harmonised legislation has seen the jurisdiction of WHS fit within criminal law. As paramedics you will encounter this element in the duty to report serious 'notifiable' incidents[48] to SafeWork NSW or the relevant state regulator. The police will now, typically, respond to serious workplace incidents.

In every jurisdiction, WHS law is governed by an Act, which sets out the broad rules of WHS, including key responsibilities, penalties and regulatory enforcement parameters. The WHS Regulations sit under the Act, and give specific instruction on key points; for example, Chapter 5 of the harmonised Regulations[49] governs construction site safety.

Australian standards and model codes of practice support the Act and Regulations by providing specific details on best practice and legal compliance. For example, the model code of practice on working at heights outlines requirements for harness use and various

Table 13.3 Occupational health and safety legislation	
Jurisdiction	**Legislation**
Australian Capital Territory	*Work Health and Safety Act 2011*
New South Wales	*Work Health and Safety Act 2011*
Northern Territory	*Work Health and Safety (National Uniform Legislation) Act 2016*
Queensland	*Work Health and Safety Act 2011*
South Australia	*Work Health and Safety Act 2012*
Tasmania	*Work Health and Safety Act 2012*
Victoria	*Occupational Health and Safety Act 2004*
Western Australia	*Occupational Safety and Health Act 1984*

other fall protection 'controls' to minimise the risk of injury. While it has been traditionally stated that codes of practice and Australian standards are 'guides' for implementation, courts have recently confirmed the weight they place on these 'guides'.[50] As WHS is heard in the criminal jurisdiction, this judicial opinion is considered *obiter dicta*, and it is therefore developing into common law practice.

Ensuring health and safety

The duties and responsibilities for health and safety attached to person conducting a business or undertaking (PCBU). This means you, if you are a contractor. It also means your employer or contracting authority. As a result, there may be several PCBUs involved in the one work arrangement. While this may seem to complicate the legal context of WHS, it is in fact very simple. Every PCBU must ensure 'as far as is reasonably practicable'—that term again—that work activities do not impact on the health and safety of workers, with 'workers' defined as anyone affected by the workplace (including direct employees, contractors, visitors, clients and members of the public).

In practice, there are several requirements for a PCBU, which are outlined below (although they are directly applicable only if you are a PCBU, and not a direct employee).

Identify risks to health and safety

A business must identify its health and safety risks. In simple terms, this means you cannot claim blissful ignorance, but must recognise the risks of the work task. For example, as a paramedic you cannot ignore the risk of being assaulted by an aggressive patient. Your breadth of potential occupational experience (you may walk onto construction sites, mines, roadways, private homes, fuel depots, etc., as part of your daily role) means you must expect and anticipate a wide variety of risks.

Eliminate risks to health and safety

The legislation is clear: its purpose is to make workplaces safe. What better way to be safe than to eliminate risks? If falling from a height is a risk, stay on the ground. Of course this is easier said than done, and a core focus of the paramedic role involves proximity to danger. This ideal is therefore impossible to implement.

Control risk which cannot be eliminated

This is where the concept of 'reasonably practicable' enters. Where we cannot eliminate risks, we can control them by minimising them as much as possible. The applied definition of reasonably practicable includes cost and practicalities.[51] For example, to remove the risk of being assaulted by a patient, we could wear military-grade armour suits, but doing so may not be cost-effective, nor conducive to providing paramedic care: reasonably practicable! There must be a balance.

So the hierarchy of controls must be followed. Essentially, where elimination is not possible, we are required to consider substituting or replacing a hazard (e.g. using mechanical lifting devices in place of manual handling), isolating people from the hazard (e.g. isolating Ebola patients in specialist hospital wings), applying administrative controls (e.g. signage and training to avoid injury), and, finally, when all else fails, providing and using PPE (personal protective equipment—including goggles, safety shoes, face masks, gloves).

As a contractor, you will have to fit in with your contracting body's requirements, which may be a private company, and its standards for PPE use, etc. It is, however, no excuse to simply follow. The law requires you to implement these practices, and have your own procedures for making your work environment safe.

Implement safe workplaces

Implementing a safe workplace is a broad concept, but boils down to the following critical aspects:[52]

- Make sure the physical environment is as safe as possible (e.g. the ambulance is well-maintained, has working brakes, lights, etc.).
- Make sure everyone is trained and competent (inexperience is a leading cause of injury).
- Develop procedures and follow them—it is important to have steps to do a job safely, but also everyone must follow them.
- Report incidents and make improvements when issues are identified (e.g. if you are always cutting yourself on a cupboard door, fix it!).
- Consult: allow workers to participate in workplace safety.

As a worker/employee, you are required to support your employer in following these steps. If you are a PCBU/contractor, you must still support the company or group that engages you (if applicable), but you must also make sure these steps are happening in your own business or operations.

Specific risks: remote and isolated work

As a paramedic, you may well be working remotely (or in isolation).[53] Even when working with a partner, you may be working outside areas of mobile phone coverage, and therefore it is important that you maintain safe procedures (having a working radio, making sure someone knows where you are).

Incidents/injuries

Incidents will always happen in a workplace, it is impossible to avoid them completely. As a paramedic, much of your work will involve responding to some form of 'incident'. It is, however, critical to recognise when you are involved in an incident yourself. This may include a patient contact that did not take place as expected, a vehicle accident, a slip or trip, or any other number of events.

When an incident occurs, and after responding to the incident (you may need to call for emergency assistance yourself!):

- Ask whether it is a notifiable incident. The WHS regulator (e.g. SafeWork NSW) may need to be notified. If so, protect the scene of the incident as if it were a crime scene.[54]
- Report it: to your employer, or to your engaging group if you are a contractor.
- Learn from it. What happened? Why?

As a worker, your duty is to report. As a PCBU/contractor, your duty is to investigate a serious incident to make sure those involved learn from it and avoid it recurring. The

WHS legislation speaks of *due diligence*,[55] which is a critical legal concept. It means that you need to do everything you should and can do to protect your safety and the safety of others. For example, if you are a fleet mechanic, you would be expected to recognise when an ambulance is not working properly. You cannot claim ignorance.

Regulation and enforcement

When things go wrong—such as serious incidents, deaths, or complaints about safety—several options may eventuate. Typically, a regulatory inspector (e.g. from SafeWork NSW) may attend a site, and issue or commence any of the following:

- *An improvement notice*—giving you a short timeframe to fix a problem (e.g. write up a safe work procedure and communicate it to your workers within 3 weeks).
- *A prohibition notice*—telling you that work must stop until you fix the issue (e.g. no work can occur until you replace your ambulance, and the regulator checks and approves it).
- *A fine*—you must pay it, or go to court to defend against it.
- *A prosecution*—you will be prosecuted, in a criminal jurisdiction, for failure to provide a safe workplace (or other offence), the result of which may be a criminal conviction and a fine.

Fines and prison sentences

As it currently stands, fines vary across states and territories. They include potential gaol time for the officers or directors of a PCBU. It is important to consult each Act directly, to be completely sure of the potential penalties. They range from maximum 5- to almost 20-year goal sentences, and fines of up to $12 million (references to NSW penalties are included for comparison,[56] along with recent Queensland penalties for industrial manslaughter).[57]

Refusal to work

As a paramedic, the highest-risk activity you will encounter is likely to be a dangerous situation, whether it be a dangerous site, a person influenced by drugs or mental illness, or the consequences of criminal activity or terrorism.

Your role as a paramedic is to provide medical assistance to your clients, and this role may conflict with the duty that you, and your employer, have to protect your own health and safety. The various safety Acts allow you to stop work when there is a safety risk. However, this may be in direct contrast to your duty to a client.

Insurances and other compliance requirements

It is important to pause to examine the implications of insurance. Insurance is not a 'fail-safe', particularly when examining business governance. Contracting is very popular in Australia, because in most jurisdictions it enables employers to limit their workers' compensation premium. Thus, you may be responsible for paying your own workers' compensation insurance. The word 'may' is important, because in some contractual relation-ships and jurisdictions, the regulators acknowledge this 'attempt to sidestep workers' compensation insurance premiums' and will determine you to be a 'direct worker' or a 'deemed worker'. In such cases your engaging body must pay your workers' compensation insurance. It is important to check this. Often the test is whether you work exclusively for the one group, or contract to a variety of organisations. You are best to seek advice from an accountant or an insurance broker.

Business consequences and structure

The way you establish your business may have many implications for you, including taxation, liability and insurance. You may establish as a sole trader, a company, a partnership, or one of several other appropriate structures. As selection of an appropriate business structure is beyond the scope of this text, it is advisable to consult an accountant or a solicitor.

Health, wellness and workplace rights

Rights and bullying, etc.

You have a number of rights in the workplace, many of which are enshrined in legislation. These include the anti-discrimination Acts, the *Fair Work Act 2009* and its provision prohibiting workplace bullying,[58] and criminal law. (See Table 13.4 for the main sources of legislation in Australia and New Zealand relevant to discrimination.) The following is a brief summary of the key types of workplace rights and responsibilities, outlining the applicable legislation and the ways of managing such issues.

Table 13.4 Discrimination legislation

Jurisdiction	Legislation
Commonwealth	*Racial Discrimination Act 1975*
	Sex Discrimination Act 1984
	Disability Discrimination Act 1992
	Age Discrimination Act 2004
Australian Capital Territory	*Discrimination Act 1991*
	Human Rights Act 2004
New South Wales	*Anti-Discrimination Act 1977*
Northern Territory	*Anti-Discrimination Act 1992*
Queensland	*Anti-Discrimination Act 1991*
South Australia	*Equal Opportunity Act 1984*
	Racial Vilification Act 1996
Tasmania	*Anti-Discrimination Act 1998*
Victoria	*Equal Opportunity Act 2011*
	Racial and Religious Tolerance Act 2001
Western Australia	*Equal Opportunity Act 1984*

Assault/violence: Can be either physical harm (battery) or the threat of physical harm. It is managed through the police and relevant state/territory criminal Acts.[59]

Harassment: Unwanted attention. Typically experienced as sexual harassment, which is a crime and managed under relevant criminal Acts. Harassment can be mistaken for discrimination or bullying, and there is often little difference between such experiences (indeed, courts often deal with them all as a similar concept).

Stalking: A defined criminal activity, aligned closely with bullying, but with distinct behavioural elements such as intimidation.

Bullying: Discussed in more detail below.

Discrimination: Being treated unfairly based on a personal characteristic, belief or other factor. Legislation outlines key discrimination contexts, including health, age, race, religion, etc.

Workplace bullying

As defined above, with the key elements being the repetition of unwanted and targeted behaviour. The volume of literature on this topic is typically focused on what is and what is not bullying. Unfortunately, the definition is ambiguous and subjective. What is considered to be bullying one workplace may be interpreted as part of a positive culture in another workplace. (For example, this is often an argument presented to defend the intensity experienced in a professional kitchen environment, where voices are raised.) This can make it difficult to identify and eradicate problem behaviour.[60]

The first step is to establish a clear definition. The *Fair Work Act 2009* outlines a definition, which has been adopted by workers' compensation courts and commissions, and then provides for the establishing of internal procedures to manage grievances, avoid (where possible) work injury developing, and resolve issues early.

Wellness

A full discussion of wellness is beyond the scope of this chapter, but exposure to trauma is an inherent component of the paramedic role. This means that maintaining wellness, physically and psychologically, is critical. There is a growing movement to prioritise workplace mental health, and relevant regulatory sources should be consulted for further information on this developing topic.[61]

Conclusion

This chapter has given a broad overview of the employment-related context of paramedic practice. It is a complicated area of law, due to the myriad legal instruments involved, and the different jurisdictions in which they operate. There is also the potential for conflict in this legal complexity, and it can be difficult to find clarity on employment issues. For example, if you experience discrimination at work, there are a number of different ways to manage it, depending on whether you are a contractor or a direct employee. There are no easy solutions, and so it may be important to seek expert advice in complicated situations.

The core of employment law is the concept of responsibilities or duties. We all have duties in the workplace, whether that be to look after our own safety and the safety of others, or to proactively manage risk and reduce injury risks. We must appreciate this, as the employment relationship, whether as a direct employee or subcontracted arrangement, invokes numerous responsibilities and requirements on both sides. It is critical that you understand what you are getting yourself into, to employ a colloquial phrase. No one option is any better than the other on paper, but some arrangements will suit your financial and family arrangements better than others. It is important that you understand the implications of your engagement, and comply with any legislated duties.

The topics introduced in this chapter that you should now understand include:

- how an employment contract is formed, and its key elements
- the operation and application of the relevant modern award and National Employment Standards
- enterprise bargaining and contractual fairness
- how a contractor relationships differs from an employment contract
- the duties and responsibilities outlined by WHS and employment laws
- your workplace rights
- how to navigate the legal complexities encountered in employment and workplace law.

Review Questions

1 An employer announces job cuts and states that *only* part-time employees will have their employment contracts terminated.

   a Could this be considered a form of discrimination?

   b Which class of person will be more affected than another?

   c What type of discrimination will this be?

   d Why?

2 A member of an ambulance crew witnesses their colleague rifling through the medicine cabinet of a patient. The paramedic leaves some of the patient's medicines, but takes other items and places them in their pocket. The paramedic who witnesses this confronts the colleague about it, as they believe the medicines have been taken for the paramedic's own use. The paramedic who takes the medicine remonstrates with their colleague and threatens them, saying that if they say anything to anyone they will 'do them in'. Identify what legislation exists to protect the paramedic who witnesses this, possibly, suspicious act.

3 A paramedic driving an ambulance under emergency conditions—lights on and sirens blaring—claims a red light as an exemption and treats the junction as a give-way. They advance through the intersection at 15 km/h. As they do so, a car collides with

Continued

Review Questions continued

the ambulance. The crew isn't injured, but the driver of the other vehicle is trapped with a fractured femur and requires freeing from the vehicle by the fire service.

   a Is the driver of the ambulance liable for the injuries sustained by the driver of the other vehicle?

   b If not, under what principle?

4 A member of a paramedic crew is continually belittled by their colleague stating such things as that they are not 'up to the job', they couldn't 'cannulate a barn door in a breeze', and they 'flap more than a frogman's flipper' at even commonplace incidents. The offended paramedic remonstrates with their colleague appropriately as to the harm these constant comments cause them. The offending officer dismisses the complaints, and states that—to the contrary—they were being supportive by 'building character'.

   a Is the stated defence of 'building character' acceptable, applied to this set of facts?

   b Why/why not?

5 Following this, the offending member of the crew stops making statements similar to the ones stated above. Unfortunately, they stop communicating altogether, good and bad, even when direct questions are asked by the previously offended crew member, making the paramedic–colleague relationship practically unworkable. Explain why this is detrimental.

6 A 64-year-old paramedic, who has given excellent service to their ambulance service, arrives back at station at the end of shift. The paramedic is met by the area manager and told that the service is restructuring and creating positions for a 'new breed of super paramedics', and the paramedic is told not to return tomorrow. They are also told that they have done nothing wrong, 'it is just the way things are'. The paramedic is thanked for their service, handed a letter with the words *Termination of Contract* in bold letters at the top, and told they will be offered some compensation but it has still to be 'worked out'. They 'should still get paid for a while', the paramedic is told. The paramedic accepts the letter and is escorted from the premises.

   a Is this lawful or unlawful dismissal?

   b Identify the section on the *Fair Work Act 2009* that deals with termination of contract.

   c Is the paramedic protected in any way?

   d If so, how?

Appendix 13.1	Industrial laws in Australia and New Zealand
Jurisdiction	**Legislation**
International	*International Convention on the Elimination of All Forms of Racial Discrimination 1965 (ICERD)* *Convention on the Elimination of All Forms of Discrimination Against Women 1979 (CEDAW)* *Convention on the Rights of Persons with Disabilities 2007* *International Labour Organization Convention No. 100—Equal Remuneration Convention 1951* *International Labour Organization Convention No. 111—Discrimination (Employment and Occupation) Convention 1958* *International Labour Organization Convention No. 158—Termination of Employment Convention 1982*
Commonwealth	*Fair Work Act 2009* *Age Discrimination Act 2004* *Equal Employment Opportunity (Commonwealth Authorities) Act 1987* *Occupational Health and Safety (Commonwealth Employment) Act 1991* *Disability Discrimination Act 1992* *Racial Discrimination Act 1975* *Sex Discrimination Act 1984* *Human Rights and Equal Opportunity Commission Act 1986* *Commonwealth Conciliation and Arbitration Act 1904* *Corporations Act 2001* *Industrial Relations Act 1988* *Privacy Act 1988* *Trade Practices Act 1975*
Australian Capital Territory	*Anti-Discrimination Act 1991* *Discrimination Act 1991* *Human Rights Act 2004* *Long Service Leave Act 1976* *Occupational Health and Safety Act 1989* *Workers Compensation Act 1951* *Work Safety Act 2008*
New South Wales	*Annual Holidays Act 1944* *Anti-Discrimination Act 1977* *Civil Liability Act 2002* *Employees Liability Act 1991* *Industrial Relations Act 1996* *Long Service Leave Act 1955* *Occupational Health and Safety Act 2000* *Privacy and Personal Information Protection Act 1998* *Public Sector Employment and Management Act 2002* *State Emergency and Rescue Management Act 1989* *Workers Compensation Act 1987* *Workplace Injury Management and Workers' Compensation Act 1998*

Continued

Appendix 13.1 Industrial laws in Australia and New Zealand continued	
Jurisdiction	**Legislation**
Northern Territory	*Annual Leave Act 1981* *Anti-Discrimination Act 1992* *Long Service Leave Act 1981* *Northern Territory Employment and Training Act 1999* *Public Sector Employment and Management Act 1993* *Workers Rehabilitation and Compensation Act 1986* *Workplace Health and Safety Act 2007*
Queensland	*Ambulance Act 1991* *Anti-Discrimination Act 1991* *Civil Liability Act 2003* *Coal Mining Safety and Health Act 1999* *Fair Work (Commonwealth Powers) and Other Provisions Act 2009* *Holidays Act 1983* *Industrial Relations Act 1999* *Public Interest Disclosure Act 2010* *Public Service Act 2008* *Workers' Compensation and Rehabilitation Act 2003* *Workplace Health and Safety Act 1995*
South Australia	*Civil Liability Act 1936* *Equal Opportunity Act 1984* *Fair Work Act 1994* *Fair Work (Commonwealth Powers) Act 2009* *Holidays Act 1910* *Law Reform (Contributory Negligence and Apportionment of Liability) Act 2001* *Long Service Leave Act 1987* *Occupational Health, Safety and Welfare Act 1986* *Training and Skills Development Act 2008* *Whistleblowers Protection Act 1993* *Workers Rehabilitation and Compensation Act 1986* *Racial Vilification Act 1996*
Tasmania	*Anti-Discrimination Act 1998* *Civil Liability Act 2002* *Industrial Relations Act 1984* *Industrial Relations (Commonwealth Powers) Act 2009* *State Services Act 2000* *Statutory Holidays Act 2000* *Workers Rehabilitation and Compensation Act 1988* *Workplace Health and Safety Act 1995*

Appendix 13.1 Industrial laws in Australia and New Zealand continued	
Jurisdiction	**Legislation**
Victoria	*Accident Compensation Act 1985* *Charter of Human Rights and Responsibilities 2006* *Equal Opportunity Act 2010* *Long Service Leave Act 1992* *Occupational Health and Safety Act 2004* *Public Administration Act 2004* *Public Holidays Act 1993* *Public Sector Management and Employment Act 1998* *Racial and Religious Tolerance Act 2001* *Whistleblowers Protection Act 2001*
Western Australia	*Civil Liability Act 2002* *Employment Dispute Resolution Act 2008* *Equal Opportunity Act 1984* *Industrial Relations Act 1979* *Occupational Health and Safety Act 1984* *Workers' Compensation and Injury Management Act 1981*
New Zealand	*Accident Compensation Act 2001* *Employment Relations Act 2000* *Equal Pay Act 1972* *Health and Safety in Employment Act 1992* *Holidays Act 2003* *Minimum Wage Act 1983* *Parental Leave and Employment Protection Act 1987* *State Sector Act 1988* *Human Rights Act 1993* *Industry Training Act 1992* *Injury Prevention, Rehabilitation and Compensation Act 2001* *Bill of Rights Act 1990* *Privacy Act 1993* *Accident Insurance Act 1998*

Endnotes

1 Australian Human Rights Commission. *Discrimination.* Online. Available: https://www.humanrights.gov.au/quick-guide/12030 (accessed 28 November 2018).

2 Australian Human Rights Commission. *The legal definition of sexual harassment.* Online. Available: https://www.humanrights.gov.au/publications/sexual-harassment-workplace-legal-definition-sexual-harassment. (accessed 28 November 2018).

3 Marx, K. and Engels, F. (1848; 1948 ed.). *Manifesto of the Communist Party.* London: Penguin Classics.

4 Stewart, A. (2015). *Stewart's Guide to Employment Law*, 5th ed. Annandale: The Federation Press, at p. 92.

5   *Fair Work Act 2009* (Cth), Pt 2-2.

6   Ibid., Pt 3-3, s 424.

7   *Johnstone v Bloomsbury Health Authority* [1991] 2 WLR 1362.

8   *Koehler v Cerebos (Australia) Ltd* [2005] HCA 15.

9   *Stevens v Brodribb Sawmilling Co Pty Ltd; Gray v Brodribb Sawmilling Co Pty Ltd* (1986) 160 CLR 16.

10 *Hollis v Vabu Pty Ltd* (2001) 207 CLR 21.

11 *Fair Work Act 2009* (Cth), Pt 2-2, Div 3.

12 Ibid., Div 4.

13 Ibid., Div 5.

14 Ibid., Div 6.

15 Ibid., Div 7.

16 Ibid., Div 8.

17 Ibid., Div 9.

18 Ibid., Div 10.

19 Ibid., Div 11.

20 Ibid., Div 11, s 119(2).

21 Ibid., Div 12.

22 Ambulance and Patient Transport Industry Award 2010, cl 7.1.

23 Ibid., cl 8.1.a and b.

24 Ibid., cl 9.1–9.3.

25 *Fair Work Act 2009* (Cth), Pt 2-2.

26 Fair Work Commission. (2016) *Resolving disputes*. Online. Available: https://www.fwc.gov.au/disputes-at-work/how-the-commission-works/resolving-disputes (accessed 28 November 2018).

27 Ambulance and Patient Transport Industry Award 2010, cl 10.

28 Ibid., cl 11.

29 Ibid., cl 14.

30 Ibid., cl 18.

31 Ibid., cl 20.

32 Ibid., cl 20.5.

33 Ibid., cl 20.6.

34 Ibid., cl 21.

35 Ibid., cl 24.1.

36 Ibid., cl 24.2.

37 Ibid., cl 24.3.

38 Ibid., cl 25.

39 Ibid., cl 26.

40 Ibid., cl 27.

41 Ibid., cl 28.

42 Ibid., cl 29.

43 Ibid., cl 30.

44 Ibid., cl 31.2.

45 *Fair Work Act 2009* (Cth), s 385.

46 *Sweeny v Boyland Nominees Pty Ltd* (2006) 226 CLR 161.

47 *Lister v Bowland Nominees Pty Ltd* [2001] 2 WLR 1311.

48 *Work Health and Safety Act 2011* (NSW), Pt 3.

49 *Work Health and Safety Regulations 2017* (NSW), Ch 5.

50 *SafeWork (NSW) v Activate Fire Pty Ltd* [2017] DCNSWDC 66, at [103].

51 *Work Health and Safety Act 2011* (NSW), s 18.

52 Ibid., s 19.

53 *Work Health and Safety Regulation 2017* (NSW), cl 48.

54 *Work Health and Safety Act 2011* (NSW), Pt 3.

55 Ibid., s 27.

56 Ibid., Div 5

57 *Work Health and Safety Act 2011* (QLD), Div 5, Pt 2a.

58 *Fair Work Act 2009* (Cth), Part 6-4b.

59 For example, *Crimes Act 1958* (Vic), s 31.

60 Ragusa, A.T. and Groves, P. (2015) Stigmatisation and the social construction of bullying in Australian administrative law: you can't make an omelette without cracking an egg. *The University of New South Wales Law Journal* 38(4), 1507–1528.

61 SafeWork Australia. (2014) *Preventing psychological injury under work health and safety laws*. Fact sheet. Online. Available: https://www.safeworkaustralia.gov.au/doc/preventing-psychological-injury-under -work-health-and-safety-laws-fact-sheet (accessed 28 November 2018).

Chapter 14
Paramedic practice in New Zealand—legal issues and current debates

Kate Diesfeld

Learning objectives

After reading this chapter, you should be able to:

- describe New Zealand's medico–legal framework
- explain the legal impact of New Zealand's accident compensation scheme for paramedics
- understand paramedics' legal obligations to the people they serve
- apply New Zealand's *Code of Health and Disability Services Consumers' Rights*
- understand the current debates regarding registration of New Zealand's paramedics.

Definitions

Accident Compensation Act 2001 Legislation defining the accident compensation system and the treatment of injury.

Code of Health and Disability Services Consumers' Rights Code defining healthcare and disability services consumers' 10 rights.

Health Practitioners Competence Assurance Act 2003 Legislation governing the registration of healthcare practitioners.

An introductory case

Terminal stages of renal failure (98HDC15374)

Mrs A, an elderly Māori woman, was in the terminal stages of renal failure. When her condition deteriorated at home, her daughter consulted the phone book and rang the New Zealand Ambulance Service (NZAS), a not-for-profit private provider. The ambulance service attempted to ascertain the patient's status over the phone, but the daughter was

An introductory case continued

only able to communicate that the patient's feet were swollen and that her doctor had instructed the daughter to call an ambulance. When the ambulance officer (the officer) entered the house, Mrs A was 'oozing' blood and mucus. He neither assessed nor took her history. The officer attempted to contact the public hospital emergency department by mobile phone. At that the time, the NZAS protocol was to contact the hospital switchboard and ask to be transferred to the emergency department receptionist. The officer reported that by the time he contacted the switchboard, the ambulance had arrived at the hospital, so he hung up.

The officer could not recall where he placed the patient in the emergency room, or what he said to the emergency department staff. He reported that his standard practice was to hand the patient record form to the receptionists, to wait for them to read and check the document, and then to leave. In this instance, he told the patient's daughter that 'someone will see you shortly', and he left.

Approximately 30 minutes later, the receptionist noticed that the patient appeared unwell. The triage nurse was unable to obtain a clear history from the patient or her daughter. The patient was taken to the resuscitation room and died within an hour.

The Health and Disability Commissioner (HDC) issued an opinion that both the NZAS and the public hospital breached the *Code of Health and Disability Services Consumers' Rights*. Both were in breach of Right 4(5): 'Every consumer has the right to co-operation among providers to ensure quality and continuity of services.'

Additionally, the NZAS was in breach because it did not provide adequate medical support. Right 4(1) states: 'Every consumer has the right to have services provided with reasonable care and skill'. The HDC observed that: 'A single medical advisor cannot be expected to provide support 24 hours a day, 7 days a week.'

The failure of the NZAS document procedures breached Right 4(2): 'Every consumer has the right to have services provided that comply with legal, professional, ethical, and other relevant standards.' Also, the NZAS consistently failed to provide information when requested during the HDC investigation, another breach of Right 4(5). Finally, the hospital was in breach of Right 4(2) for failure to provide immediate triage. In other countries, this conduct might result in a malpractice lawsuit. However, New Zealand's novel legal framework provides for an alternative legal pathway, starting with the Health and Disability Commissioner.

This chapter introduces New Zealand's medico–legal framework, and an overview of the relevant law for paramedic practice in New Zealand.

Introduction

Paramedics in New Zealand face many of the dilemmas encountered by paramedics abroad. Universal legal issues include patients' capacity to provide informed consent, privacy, paramedics' duty of care and, in some instances, criminal proceedings. New Zealand has specific legislation and case law related to these medico–legal issues. Of note, paramedics are not registered in New Zealand.

This chapter introduces New Zealand's novel accident compensation system, and the broader legal framework that applies to paramedics. To safeguard patients, New Zealand has also created an enforceable code of rights with avenues for redress. Also, New Zealand has reformed its legislation to address the competence of *registered* health practitioners; this regime may apply to paramedics in the future.

In 2008, the Health Committee initiated an inquiry into the provision of ambulance services at the request of the New Zealand Ambulance Association ('the Association'), which is an ambulance union. The committee's chair presented a report, *Inquiry into the Provision of Ambulance Services in New Zealand*, to the House of Representatives.[1]

The Association was concerned about public safety because the under-resourced services resulted in significant inconsistencies across the sector and regions. Issues included single-crewing, funding, training and competence standards. The Association expressed that 'the provision of emergency ambulance services is inadequate and *ad hoc*'.[2] Paramedic registration was, and remains, a live issue in New Zealand.

The history of New Zealand paramedics and ambulance services

New Zealanders have enjoyed the benefits of emergency care services for many years. The first reported 'ambulance' response was by an 'Ashford litter' in Christchurch in 1885, a horse-drawn ambulance was used in 1898, and the first motor ambulance was used in Timaru in 1916.[3] Between then and now, the occupation has undergone substantial change and faced many challenges. Al-Shaqsi's history of New Zealand's ambulance services and paramedic practice provides an informative overview.[4] For example, New Zealand's emergency medical services are currently contractual and funded both privately and publicly.

New Zealand ambulance funding

Private funding is generated from a range of sources. This chapter will refer to data regarding St John New Zealand, the largest provider. Its ambulance service is the emergency arm of the health sector. According to its 2017/2018 annual report, it 'responded to more than 533,000 [emergency] 111 calls for an ambulance in the last year [and its] 3,228 paid staff, 9,389 volunteers and 7,202 youth members touch more than one million people each year'.[5]

For 2017/2018, 'St John NZ's reported performance was a deficit of $1.7 million[6] with an underlying deficit (after taking account of significant or one-off items) of $4.4 million for the financial year July 2017– June 2018' (2017/18), 'compared with the $9.9 million underlying deficit for the previous year'.[7] On a positive note, St John will 'receive more than $100 million over the next four years commencing 2017/18 to double crew all emergency ambulances, along with a sustainable funding model to increase baseline funding and support future growth'.[8]

'Investment from government and community contracts with the Ministry of Health (to respond to medical emergencies), the Accident Compensation Commission (ACC) (to respond to personal injuries), and district health boards (for patient-transfer services) fund around 72% of (St John's) ambulance service operating costs.'[9] Donations reached almost $36 million in 2017/2018.[10]

The service does charge patients who are treated by an ambulance officer or are transported in an ambulance because of a medical emergency. The part-charge is $98 (including GST), while 'the cost to St John of a typical emergency ambulance call out is around $620 (incl GST)',[11] based on 2017/18 data.

None of the funders monitor the service's non-mandatory standards. Providers are only required to show 'reasonable endeavours' to comply with the 'very non-specific' standards.[12] The need for national competence standards was highlighted by a coroner's recommendation in 2008 for stringent national paramedic guidelines after the death of a patient wrongly assessed by paramedics as having a virus, and this was supported by the Kedgley Report.[13] The emphasis on patients' safety reflects the primary purpose of, and a justification for, the registration of paramedics under the *Health Practitioners Competence Assurance Act 2003*, which currently governs occupations including medicine and nursing.

A volunteer workforce
Importantly, volunteers make a significant contribution in New Zealand. In 2017, a remarkable 3519 clinically trained volunteers provided vital, frontline service.[14] Anecdotally, the relatively low rate of complaints regarding volunteers may be explained by the public's appreciation of the volunteers' dedication. Also, the low rate may indicate that ambulance services effectively manage complaints, while reporting salient details to the Ministry of Health. (However, Al-Shaqsi[15] discussed the wider impact of volunteerism, including the potential impact on the quality of service by high workforce turnover.) Clearly, volunteers play an essential role in New Zealand.

New Zealand's medico–legal landscape
Both healthcare and paramedic practice in New Zealand are governed by a wide array of legislation. As elsewhere, New Zealand health providers are legally required to perform their duties to the standard of reasonable care and skill. 'At common law, a health provider may be held liable in the tort of negligence for failing to exercise reasonable care and skill when death, injury or other damage is caused to the patient by that failure.'[16] However, New Zealand's accident compensation scheme distinguishes it from other countries like Australia.

For a listing of select legislation and select cases in New Zealand and Australia, see Appendix 14.1. New Zealand's two distinguishing features are its 'treatment injury' provisions under the compensation scheme, and the *Code of Health and Disability Services Consumers' Rights* (the Code).[17]

No-fault compensation

Since 1974, New Zealand has implemented a compensation system for victims of accident and injury that almost entirely bars personal injury litigation, including medical malpractice.[18] Scholars have identified both the benefits and the harms that flow from malpractice litigation.[19] The merits include potential damage awards for the injured, which may deter the provider (and others) from further negligence or misconduct. Also, malpractice litigation aims to identify fault and hold people accountable.

While litigation does attribute blame, it is an adversarial process that may be accompanied by shame or embarrassment for those who breach professional standards.[20] There can also be significant employment impacts. Consequently, providers may resist disclosure: 'Doctors and nurses in the shadow of litigation clam up [because] they are naturally wary of admitting any doubts'[21] about their practices. The Australian system has attempted to limit this negative effect by requiring disclosure by professionals who cause harmful medical errors, without an admission of liability.[22, 23] This approach recognises that providers do make mistakes, and promotes a culture of truth-telling. Importantly, in Australia, practitioners have a *legal duty* to inform so that the harm can be remedied.

Unfortunately, the possibility of litigation may also increase defensive practices. For example, Australian research revealed how doctors' concerns about litigation impacted on their practices, particularly for those who have previously experienced a medico–legal dispute.[24] In a survey, 2999 respondents reported changes in practice due to medico–legal concerns: 43% of doctors reported that they referred patients more than usual; 55% stated that they ordered more tests than usual; and 11% stated that they prescribed medications more than usual.[25]

Also, lawsuits are financially and emotionally costly for all parties. The conflict may damage the relationships between health providers, patients and the public.[26]

However, while a no-fault system may diminish some of these effects, it is not without flaws. Arguably, if litigation is barred, there must be a rigorous system to ensure accountability and public safety.[27] The reality of this danger was demonstrated by the notorious experiment conducted at the National Women's Hospital in New Zealand by a prominent medical academic.

> Without gaining his patients' consent, he withheld standard treatment for patients with cervical carcinoma in situ, in the belief and hoping it was unnecessary. Some patients benefitted in consequence, but for others the outcomes were disastrous.[28]

Subsequently, the Commission of Inquiry in 1987–88 led to the famous Cartwright Report.[29] In response, New Zealand's government established legal and ethical protections that are relevant to paramedicine. Part of New Zealand's response was amending the accident compensation scheme to provide cover for what is now referred to as 'treatment injury', and establishing the enforceable Code. In rare instances, serious code breaches may progress to the Human Rights Review Tribunal (the HRRT).

> Thus, rare claims for exemplary damages and other exceptional situations aside, patients who have died or suffered physical injury as a result of a health practitioner's failure to exercise reasonable care and skill cannot bring a civil claim for negligence for damages for a practitioner in respect of that injury.[30]

While there is evidence that some injured persons are dissatisfied with non-monetary remedies,[31] New Zealand's regime has endured, and the title of the current legislation is the *Accident Compensation Act 2001.*

'Treatment injury' under the *Accident Compensation Act 2001* and paramedics

In New Zealand, patients injured as a result of their medical treatment may make a claim for compensation under the *Accident Compensation Act 2001* (the ACA). However, the provision for treatment *injury* compensation applies only to injuries suffered by a person who has sought or received that treatment from a *registered health professional,* or *received treatment at the direction of a registered health professional.* Section 32 of the ACA states:

> Treatment injury means personal injury that is—
>
> (a) suffered by a person—
>   (i) seeking treatment from 1 or more registered health professionals; or
>   (ii) receiving treatment from, or at the direction of, 1 or more registered health professionals; or
>   (iii) referred to in subsection (7); and
>
> (b) caused by treatment; and
>
> (c) not a necessary part, or ordinary consequence, of the treatment, taking into account all the circumstances of the treatment, including—
>   (i) the person's underlying health condition at the time of the treatment; and
>   (ii) the clinical knowledge at the time of the treatment.

(See Appendix 14.2 for more details.)

As noted, the role of the 'registered health professional' is relevant for 'treatment injury' cover under section 32(1)(a)(i) and (ii) of the ACA. Ambulance officers do not fall within the section 6 definition of 'registered health professional'. 'Treatment given by these providers cannot fall within cover for treatment injury, unless given under the direction of another registered health professional.'[32] If a person cannot obtain cover under section 32, the person could attempt to obtain cover for 'personal injury caused by an accident' or another head of cover under section 20(2) of the ACA. Also, patients may find an alternative route for a remedy, as described above, through the HRRT for breach of the Code.

Health and Disability Commissioner Act 1994

A significant outcome of the Cartwright Inquiry was the establishment of the Health and Disability Commissioner (HDC). Pursuant to the *Health and Disability Commissioner Act 1994* (HDCA), the HDC promotes and protects the rights of people who are receiving health or disability services. These protections are defined as 10 rights within the Code (see Appendix 14.3). Any persons who hold themselves out as providing a health or disability service, whether they are registered or unregistered, or providing a service for payment or voluntarily, must abide by the Code according to section 3(k) of the HDCA. More specifically, any person who provides ambulance services to the public is bound by the Code under section 3(i). The onus is on the provider to prove that they took reasonable actions, according to clause 4 of the Code. It is very important for New Zealand ambulance services to understand that they must abide by New Zealand law and refer to current New Zealand scholarship, such as the texts on health law by Keenan[33] and by Skegg and Paterson.[34]

If paramedics fail to abide by the Code, a complaint may be made by the consumer or other concerned person, then investigated, resolved between parties or referred to the HDC for a determination of whether a breach occurred. If the Commissioner determines there was a breach, they may make recommendations and may refer it to the independent Director of Proceedings.[35] In the year ending 30 June 2018, of the 2498 new complaints filed with the HDC, 102 were formally investigated, and breaches found in 70.[36] Very few were referred to the Director of Proceedings; there were 28 referrals in progress during 2017/18, including 11 referrals received during the course of the year. One involved an ambulance service.[37]

The Director may refer the case of a serious breach of the Code to the relevant registration body or disciplinary tribunal (for registered practitioners), or to the HRRT.[38] Of note, the HRRT is not a disciplinary body; it reviews breaches of the Code (as well as of the *Privacy Act 1993* and the *Human Rights Act 1993*). Thus, it is very important for paid and volunteer paramedics to appreciate that serious breaches may be heard by the HRRT.

Several claims have been made about this regime. Historically, there was a lack of accountability under the accident compensation scheme when providers engaged in misconduct and malpractice. Also, the accident compensation and HDC system was described as 'cumbersome' and 'confusing' within the Cull Report,[39] which analysed the processes concerning adverse medical events. The Cull Report recommendations influenced the creation of the *Health Practitioners Competence Assurance Act 2003* (HPCAA).

The HPCAA applies to registered practitioners, but not to paramedics. Depending on the type and seriousness of the breach by a *registered* practitioner, an HDC case may proceed to the Director of Proceedings and be referred to the Health Practitioners Disciplinary Tribunal (HPDT). There may be a low-level resolution by the regulatory body or, ultimately, a hearing before the HPDT. Importantly, the HPDT's penalties do *not* include compensation to the patient, due to the accident compensation scheme. In contrast, exemplary damages may be awarded to aggrieved persons by the HRRT. *Registered* practitioners may be held accountable by both tribunals.

As paramedics do not have a registration body or disciplinary tribunal, serious breaches involving consumers may only proceed to the HRRT. As noted above, in extraordinary (and rare) cases the HRRT may award exemplary damages[40] up to $350,000 for 'flagrant disregard' of rights.[41] However, the HRRT has not yet awarded damages of this amount for a breach of the Code. More commonly, the HRRT makes a declaration regarding whether there has been a breach. Paramedics may, of course, be accountable to their employers and subject to criminal proceedings.

Code of Health and Disability Services' Consumers Rights

The purpose of the HDCA is, according to section 6, 'to promote and protect the rights of health consumers and disability services consumers, and, to that end, to facilitate the fair, simple, speedy, and efficient resolution of complaints relating to infringements of those rights'. The HDC is an independent, statutory ombudsman with authority to investigate any action of a provider where an action is, or appears to be, a breach of the Code. The rights have direct application to paramedics.

The Code places obligations on providers of health and disability services (*providers*) and confers rights on people who use health and disability services (*consumers*). Duties apply to health professionals, unregistered healthcare providers (e.g. paramedics) and institutional providers such as hospitals and rest homes.[42] The Code addresses rights relating to: respect and privacy; fair treatment; dignity and independence; appropriate standards; effective communication; information; choice; consent; support; rights during teaching and research; and complaints procedures.

Importantly, the Commissioner's jurisdiction is restricted to quality of service, and does not include issues of funding or *entitlement* to a particular service.[43] According to the previous Commissioner, Professor Ron Paterson, the Code and the resulting Commissioner's opinions have been described as 'tools for quality improvement'.[44] The Commissioner issues an opinion, not a decision. Those opinions are the concrete foundation for any potential referral to the two tribunals described above. The HDC opinions also have preventive potential, because they demonstrate the boundaries of acceptable practice for other providers.[45]

Historical research on paramedic breaches is informative. Between February 2004 and April 2009, the HDC received 46 complaints about ambulance services, of which 25 referred to Right 4, regarding the appropriate standard of care.[46] In the majority of cases, the HDC took no further action. Of the 31 complaints filed between January 2008 and June 2011 regarding ambulance services, one was resolved by the HDC, 16 received no further action and 9 were still open.[47] In the majority of those cases, the HDC took no further action.[48]

The HDC selectively publishes decisions of educational value and currently a search for 'ambulance service' detected 13 opinions (Appendix 14.1).

Right 4 is the mostly frequently breached right, across occupations. Right 4 establishes that:

(1) Every consumer has the right to have services provided with reasonable care and skill.

(2) Every consumer has the right to services provided that comply with legal, professional, ethical, and other relevant standards.

(3) Every consumer has the right to services provided in a manner consistent with his or her needs.

(4) Every consumer has the right to have services provided in a manner that minimises the potential harm to, and optimises the quality of life of, that consumer.

(5) Every consumer has the right to co-operation among providers to ensure quality and continuity of services.

The following three cases are representative of the issues that paramedics encounter, beginning with Case 14.1—13HDC01190. In this case, in the HDC's opinion, the paramedic's assessment and treatment was 'seriously inadequate', which was a breach of Right 4(1) for failing to provide services with reasonable care and skill. The substandard

Case 14.1 Care provided by paramedic during patient transfer (13HDC01190)

The consumer lived in her own home and had diabetes, ischaemic heart disease, and chronic obstructive airway disease. The woman was reliant on oxygen, and experienced shortness of breath and pain. Her daughter activated the medical alarm and called 111. Based on the medical officer's advice, the woman was not transported to hospital by the paramedic. Two hours later, the daughter called the ambulance again. The paramedic could not rouse the volunteer from sleep, so attended the call-out alone. The medical officer advised the paramedic to transport the consumer to hospital. The paramedic did not bring portable oxygen up to the consumer's house. While being wheeled to the ambulance, the chair tipped over and the consumer collapsed. The paramedic attached an acute mask for oxygen and put the consumer on a monitor. Despite the alarms sounding because of the low oxygen levels, the paramedic did not stop until they reached the hospital. The woman died during the journey.

documentation was a breach of Right 4(2) for failing to provide services that comply with legal, professional, ethical, and other relevant standards.

Of note, providers do have protections, although the Code's focus is clearly dedicated to safeguarding consumers. Clause 3 of the Code provides that:

(1) A provider is not in breach of this Code if the provider has taken reasonable actions in the circumstances to give effect to the rights, and comply with the duties, in this Code.

(2) The onus is on the provider to prove that it took reasonable actions.

(3) For the purposes of this clause, 'the circumstances' means all the relevant circumstances, including the consumer's clinical circumstances and the provider's resource constraints.

In this opinion, the HDC noted that the paramedic's scope of practice was reduced from paramedic to emergency medical technician. The HDC recommended that the paramedic apologise to Mrs A's family, that he review relevant aspects of his practice, and document these to the HDC. The recommendations included that the ambulance service provide evidence of specific staff training on specific processes, as well as the *Updated Clinical Procedures and Guidelines 2013–2015*. Staff were to be trained on those and ongoing refresher updates delivered. The service was advised to use the anonymised case in its internal publication, and to audit its rate of pager failures. Of note, although the doctor and service were not found in breach, the HDC made adverse comments regarding both.

This case demonstrates how the Code applies to paramedics and how the HDC functions. It also illuminates the relatively low cost and less adversarial nature of the HDC system, in comparison with ordinary litigation. The simple language of the HDC opinion expresses how the HDC aims to educate and does not aim to punish. Also, the opinion indicates

Case 14.2 Toxic shock syndrome (09HDC02269)

This complaint alleged that ambulance staff failed to treat a consumer with the appropriate standard of care when attending him at his home. In addition, the staff did not relay information to the hospital that had been reported to them by the consumer's partner, instead advising the hospital staff that his condition was psychosomatic. On the same day, the hospital medical staff failed to appropriately examine the consumer and diagnose his group A streptococcal toxic shock syndrome, instead supplying him with painkillers and sending him home in a taxi still in pain. He died at home later that day.

some of the range of remedies available to seriously injured consumers in New Zealand under the HDC's limited powers.

Case 14.2: 09HDC02269 provides another example of the preventive and educative value of the HDC's opinions. According to the HDC, in this case the ambulance officer had breached Right 4(2) and (5). In assuming the consumer's condition was psychosomatic, the officer did not pay adequate attention to other symptoms and signs reported by the consumer's partner. This interfered with the officer's ability to provide an objective, professional assessment.

Consequently, in recording his subjective judgement, the officer may have contributed to the 'less than satisfactory treatment' subsequently given by the medical and nursing staff. Also, the officer was negligent during the hand-over to the emergency department staff, because he failed to inform staff, and document, the consumer's condition.

The conduct of other staff was also scrutinised. While there was no breach by the ambulance driver, the ambulance service or the hospital, there was a breach of Right 4 by the senior house officer.

The HDC recommended that the ambulance officer apologise to the consumer's surviving partner. The officer was directed to refrain from making and documenting personal, subjective judgements when assessing patients. The senior house officer was found in breach of Right 4(1) for failing to provide services in the emergency department with reasonable care and skill. The HDC recommended that she study the diagnosis and treatment of lower back pain, and approach diagnosis in a systematic manner, eliminating serious systemic illnesses before diagnosing mechanical back pain. She was also directed to undertake peer review of her note-taking.

This opinion demonstrates how the HDC manages a complaint where an incident involves multiple providers. Due to the HDC's limited powers, even though the case concerned the consumer's death, it resulted in relatively lenient recommendations. Even when a death has occurred, a paramedic cannot be referred to a disciplinary tribunal, the HPDT. However, if the paramedic was found in breach, the matter could be referred to the HRRT, with the paramedic being liable for up to $350,000 exemplary (not compensatory) damages for the aggrieved person or their representatives.

Case 14.3 Reflux (03HDC00153)

In this case, the consumer's wife complained that an ambulance officer did not appropriately review and assess the consumer. The 55-year-old consumer woke with pain in his chest and stomach area. The ambulance officer diagnosed unrelieved reflux exacerbated by hyperventilation. He reported that he gave the consumer the option of going to hospital, but the consumer was reluctant. Therefore, after the officer suggested that the consumer drink a hot Milo to settle his stomach and to consult his general practitioner, the officer left. The consumer's partner did not recall the discussion regarding the hospital option. Approximately 10 minutes later, the consumer collapsed. The ambulance returned, the officer commenced CPR and defibrillation, and the consumer was transferred to the hospital. After being in a coma for 36 hours, the consumer suffered brain damage that resulted in severe impairment.

Case 14.3: 03HDC00153 relates to the clinical assessment of a consumer. Although there was disagreement about the ambulance officer's conduct, the first time he visited the consumer's residence the officer concluded that the consumer had suffered an anxiety attack that had resolved. There was no documentation that transport to hospital had been offered and was refused. According to the HDC, the officer did not further enquire into the consumer's condition, and did not transport him to hospital for a full assessment. This breached Right 4(1). Also, his failure to fully document details for an appropriate assessment breached Right 4(2).

However, the ambulance service avoided a breach for vicarious liability under section 72(2) of the HDCA because it employed Mr B, who was a trained and experienced ambulance officer and team leader. Mr B had completed an advanced life support course through the service, which provides training on the assessment, diagnosis and treatment of cardiac patients. The service provided training on, and required staff compliance with, the requirements of the Ambulance Education Council's 'Authorised Patient Care Procedures'. Accordingly, the service had taken reasonable steps to ensure that its officers assess and respond appropriately.

This opinion reveals how ambulance services may avoid breaches through stringent employment standards, routine updating of policies, and zealous monitoring of their implementation. Regarding the ambulance officer, the HDC's sole recommendation was that he 'review his practice in light of this report', and a copy of the report was sent to the New Zealand Ambulance Board. Had paramedics been registered, this officer might have been disciplined by the HPDT in the interests of public safety. This officer might have received a range of penalties, such as de-registration, suspension, fines, 'rehabilitation' through advanced training,[49] the payment of costs, and censure. However, currently paramedics do not have a national disciplinary body.

Case 14.4 refers to the final opinion (00HDC06794) which has universal application, although it related to a radiologist. The issue is relevant to paramedic students, educators

Case 14.4 Radiologist did not obtain consent for registrar to observe ultrasound at teaching hospital (OOHDC06794)

A woman complained about the conduct of a provider who did not obtain her informed consent to have another professional present during a medical procedure. The woman received a pelvic ultrasound at a public teaching hospital. The radiologist authorised a registrar to observe, and introduced the registrar as a colleague. The radiologist did not explain to the woman why the registrar was present or that the registrar was in training.

and employers. Also, it clarifies a common myth regarding the obligations of students (or trainees) and their supervisors. The HDC determined that the radiologist breached Right 6(1)(d) for failing to notify the patient of the proposed participation in teaching. Also, in failing to explain why the registrar was present, the radiologist did not obtain the woman's *informed* consent, a breach of Right 7(1). The radiologist erroneously believed that consent was only required when the trainee was *undertaking an intervention*. However, this case clarified that the consumers' right to an explanation includes *observational* teaching. Right 9 expresses that the Code applies to consumers who are participating in, or when it is proposed that they participate in, teaching or research. This opinion is a potent reminder that lessons for practice may be derived from cases that involve other occupations.

As noted above, consumers are generally barred from bringing a civil action in medical malpractice in New Zealand. Although serious breaches of the Code may be referred to the Director of Proceedings and progress to the HRRT, only one has done so as of the date of publication. Nonetheless, the above cases illustrate paramedics' duties to their patients, which is central to the HPCAA and to debates regarding paramedic registration in New Zealand.

The registration debate

The registration of paramedics has been an enduring the subject of debate in New Zealand. If registered, paramedics would be regulated under the HPCAA. They would join the ranks of 22 registered occupations, including nurses, midwives, dentists and doctors. Given the training and expertise that competent paramedic practice requires, entry into the community of registered professionals and the corresponding recognition may be long overdue.[50]

Members of the paramedic workforce believe they meet the primary criteria for regulation under the HPCAA because they offer a health service that may pose a risk of harm to the public's health and safety. As of 2017, the Ministry of Health estimated that the paramedic workforce has approximately 1000 individuals in scope for registration.

These have authority to practice (ATP) as granted by their employer of 'Paramedic' or higher as well as a minimum of a Bachelor's Degree, or professional service equivalent. The overall workforce, including volunteers, is the order of 4500, 48% of whom are 'First Responders'. Also, 1300 (29%) are 'Emergency Medical Technicians' (EMT, NCEA Level 5) who although able to administer 16 medications, are not normally able to provide 'high risk' interventions, as defined by the Ministry of Health. Increasingly the paid EMT workforce are degree qualified and such degree qualified EMTs are able to practise. Paramedic-level interventions when crewed with a Paramedic or higher Authority to Practice, even though the Paramedic may not have a degree.[51]

The workforce welcomes registration. According to the New Zealand stakeholder feedback published in 2017, the vast majority (90%) of the workforce believed that it is in the public interest to regulate paramedics under the HPCAA, with 80% believing it is practical and cost-effective to do so. Of the 12% who were unsure, free text comments indicate that they lack information regarding how registration would be implemented.[52]

The HPCAA aims to deliver a consistent system for protecting public safety through the provision of standards and by the monitoring of professional competence. Its purpose is to 'protect the health and safety of members of the public by providing for mechanisms to ensure health practitioners are competent and fit to practise their professions' according to section 3(1). The HPCAA explicitly places public safety at the forefront of professional regulation. Public safety was also a core concern of the Kedgley Inquiry[53] in 2008, regarding the standards, qualifications and potential registration of paramedics.

The first application for registration by Ambulance New Zealand cited research conducted during the second half of 2010 among ambulance officers and New Zealand Defence Force medics.[54]

Some additional form of regulation is needed in New Zealand to improve public health and safety,[55] and regulation of paramedics under the Act would be the most efficient and effective at this point in time.[56]

Ambulance New Zealand identified many benefits of registration, and reported that 'implementation of regulation is possible'.[57] Benefits included:

1 Paramedics deliver health services that do have the very real potential to cause patient harm.

2 There is a trend to regulate paramedics as health practitioners in jurisdictions similar to New Zealand.

3 Registration would ensure consistent, professional development requirements across New Zealand.

4 The sector would have one registering authority that would be independent of employers, unions and education providers.

5 It is likely that the public would view paramedics as 'trained and registered health practitioners'.

6 The authority would have a more robust process for assessing foreign providers.

Again, the primary purpose of registration under the HPCAA is patient safety. Research indicates that patient safety is of vital concern to this sector and the people they serve.

The stakeholders' report by Paramedics Australasia to the New Zealand inquiry into registration was very informative. It identified that 'over 50% of respondents are directly aware of harmful incidents' within paramedic practice.[58] The level of awareness corresponded with the higher level of paramedic ATP. The rates reported by non-ambulance sector participants and members of the New Zealand Defence Force were as high as 70%.[59] Of the respondents who believed paramedics pose a potential harm to the health and safety of the public, almost 96% believed these risks to be life-threatening.[60]

Another protective measure is access to the pan-professional disciplinary body, the HPDT. It hears cases involving misconduct (including malpractice and negligence), unfitness to practise, bringing the profession into disrepute, and practising outside the designated scope of practice. The potential penalties range from censure, fines and payment of costs, to having conditions upon practice and de-registration. If registered, paramedics would enjoy a consistent, national, transparent disciplinary regime, but also potentially be subject to these penalties. Cases of serious breaches of the Code by paramedics, arguably evident within the above HDC opinions, and other conduct could result in formal discipline by the HPDT.

The impact on volunteers is a crucial factor, too. In 2011, Ambulance New Zealand reported volunteers' perspectives on registration: 'nearly 75% of the respondents who identified themselves as volunteers agreed there was high risk that the sector would lose large numbers of volunteers if they were required to be registered',[61] and '84% of people working in remote areas thought regulation would stop volunteers from practising'.[62]

However, the result of a questionnaire sent out by Ambulance New Zealand in 2008 reported that 28% of volunteers would definitely consider a career as a paid staff member, and 31% might do so.[63] It was not clear whether more volunteers would pursue the necessary qualifications to become registered. However, registration could offer an attractive career pathway for volunteers. Volunteer status remains a challenging issue in the debates regarding registration.

Likewise, the cost of registration is central to the debate. Historically, unions negotiated into industrial agreements the payment of annual practising certificate fees, and at least a portion of the cost of maintaining competence.[64] This arrangement might be altered by the registration regime. For other providers, such as nurses, registration costs are often borne by the employer; however, this may not be the case for paramedics. It was proposed in the Ministry of Health consultation document in 2017 that there would be no fee in the first year, but an annual cost of $425 if 1000 paramedics registered.[65] Historically, Ambulance New Zealand reported that, although the costs of registration are a concern, 'the majority of those consulted accepted that the costs were outweighed by the benefits'.[66]

The first consultation exercise also revealed that paramedics strongly preferred a paramedic-specific registration authority. The notion of a blended board with, for example, nurses or doctors, was rejected because 'there was little synergy in scope or in the way the sector is organised or the training of the professions and paramedicine'.[67]

Additional challenges to the future of New Zealand paramedicine were identified by Al-Shaqsi.[68] For example, New Zealand and most other countries must anticipate the impact of ageing populations. Many older people are resorting to emergency services for primary health service; however, if routine healthcare was better resourced, older people might enjoy 'better quality (care), greater dignity and lower costs'.[69] Thus, New Zealand's ability to deliver competent paramedic services depends on wider, preventive public health strategies.

More recently, the Minister of Health agreed that Ambulance New Zealand's application for registration could proceed.[70] In April 2016, it convened an expert panel, which reported that the profession meets the criteria for being considered for regulation. The Ministry was advised it should undertake stakeholder consultation,[71] and stakeholder feedback was submitted in June 2017.[72] The Minister accepted the proposal that a stand-alone Paramedic Board would work with the Nursing Council, thereby minimising costs to the ambulance sector and keeping paramedic registration fees as low as possible.[73] The remaining stages are as follows. The Ministry provides advice to the Minister regarding whether the profession should be regulated. If the Minister agrees that the profession should be regulated, the Minister seeks agreement from Cabinet. Subject to the Cabinet's agreement, an Order in Council is prepared by the Parliamentary Counsel Office. For the final stage, the Minister recommends to the Governor-General that the profession be designated under the Act.[74]

Conclusion

Paramedics face some of the most challenging medical crises, often under extreme conditions and time limitations. Their responses may have life-sustaining (and life-threatening) impacts. The wider legal, political and economic contexts may profoundly impact on paramedic practice. In part, public safety is guarded by the HDC and the Code. However, as demonstrated by the Cartwright,[75] Cull[76] and Kedgley[77] reports, New Zealand remains very concerned about the safety of health consumers. These concerns were intimately understood and shared by many paramedics, according to reports by Tunnage, Swaine and Waters,[78] Costa-Scorse,[79] Al-Shaqsi,[80] Tye[81] and Ambulance New Zealand.[82] Likewise, the paramedic and ambulance workforce made strong submissions in support of registration in 2017.[83]

The sector has experienced a marked shift, from providing emergency transport in the 1970s to expert healthcare in the community. Consequently, the profession is poised for registration.[84] While this may be a partial solution, serious concerns remain regarding the future of New Zealand's dedicated volunteers. Their contributions to New Zealanders' health is profound, and was recognised in the registration debates.

More broadly, New Zealand attempted to stem litigation through its accident compensation scheme. For *registered* health practitioners, the gaps in accountability have been partly addressed through legislation and the professional disciplinary tribunal. For paramedics and members of other *unregistered* occupations, accountability and public safety remain a serious issue. For these reasons, and because of the multiple benefits to paramedics, registration is the most prominent legal debate paramedics currently face in New Zealand.

Acknowledgement

The author thanks Dr Bronwyn Tunnage and Brendan Wood CSt.J, DSD, for their insights.

Review Questions

1 What is the title of the key legal code for protection of patients' rights in New Zealand?
2 Which right is most frequently breached by providers?
3 If a paramedic breaches a right, what is the legal impact for the paramedic?
4 How is the Human Rights Review Tribunal (HRRT) relevant to paramedics? What are the potential outcomes of a finding of breach by the HRRT?
5 What is the current legal impact of New Zealand's *Accident Compensation Act 2001* for patients who suffer physical harm from negligent treatment by a paramedic?
6 What are the arguments for, and against, registration of paramedics in New Zealand?
7 What legal impact will registration have on New Zealand paramedics and their patients?

Appendix 14.1 Legislation and cases relevant to paramedics in New Zealand and Australia		
	New Zealand	**Australia**
Legislation	*Accident Compensation Act 2001* *Health and Disability Commissioner Act 1994* *Health and Disability Commissioner (Code of Health and Disability Services Consumers' Rights) Regulations 1996* *Health Practitioners Competence Assurance Act 2003* (Available: http://www.nzlii.org/nz/legis/consol_act/toc-H.html)	*Civil Law (Wrongs) Act 2002* (ACT), Pt 2 *Civil Liability Act 2002* (NSW), Pt 10 *Personal Injuries (Liabilities and Damages) Act 2003* (NT), Pt 2, Div 2 *Civil Liability Act 2003* (Qld), Ch 4, Pt 1 *Civil Liability Act 1936* (SA), Pt 9, Div 12 *Civil Liability Act 2002* (Tas), Pt 4 *Wrongs Act 1958* (Vic), Pt IIC *Civil Liability Act 2002* (WA), Pt IE
Cases	Health and Disability Commissioner cases: 97HDC5922 97HDC9983 98HDC15374 99HDC02269 00HDC06794 (radiologist) 01HDC15000/02HDC00077 03HDC00153 04HDC00658 12HDC01019 13HDC01190 14HDC01598 15HDC01841 16HDC01960 (Available: http://www.hdc.org.nz/decisions—case-notes)	

Appendix 14.2 Definition of 'treatment injury' under the *Accident Compensation Act 2001*

Section 32 Treatment injury

(1) **Treatment injury** means personal injury that is—
- (a) suffered by a person—
    - (i) seeking treatment from 1 or more registered health professionals; or
    - (ii) receiving treatment from, or at the direction of, 1 or more registered health professionals; or
    - (iii) referred to in subsection (7); and
- (b) caused by treatment; and
- (c) not a necessary part, or ordinary consequence, of the treatment, taking into account all the circumstances of the treatment, including—
    - (i) the person's underlying health condition at the time of the treatment; and
    - (ii) the clinical knowledge at the time of the treatment.

(2) **Treatment injury** does not include the following kinds of personal injury:
- (a) personal injury that is wholly or substantially caused by a person's underlying health condition:
- (b) personal injury that is solely attributable to a resource allocation decision:
- (c) personal injury that is a result of a person unreasonably withholding or delaying their consent to undergo treatment.

(3) The fact that the treatment did not achieve a desired result does not, of itself, constitute **treatment injury**.

(4) **Treatment injury** includes personal injury suffered by a person as a result of treatment given as part of a clinical trial, in the circumstances described in subsection (5) or subsection (6).

(5) One of the circumstances referred to in subsection (4) is where the claimant did not agree, in writing, to participate in the trial …

Appendix 14.3 *Code of Health and Disability Services Consumers' Rights*

Right 1: Right to be treated with respect

Right 2: Right to freedom from discrimination, coercion, harassment, and exploitation

Right 3: Right to dignity and independence

Right 4: Right to services of an appropriate standard

Right 5: Right to effective communication

Right 6: Right to be fully informed

Right 7: Right to make an informed choice and give informed consent

Right 8: Right to support

Right 9: Right in respect of teaching or research

Right 10: Right to complain

(Full text available at: https://www.hdc.org.nz/your-rights/about-the-code/code-of-health-and-disability-services-consumers-rights/)

Endnotes

1 Kedgley, S. (2008) *Inquiry into the Provision of Ambulance Services in New Zealand*. Report of the Health Committee. Presented to the New Zealand House of Representatives. Online. Available: https://www.parliament.nz/en/pb/sc/business-before-committees/document/00DBSCH_INQ_8235_1/inquiry-into-the-provision-of-ambulance-services#RelatedAnchor (accessed 5 February 2018).

2 Ibid., at p. 3.

3 Wright-St Clair, R. (1985) *St John New Zealand: A History of the Most Venerable Order*. Wellington: Millwood Press.

4 Al-Shaqsi, S. (2010) Current challenges in the provision of ambulance services in New Zealand. *International Journal of Emergency Medicine* 3(4), 213–217, citing Hodgson, H. (2008) Ambulance Services Sustainable Funding Review. Wellington: Ministry of Health.

5 St John New Zealand. (2018) *Annual Report 2018 Pūrongo-ā-tau o Hato Hone*, at p. 1. Online. Available: https://www.stjohn.org.nz/globalassets/documents/publications/annual-report/stj-annual-report_2018_hq.pdf (accessed 10 December 2018).

6 Please note that all dollar amounts are New Zealand dollars (NZ$).

7 St John New Zealand, *Annual Report 2018*, at p. 34.

8 Ibid.

9 Ibid., at p. 38.

10 Ibid., at p. 19.

11 Ibid., at p. 38.

12 Al-Shaqsi, Current challenges in the provision of ambulance services in New Zealand, at p. 215.

13 Coroner, G.L. *Evans's reference to an inquest into the death of Melfyn Wynne-Williams, Decision No. 13/08,* cited in Kedgley, *Inquiry into the Provision of Ambulance Services in New Zealand*, at p. 11.

14 St John New Zealand, *Annual Report 2018,* at p. 13.

15 Al-Shaqsi, Current challenges in the provision of ambulance services in New Zealand, at p. 215.

16 Manning, J. (2015) The required standard of care for treatment. In: P. Skegg and R. Paterson (eds), *Health Law in New Zealand* (pp. 95–133). Wellington: Thomson Reuters, at p. 95.

17 Skegg, P.D.G. (2011) A fortunate experiment? New Zealand's experience with a legislated code of patients' rights. *Medical Law Review* 19(2), 235–266.

18 Paterson, R. (2015) Regulation of health care. In: P. Skegg, and R. Paterson (eds), *Health Law in New Zealand* (pp. 3–25). Wellington: Thomson Reuters.

19 Brazier, M. (1992) *Medicine, Patients and the Law*, 2nd ed. London: Penguin.

20 Merry, A. and Brookbanks, W. (2017) *Merry and McCall Smith's Errors, Medicine and the Law*, 2nd ed. Cambridge: Cambridge University Press.

21 Brazier, *Medicine, Patients and the Law*, at p. 221.

22 *Civil Law (Wrongs) Act 2002* (ACT), Pt 2; *Civil Liability Act 2002* (NSW), Pt 10; *Personal Injuries (Liabilities and Damages) Act 2003* (NT), Pt 2 Div 2; *Civil Liability Act 2003* (Qld), Ch 4, Pt 1; *Civil Liability Act 1936* (SA), Pt 9, Div 12; *Civil Liability Act 2002* (Tas), Pt 4; *Wrongs Act 1958* (Vic), Pt IIC; *Civil Liability Act 2002* (WA), Pt IE; *Wighton v Arnott* [2005] NSWSC 637.

23 See further, Madden, B. and Cockburn, T. (2007) Bundaberg and beyond: duty to disclose adverse events to patients. *Journal of Law and Medicine* 14(4), 501–527.

24 Nash, L.M., Walton, M.M., Daly, M.G. et al. (2010) Perceived practice change in Australian doctors as a result of medicolegal concerns. *Medical Journal of Australia* 193(10), 579–583.

25 Ibid.

26 Brazier, *Medicine, Patients and the Law*, at p. 219.

27 Ibid., at p. 430.

28 Skegg, A fortunate experiment?, at p. 235.

29 Cartwright, S. (1988) *The Report of the Committee of Inquiry into Allegations Concerning the Treatment of Cervical Cancer at National Women's Hospital and into Other Related Matters*. Available: http://www.moh.govt.nz/notebook/nbbooks.nsf/0/64D0EE19BA628E4FCC256E450001CC21/$file/The%20Cartwright%20Inquiry%201988.pdf (accessed 30 November 2018).

30 Manning, The required standard of care for treatment, at p. 95. See section 317(1) of the *Accident Compensation Act 2001*. For exceptions where a civil action for personal injuries suffered in the health setting may still be brought despite section 317(1), see Manning, J. (2015) Civil proceedings for personal injury cases. In: P. Skegg and R. Paterson (eds), *Health Law in New Zealand* (pp. 1061–1114). Wellington: Thomson Reuters.

31 Bismark, M., Dauer, E., Paterson, R. et al. (2006) Accountability sought by patients following adverse events from medical care: the New Zealand experience. *Canadian Medical Association Journal* 175(8), 889–894.

32 Manning, The required standard of care for treatment, at p. 1019.

33 Keenan, R. (ed.) (2016) *Health Care and the Law*, 5th ed. Wellington: Thomson Reuters.

34 Skegg, P. and Paterson, R. (eds). (2015) *Health Law in New Zealand*. Wellington: Thomson Reuters.

35 Health and Disability Commissioner. (2018) *Health and Disability Commissioner Annual Report Ending 30 June 2018*. Auckland: Health and Disability Commissioner, at p. 34. Available: https://www.hdc.org.nz/resources-publications/search-resources/annual-reports/annual-report-for-the-year-ending-30-june-2018/ (accessed 7 December 2018).

36 Ibid., at pp. 16–18.

37 Ibid., at p. 34.

38 Health and Disability Commissioner. (2017) *Health and Disability Commissioner Annual Report Ending 30 June 2017*. Auckland: Health and Disability Commissioner, at p. 7. Available: http://www.hdc.org.nz/media/4540/hdc-annual-report-for-the-year-ending-june-2017.pdf

39 Cull, H., QC. (2001) *Review of Processes Concerning Adverse Medical Events*. Wellington: Ministry of Health.

40 Baker, T. (2008) The Human Rights Review Tribunal and the rights of health and disability consumers in New Zealand. *Journal of Law and Medicine* 16(1), 85–102.

41 Human Rights Review Tribunal. *Home page*. [website]. Online. Available: https://www.justice.govt.nz/tribunals/human-rights/

42 Paterson, R. (2001) The patients' complaint system in New Zealand. *Health Affairs* 3(21), 70–79.

43 Diesfeld, K. (2003) Patients' rights and procedures: international perspectives. *International Journal of Therapy and Rehabilitation* 10(11), 497–503.

44 Paterson, The patients' complaint system in New Zealand.

45 Diesfeld, Patients' rights and procedures: international perspectives.

46 Ambulance New Zealand. (2011) *Application for the Regulation of Paramedics under the Health Practitioners Competence Assurance Act 2003*. Wellington: Ambulance New Zealand.

47 Ibid., at p. 8.

48 Relevant opinions of the Health and Disability Commissioner are: 97HDC5922; 97HDC9983; 98HDC15374; 99HDC02269; 01HDC15000/02HDC00077; 03HDC00153; 04HDC00658; 12HDC01019; 13HDC01190; 14HDC01598; 15HDC01841; 16HDC01960.

49 See Diesfeld, K. and Godbold, R. (2010) Legal rehabilitation of health professionals in New Zealand. *International Journal of Therapy and Rehabilitation* 17(4), 40–47.

50 Reynolds, L. and Adelaide, S. (2004) Is prehospital care really a profession? *Journal of Emergency and Primary Health Care* 2(1–2), art. No. 990086. Online. Available: http://www.jephccom/uploads/ 9908opdt2004 (accessed 10 October 2011).

51 Paramedics Australasia. (2017) *New Zealand paramedic and ambulance workforce opinions regarding regulation under the Health Practitioners Competence Assurance Act 2003: Stakeholder feedback from Paramedics Australasia, New Zealand, 27 June 2017*, at p. 2. Online. Available: https://www.paramedics .org/wp-content/uploads/2017/07/Paramedics-Australasia-New-Zealand-Response-to-MoH-Paramedic-Regulation-Consultation.pdf (accessed 10 December 2018).

52 Ibid., at p. 11.

53 Kedgley, *Inquiry into the Provision of Ambulance Services in New Zealand*.

54 Tye, S. (2011) *Final Report: Registration of Ambulance Officers and New Zealand Defence Force Medics under the HPCA Act 2003, Consulting the Profession*, cited in Ambulance New Zealand. (2011) *Application for Regulation of Paramedics and New Zealand Defence Force Medics under the Health Practitioners Competence Assurance Act 2003*. Wellington: Ambulance New Zealand, at p. 4.

55 Tunnage, B., Swain A. and Waters, D. (2015) Regulating our emergency care paramedics. *New Zealand Medical Journal* 128(1421): 55–58.

56 Ambulance New Zealand, *Application for the Regulation of Paramedics under the Health Practitioners Competence Assurance Act 2003*, at p. 16.

57 Ibid.

58 Paramedics Australasia, *New Zealand Paramedic and Ambulance Workforce Opinions Regarding Regulation Under the Health Practitioners Competence Assurance Act 2003*, at p. 9.

59 Ibid.

60 Ibid., at p. 8.

61 Ambulance New Zealand, *Application for the Regulation of Paramedics under the Health Practitioners Competence Assurance Act 2003*, at p. 5.

62 Ibid., at p. 6.

63 Ibid., at p. 25.

64 Ibid., at p. 24.

65 Ministry of Health. (2017) *Regulating the Paramedic Workforce Under the Health Practitioners Competence Assurance Act 2003: Consultation document*. Wellington: Ministry of Health, at p. 7. Available: https:// www.paramedics.org/wp-content/uploads/2017/05/New-Zealand%E2%80%93Consultation -document-regulating-paramedics-under-the-HPCA-Act.pdf

66 Ambulance New Zealand. (2011) *Application for the Regulation of Paramedics under the Health Practitioners Competence Assurance Act 2003*, at p. 27.

67 Ibid., at p. 26.

68 Al-Shaqsi, Current challenges in the provision of ambulance services in New Zealand, at p. 213.

69 Ibid.

70 Ministry of Health. (2017, 17 October) *Regulating a new profession*, Online. Available: https:// www.health.govt.nz/our-work/regulation-health-and-disability-system/health-practitioners-competenc e-assurance-act/regulating-new-profession (accessed 30 November 2018).

71 Ibid.

72 Paramedics Australasia, *New Zealand paramedic and ambulance workforce opinions regarding regulation under the Health Practitioners Competence Assurance Act 2003*.

73 Ambulance New Zealand. (2017) *Minister of Health agrees to paramedic registration consultation—May 2017*. Online. Available: http://www.ambulancenz.co.nz/104/latest-news-on-registration/ (accessed 30 November 2018).

74 Ministry of Health, *Regulating a new profession*.

75 Cartwright, *The Report of the Committee of Inquiry into Allegations Concerning the Treatment of Cervical Cancer at National Women's Hospital and into Other Related Matters*.

76 Cull, *Review of Processes Concerning Adverse Medical Events*.

77 Kedgley, *Inquiry into the Provision of Ambulance Services in New Zealand*.

78 Tunnage et al., Regulating our emergency care paramedics.

79 Costa-Scorse, B. (2008) Submission on the provision of ambulance services in New Zealand. *Emergency Primary Health Care* 6(3), art. no. 990321. See also Diesfeld, K. (2008) Commentary on the AUT submission and inquiry into the provision of services in New Zealand. [Guest Editorial]. *Journal of Emergency Primary Health* 6(3), 9–10.

80 Al-Shaqsi, Current challenges in the provision of ambulance services in New Zealand, citing Hodgson.

81 Tye, *Final Report*.

82 Ambulance New Zealand, *Application for the Regulation of Paramedics under the Health Practitioners Competence Assurance Act 2003*.

83 Paramedics Australasia, *New Zealand paramedic and ambulance workforce opinions regarding regulation under the Health Practitioners Competence Assurance Act 2003*, at p. 19.

84 Tunnage et al., Regulating our emergency care paramedics.

Chapter 15
Paramedic research

Wendy Bonython

Learning outcomes

After reading this chapter, you should:

- understand why research is a critical activity for paramedicine as a profession
- understand the stages of research design
- understand the ethical principles governing the conduct of research.

Definitions

Ethics The study of what it means for something to be morally right or wrong.

Human research 'Research conducted with or about people, their data or tissue.'[1]

Research '... the creation of new knowledge and/or the use of existing knowledge in a new and creative way so as to generate new concepts, methodologies, inventions and understandings.'[2]

Research misconduct 'Includes fabrication, falsification, plagiarism or deception in proposing, performing or reporting the results of, research.'[3]

An introductory case

Smallpox infection

it now becomes too manifest to admit of controversy, that the annihilation of the smallpox, the most dreadful scourge of the human species, must be the final result of this practice.

—Edward Jenner, *On the Origin of the Vaccine Inoculation*[4]

In 1796, Edward Jenner, an English surgeon and physician, made an incision in the arm of 8-year-old James Phipps, his gardener's son. He introduced into the incision pus

> ## An introductory case continued
>
> isolated from cowpox blisters on the hands of a milkmaid, Sarah Nelmes. Jenner was testing a theory based on his own observations and rural wisdom: that milkmaids were generally immune to smallpox, a disease that at the time killed around 10% of the population.
>
> After inoculating Phipps with cowpox, Jenner then attempted on several occasions to infect him with pus derived from smallpox—the standard for inoculation at the time, known as *variolation*—without success.
>
> Jenner's experiments proved that cowpox inoculation could protect against smallpox, and was safer than variolation, which produced a smallpox infection that was milder than naturally acquired smallpox, but still carried the risk of infecting others, and could potentially kill the recipients or leave them exposed to natural infection if not performed properly.[5]
>
> *This chapter will provide you with some context in which to consider and reflect on this case.*

Introduction

Sometimes referred to as the 'Father of Immunology', Edward Jenner's experiments are a classic example of the power of research to change the practice of healthcare. His findings were initially regarded with scepticism; yet in 1980 the World Health Organization was able to declare the eradication of smallpox as a result of a global vaccination campaign.[6]

Would Jenner have been able to achieve the same results in a modern research environment? Bioethicists have conflicting views on this: the experiments as he performed them would be unlikely to receive ethics approval from any ethics committee today, yet the benefits to humankind of the work are evident.

We are all users of research, whether we realise it or not. Research in its various forms tells us, among other things, how to more effectively treat our illnesses, how to develop our economies and societies, and how to harness our technologies.

As paramedics, research relevant to the practice of paramedicine will shape the way you do your jobs. What may be standard—or even best—practice now may be discarded or modified by the time you graduate and enter practice, as research uncovers more data about the risks and benefits of particular activities, or results in the development of new equipment and processes. Some paramedics will transition from being professional consumers of research into producers of research, undertaking their own experiments and evaluations for the purpose of improving the knowledge base underpinning paramedicine, and better informing its practice.

In this chapter, we will consider what research is, why professionals engage in research, how we go about doing research, and why the way we do research matters.

What is 'research'?

The Australian Research Council defines 'research' 'as the creation of new knowledge and/or the use of existing knowledge in a new and creative way so as to generate new concepts, methodologies, inventions and understandings'. So, as well as completely new research, it includes the synthesis and analysis of previous research to the extent that it is new and creative. This definition of research is consistent with a broad notion of research and experimental development (R&D) as comprising 'creative work undertaken on a systematic basis in order to increase the stock of knowledge, including knowledge of man [human-kind], culture and society, and the use of this stock of knowledge to devise new applications'.[7]

Despite the definition's high level of abstraction, there are several critical characteristics of research identified within it. Activities claiming to be research activities in some way *advance or develop knowledge*—more than merely generating data, research requires *analysis or interpretation* in order to make sense of that data. Healthcare research typically follows what is known as the *scientific method*: 'a method or procedure that has characterized natural science since the 17th century, consisting in systematic observation, measurement, and experiment, and the formulation, testing, and modification of hypotheses'.[8] This process is typically *iterative and cyclical*: researchers make an observation, formulate a question related to that observation, develop a hypothesis which answers that question, perform experiments to test the hypothesis, collect the results of the experiments, analyse those results, and draw conclusions, including whether or not the hypothesis is true. Using those conclusions, the researcher (or another researcher) will make new observations contextualising the original conclusions, and the process will start again, generating a body of knowledge over time.[9,10]

Consequently, activities need not be entirely novel in order to qualify as 'research': something that looks at existing research in a different way, and produces different conclusions, may be characterised as research: *meta-analyses* (the grouping together of multiple similar previous studies, and re-analysis of the data across those studies) are a common example of this type of research; or a re-analysis of existing observations and results from a different perspective.

Several important theoretical concepts underpin any discussion of research. First, research leads to knowledge. Importantly, however, knowledge is gathered and constructed in different ways by different people, and the validity of different types of knowledge may be contestable.

As health practitioners, we tend to think of research in several ways that are reflective of scientific method. We think of knowledge in terms of *positivism*: the world exists in a certain way as a series of phenomena, capable of external objective observation, and whose properties are not affected by the identity of the observer—rocks are hard, the sun is hot, or water is wet. We assume that those phenomena will follow certain laws, and, once we have identified what those laws are, we can use them to predict future phenomena: the apple will always fall towards the Earth from the tree, for example. We are sceptical: we ask for evidence to explain why those phenomena should occur in the way they do; and we gather that evidence through empiricism: we systematically observe those phenomena using (primarily) our unaided senses, to generate evidence to support our explanation of them. Ultimately, we use this knowledge to develop theories which explain the world around us; those theories remain valid until they are disproven by subsequent experimentation.

In other contexts, however, knowledge may arise in other ways. Traditional Chinese medicine, for example, combines what we might recognise as phenomenologically-derived knowledge of the type described above, with philosophical and cultural beliefs and practices that may not be so easily verified by empirical observation. Other traditional practices may similarly incorporate spiritual beliefs and cultural values and practices into their knowledge base.

While positivism explains much of how we gain or collect knowledge in healthcare, it does not necessarily account for how we construct, or make sense of, that knowledge. *Post-positivism* challenges many of the underlying principles of positivism in the scientific method. Drawing on examples such as the theory of relativity or quantum mechanics, which can't adequately be explained by the normal operation of laws and scientific method, it recognises that some theories may be *probabilistic* rather than *absolute* ('likely to' rather than 'will'), and questions the externality of the observer to the phenomenon they are observing (if a tree falls in a forest when there's no one around, does it make any sound?).

Critics of positivism note that even when an observer appears to be independent of the phenomena they are observing, their own theoretical beliefs and knowledge will influence their observations: if theory suggests to them that a phenomenon is more likely to be reflected in one set of observations than another, they may focus their efforts on the former, thereby missing any effects that do manifest in the latter, and thereby skewing or biasing their results. Alternatively, positivism accepts that researchers may approach a particular question from different perspectives depending on their disciplinary background: a social worker, a psychologist, a doctor, a dietician and a biochemist approaching obesity as an issue will each adopt different approaches, influenced by their differing disciplinary backgrounds. Post-positivism recognises these differences in the perspective of the researcher, and accommodates them.

Post-positivism also allows us to modify the scope of operation of theories by developing *auxiliary or supplementary theories* to accommodate non-corroborating evidence, rather than discard the theory in its entirety. If, for example, we propose 'insulin helps diabetics' as a theory, and evidence emerges that it does not help some diabetics, positivism would require we abandon the theory entirely; post-positivism enables us to retain it and reformulate it, on the basis of evidence, to 'insulin helps diabetics who have inadequate insulin production; that is, not diabetics whose insulin production is adequate, but who are insulin-resistant'.

A further limitation of the positivist approach to human research is that it overlooks the impact of human behaviour. In the health context, this means recognising that patients are people, rather than just an embodiment of a particular illness or health condition. This means that they may have other confounding conditions that obscure the study; but it also means that they may have behavioural or other attributes that influence the conclusions drawn from research. By way of example: an aggressive novel treatment may be remarkably successful at targeting and destroying cancerous cells; however, that efficacy needs to be contextualised against its effect on the patient. If it kills or severely interferes with the patient's quality of life, patients may ultimately refuse to take it, and as such it is likely to be a poor choice of treatment.

This example highlights another important aspect of research: there are differences between *quantitative data* (data that can be quantified or counted in some way) and *qualitative data* (data that describes or evaluates phenomena, usually using words or themes). Quantitative data can be derived from all sorts of sources: demographic data, cell counts, costings—in essence, anything that is reported along a scale. Notably, some simple data collections whereby data is provided in words can be converted into quantitative data: a common example is the Likert scale ('Rate the following on a scale of 1 to 5, where 1 means extremely like, and 5 means extremely dislike')—even if the question omits the numbers, by asking the participant to rate something from 'extreme dislike' to 'extreme like', its scalar qualities make it quantitative rather than qualitative data.

In our example above, quantitative data in the form of cancer cell counts over a period of treatment might tell us that our new drug is effective. Without qualitative data, however, we might fail to detect a problem with side effects. We might use a patient survey, with questions like the one shown above; however, these questions are 'closed', and as such we will only get the answers we have already anticipated getting in response to them, potentially introducing another source of researcher bias into the research. A better approach would be to include some 'open' questions in our survey, or to conduct some patient interviews, asking patients taking the novel drug for their impressions and experiences of it: do they feel better or worse? What side effects have they noticed? Would they be likely to continue taking the drug? The structure of these questions is qualitative: it enables participants to use their own words to express their answers, thereby better reflecting their views, rather than restricting them only to the answers the researcher has anticipated they might want to give. Quantitative data is often analysed and interpreted using statistics, whereas analysis of qualitative data is thematic, requiring researchers to read and interpret the responses to identify the common or dominant themes emerging from those responses.

Qualitative and quantitative methodological approaches serve different purposes and come from different disciplinary perspectives. Quantitative data is *reductionist* in nature—it tries to simplify and reduce complexity, by focusing on specific variables, enabling the research to focus on the relationship(s) between those variables without confounding 'noise'. It is theory-driven, insofar as the hypotheses being tested will be derived from a specific theoretical basis, and the results can therefore only be expressed in terms of that particular theory basis: if they discredit one hypothesis, they cannot be inferred as offering support for an alternative theory, unless that alternative theory is itself reflected in one of the other hypotheses being tested. Quantitative data is also *normative*, in that they enable the researcher to make predictions about what should happen, based on their observations of what has happened previously. Perhaps unsurprisingly, it is heavily influenced by the natural sciences and scientific method.

Qualitative data, in contrast, seeks to *contextualise* phenomena, and provide insight into their meaning and interpretation. Post-modernist theories of research provide more scope for the incorporation of qualitative data into research frameworks. Qualitative approaches are more commonly associated with the social sciences, and are influenced by disciplines including anthropology, sociology and philosophy.

Healthcare research encompasses both approaches, frequently in the same study. Sometimes described as *mixed-methods*, research projects might consist of several data collections activities directed towards the same research question; for example, a *literature survey* to identify a theoretical basis, a *quantitative study* examining a set of demographic data against a particular phenomenon, and a *qualitative survey* or interview to contextualise the findings of the quantitative limb of the study. Frequently research of this type will be carried out by multidisciplinary teams, consisting of researchers with a variety of disciplinary backgrounds. These may include, but not be limited to, natural and clinical scientists, health practitioners, social and counselling practitioners, and social scientists. In studies where there is a lot of complex quantitative data analysis, the research team may also include expert statisticians.

Who does research, and why?

As mentioned earlier, we are all consumers of research. Research shapes and informs the policies and laws governing our lives: it tells manufacturers what we buy, it tells politicians who we think we will vote for, it tells clinicians which drugs are most likely to be successful, and it tells us about the past, and makes predictions about the future, of the world around us. As healthcare practitioners, paramedics are professional consumers of research. Research undertaken by other paramedics or health professionals, and reported in peer-reviewed scholarly journals, tells us whether the treatments and interventions we provide are optimal, or whether they may cause unintended consequences for patients. Ultimately, such research may result in changes to the policies and procedures governing the way we do our jobs on a daily basis.

We may also be involved in evaluating those policy changes—recording our professional experiences of them, and reporting them to others, or compiling them ourselves, into research which in turn is fed into the knowledge base of the profession. Evaluation activities of this type are themselves a form of research, enabling us to determine how well something translates from a laboratory or hospital setting into the paramedicine context. In this way, a research consumer may become a research contributor or producer.

Research is often described as falling into two broad categories: *basic research*, sometimes referred to as *foundational research*, which is undertaken for the purpose of developing theory, filling gaps in knowledge, or even be driven by intellectual curiosity;[11] and *applied research*, which seeks to provide solutions to existing real-world problems in order to effect change.[12] The reality, however, is more scalar: basic research is often foundational to later applied research, and basic research may inadvertently generate knowledge that provides solutions to real-world problems.

Research funding is a political issue in many countries. Economic constraints frequently result in researchers being unable to secure public funding for potentially beneficial research activities. Often, governments will prioritise investment in research that they see as likely to result in a more immediate societal benefit, at the expense of more basic research with fewer immediate opportunities for commercialisation, or immediately deliverable public goods. Other sources of funding for research include various philanthropic organisations, which may fund research in a particular area, on a particular topic, or for the benefit of a particular sector of the community; or commercial organisations, which may fund research with strong commercialisation prospects, or to address a particular problem they are struggling with. On the whole, however, funding of research is dependent on being able to identify and articulate a particular research problem or knowledge gap that the researcher proposes to solve, or contribute to filling by developing further relevant knowledge.

Traditionally, universities generated a lot of basic research, and were able to do so on the basis that their funding permitted them to pursue research with fewer commercial imperatives. That is no longer the case: most Australian and New Zealand universities now have commercialisation and funding targets, which require them to redirect their research efforts towards applied research activities with the objective of securing their financial positions. Other areas where research is traditionally done include hospitals (noting that they are typically affiliated with university medical schools), industry and some government departments. Researchers in the latter two institutions, in particular, have traditionally focused their efforts on applied research, generally addressing problems directly confronting their employers or employers' stakeholders.

Increasingly, however, research is being undertaken by people throughout the community. Not-for-profit organisations, commercial—as opposed to industrial—entities, and even citizens groups are increasingly commissioning and even undertaking research. Further, the rise of so-called 'citizen science' has led to more people participating in research, including collecting and contributing data on large-scale health and environmental research projects, to name but a couple of examples.

Additionally, undertaking research is increasingly being viewed as a professional obligation. A commitment to ongoing education and practice improvement is a characteristic of the professions, and while professional standards have long required that members consume research, through implementation of evidenced-based changes to practice, many professional codes now set out minimum standards for members to abide by when carrying out research, and also may tacitly or overtly encourage members to engage in research. The Paramedics Australia *Code of Conduct* states:

> Members shall promote, support, and where possible participate in research of pre-hospital care practices and ambulance service management and technical service support systems.[13]

For most professions, professional obligations regarding research consist of supporting research activities through the contribution of data, or other forms of participation; it is unlikely, for example, that professional disciplinary bodies will begin targeting members who fail to actively undertake research, nor is it necessarily the case that penalties could be applied to any member who did not undertake research. Many codes do, however, require that members of a profession who do undertake research commit to abiding by the relevant ethical and legal standards governing research.

As a regulated profession under the oversight of the Australian Health Practitioner Regulation Agency (AHPRA) from 2018 onwards, Australian paramedicine professionals are subject to the professional standards proscribed by AHPRA, which were formulated in conjunction with their regulatory board. While not overtly stating a requirement for all paramedicine professionals to actively engage in research, the AHPRA codes require health professionals to comply with National Health and Medical Research Council (NHMRC) guidelines in conducting research. Note, however, that the AHPRA codes also require practitioners to update and maintain their professional knowledge standards, including keeping abreast of changes in practice. As such, practitioners are necessarily required to be consumers of research under the code, even if they are not actively engaged in conducting research.[14]

Reflecting this emphasis on research within the professions, many university courses now require students to undertake a research project and/or formal training in research in order to fulfil the requirements of their degree, which is typically a precondition for practitioner registration. Additionally, many universities offer high-performing students the opportunity to undertake further studies at the graduate or post-graduate level; these will often consist in large part or entirely of research work.

Identifying the problem; designing the research

In the first part of the chapter, we identified the various stages of the scientific methodology process, noting that as a starting point we need observations to assist us in identifying a problem or an area we would like to research. Identifying that research problem, and refining it into an articulated research question, is a fundamental part of research design. If you get the question wrong, the chances of your research project yielding meaningful data are greatly diminished. The question determines the remainder of your research plan: what your hypotheses are; how you will test them; how you will analyse the data you collect; and what conclusions you will be able to draw.

Designing and planning the research is, therefore, a critical activity. The design of the research will typically be documented in a research protocol or proposal. Before the first experiment is conducted, before the first question is asked of a participant, before any activities forming the practical aspect of the research are undertaken, the researcher needs to have in place a clearly articulated research question, a hypothesis, an experimental method, and an analytical strategy, all of which will ordinarily be supported by a comprehensive review and summary of the relevant academic literature on both the topic and the proposed methodological approach. It is at this stage of the process that the researcher needs to ensure their proposed research complies with any ethical and governance requirements imposed either by law or by their institution—a subject we will return to in the next section.

Often, experienced practitioners or researchers will have a clear idea of the problem they want to research, based on their own prior observations and knowledge. They may have noticed something that occurs in the course of practice, for example, or they may be aware of a pre-existing gap in the knowledge base of a particular topic, which directs them towards a research area, and may even provide them with an express research question they want to answer.

For the student who is asked to come up with their own research project, it might be a little harder. Research problems are generally based on observation—but those observations need not be your own, nor do they need to be first-hand. You might decide to read up on a topic of interest and approach your reading with the purpose of identifying what it doesn't say, rather than simply considering what it does. Alternatively, you might find other researchers have identified unanswered questions in the course of their research, and you might consider developing a research activity to answer some of those questions.

Once you have identified a problem or a gap, you need to think about how you can articulate it as a question. 'Researching obesity', for example, is hopelessly broad, and provides you with no guidance in designing your research, nor any clear objectives for the research. 'Does (the hypothetical) vitamin Z reduce obesity?', on the other hand, gives you a clearer objective ('Yes, it does, because …', or 'No, it doesn't, because …'), and enables you to start thinking about what your hypothesis (vitamin Z does reduce obesity) and the accompanying *alternative (or null) hypothesis* (vitamin Z does not reduce obesity) might be; and also to start designing experiments to test this hypothesis (collecting data on obesity and vitamin Z from a population of people, known as the *research participants*, and comparing them on the basis of these two variables, for example).

We need to consider carefully who we are going to collect the data from, for several reasons. First, there is the practical matter of ensuring that the data are actually capable of answering the question. If we are looking for a linkage between two variables, we need to make sure we have included enough people who are obese in our study to have a reasonable chance of identifying any linkage or excluding one in the event our null hypothesis is correct. We also need to think about how we are going to test them, and about any external factors we need to control for.

In an ideal world, we would sample a really large number of people at random, providing us with a large data set we could use to test our hypotheses. In reality, researchers seldom have this luxury: often there are budgetary limits on the number of people you can sample, or it may simply be too much work to collect all of those samples from a large group of people, when you only need a smaller number to verify your hypothesis. A better approach might instead be to target particular groups, by, for example, specifically recruiting people with the characteristics you are looking to examine. If you know that one of those characteristics is really rare within the population, you might need to sample additional people from certain groups to ensure that the characteristic is included in your data set.

Working out the size and criteria for your sample population becomes increasingly complicated as the research question you want to answer increases in complexity. Working out who you want to include in your population also has implications for ethics: as we will see shortly, you need to obtain consent from all of your participants, and the benefits of the research have to justify the inconvenience of participation. Without a clear idea of who you want to recruit, you will not get ethics approval.

Inherent in identifying who you want to collect data from is consideration of what data you want to collect, and how you want to collect it. You could, for example, randomly survey 1000 people and ask them what their vitamin Z status is, and whether they are obese. The results, however, would not be very good, as many people are unlikely to know what their vitamin Z status is; and there is a possibility that they may either use different criteria for defining obesity than you, or flat-out lie, when answering the obesity question. If vitamin Z status is routinely tested in pathology labs under consistent conditions, and patient weight is concurrently recorded, you might be able to access existing data holdings, although this raises a separate set of ethical challenges. Providing participants with controlled doses of vitamin Z to take over a certain period of time, and taking blood samples and weighing each participant at the beginning and end of the period, is likely to give you more accurate data, but is more intrusive to participants, and involves a greater financial and human resources burden for the researcher. That burden might be offset by reducing the number of participants to something far smaller and manageable, while still being sufficient to enable you to detect the phenomenon you are looking for, if it exists.

For other types of research question, other methods of collecting data may well provide better answers. If you are interested in patient perceptions of quality of care, a better approach would be to survey or interview participants; if you are considering a very rare phenomenon, you may have one only participant (e.g. a case study); in extreme cases, you might even be that one participant, in an approach known as *auto-ethnography*.

Once you have decided what data you are going to collect, you need to consider how you are going to analyse it. Our example of vitamin Z and obesity, as a quantitative study, will necessarily require quantitative analysis—typically some simple statistics. If we use a qualitative approach, our analysis is likely to take the form of thematic analysis—analysing what our research participants have said, to identify particular themes.

When designing your research plan, it is a good idea to also think about how you are going to communicate your research to a wider audience. In many instances this will consist of writing an article or a report for publication in a journal or elsewhere, or presenting a talk or a poster at a conference. Occasionally there might be restrictions on where and how you can publish, imposed as a condition of the funding—you need to check what these are prior to starting your research. Similarly, you should also find out what your institution's policies are on data storage and retention. How long do you keep data for once you have finished the research? What happens to it if you leave? Who takes responsibility for it? Can it be shared with other researchers? You need to consider all of these matters before you start your application for ethics approval.

'Good' research vs 'ethical' research

Historically, a distinction has been drawn between *good research*—research that is well designed, verified, reproducible, etc.—and *ethical research*—research that is conducted in accordance with ethical principles. That distinction has largely disappeared: journals will not publish research that is clearly unethical, funding is generally contingent on obtaining ethics approval, and most institutions have their own ethics committees who are responsible for determining whether research meets ethical standards. That said, those processes typically focus on ethical research with respect to the protection of participants; other forms of unethical research, involving plagiarism or fabrication of results by researchers, misappropriation of funds etc., do still occur from time to time. While they do result in research that is unethical, they are generally more broadly treated as instances of researcher misconduct, potentially attracting disciplinary or even criminal sanction.[15]

That has not always been the case. In the aftermath of World War II, the world became aware of research programs carried out in both Nazi Germany and Japan. In the 'Doctors' Trial'[16]—the first of the Nuremberg War Crimes Tribunals—20 of the 23 defendants were doctors who were being tried for their part in the German program on non-consensual medical experimentation performed on prisoners of war, citizens of German occupied nations, and German nationals during World War II.[17] The Nazi Program in World War II is by no means the only example of unethical research: the Japanese military also had active research programs using unconsenting prisoners of war during World War II, and there are many more instances of vulnerable populations being exploited by unethical researchers. Of particular note are research programs into mental illness, infectious disease, radiation exposure and intellectual disability carried out on prisoners, people with intellectual disability or mental illness, migrants and racial minorities, and people who are economically vulnerable, including in the United States and Europe.

As recently as 2010, then US president Barack Obama formally apologised to the people of Guatemala for US involvement in the Guatemala syphilis study,[18] a study undertaken in Guatemala by American researchers that was similar to the ethically discredited Tuskegee Syphilis Study, in which impoverished black sharecroppers in Alabama were intentionally denied proven treatment for syphilis.[19] Common ethical defects in all of these studies are their exploitation of vulnerable populations, and their failure to obtain meaningful informed consent from participants, demonstrating that participants understand what the researchers propose to do to them, what the risks and benefits to them of participating are, and enabling them to refuse to participate without fear of retribution.

In response to the evidence presented at the Doctors' Trial, the judges of the Nuremberg trial released the *Nuremberg Code*, which outlines 10 principles for the conduct of ethical human research. They are as follows:

1 The voluntary, well-informed, understanding consent of the human subject in a full legal capacity is required.
2 The experiment should aim at positive results for society that cannot be procured in some other way.
3 The experiment should be based on previous knowledge (e.g. an expectation derived from animal experiments) that justifies the experiment.
4 The experiment should be set up in a way that avoids unnecessary physical and mental suffering and injuries.
5 The experiment should not be conducted when there is any reason to believe that it implies a risk of death or disabling injury.
6 The risks of the experiment should be in proportion to (i.e. not exceed) the expected humanitarian benefits.
7 Preparations and facilities must be provided that adequately protect the subjects against the experiment's risks.
8 The staff who conduct or take part in the experiment must be fully trained and scientifically qualified.
9 The human subjects must be free to immediately quit the experiment at any point when they feel physically or mentally unable to go on.
10 Likewise, the medical staff must stop the experiment at any point when they observe that continuation would be dangerous.

Case 15.1 Nazi research

Beginning in the early 1930s, University of Vienna anatomist and Nazi Eduard Pernkopf began compiling *The Topographical Anatomy of Man*, an anatomical atlas whose illustrations remain unsurpassed to the present day.[20] In 1998, the University of Vienna undertook an investigation which revealed that the university's Anatomy Department received the bodies of prisoners executed by the Gestapo and the assizes court during the period Pernkopf was compiling his atlas, and that there was a reasonable chance that some of the remains depicted in the atlas were those of executed prisoners.[21]

The code was never formally adopted into international law. Indeed, its scope of operation was controversial, with some critics arguing that it applied only to barbaric or egregious acts purportedly carried out in the name of research. However, the code did inform the subsequent World Health Organization's *Declaration of Helsinki*.[22] That declaration has been updated a number of times since its release in 1964, and its contents and revisions, like the Nuremberg Code, have been controversial. Many of the principles contained in it have been incorporated into the domestic legislation which forms the basis of the research ethics frameworks found in many nations, including Australia. However, nations have not been uniform in deciding which parts of the declaration to adopt or reject, and some have adopted principles but not attributed them to the Helsinki Declaration. It would therefore be wrong to assume that all countries abide by a universal standard of human research ethics.

To illustrate these points, consider the situation explored in Case 15.1.

There is no question that, if true, the consent of the research subjects to be included in the atlas would not have been sought; furthermore, it is clear that research conducted on people obtained in this way is unethical. The ethical dilemma, therefore, is this: should Pernkopf's atlas continue to be used, noting that some subjects are unidentified, all subjects are deceased, and consent from participants or their descendants is unobtainable? Or is it ethically more problematic to deny the benefits the atlas potentially gives to practitioners and students by banning it, noting that to do so won't reverse the harms already done to those people?

Research ethics in Australia

In Australia, human research is governed by the joint National Health and Medical Research Council (NHMRC), Australian Research Council (ARC) and Australian Vice Chancellors' Committee (Universities Australia), which developed the *National Statement on Ethical Conduct in Human Research* (the 'National Statement'), in accordance with the *National Health and Medical Research Council Act 1992* (Cth). The National Statement applies to any research funded by, undertaken by, or conducted under the auspices of the NHMRC, the ARC or any Australian university. It also provides the standards for all research undertaken in Australia involving humans, including research by 'governments, industry, private individuals, organizations, or networks of organisations'.[23]

Human research is defined as research with or about people, their data and their tissues. Note also that Australia has a regulatory framework governing animal research. For reasons associated with Australia's federal political structure, that framework is not nationwide. This means that if you plan to do any research involving animals, make sure you have familiarised yourself with the ethics standards and procedures applying to animal research in your state or territory.

The values underpinning ethical research as outlined in the National Statement are: respect for human beings, research merit and integrity, justice, and beneficence.

Respect for human beings requires that researchers respect the inherent value of all people, including respecting their autonomy—their right to self-determination. This includes recognising that research participants are entitled to choose whether or not they want to participate in research without fear of coercion or retribution, and ensuring that even people who may be limited in their ability to exercise their autonomy are treated with respect and given the opportunity to make their own decisions wherever possible. This is reflected in particular in Chapters 2.2 and 2.3 of the National Statement, which, respectively, set out the general requirements for valid informed consent by research participants, and identify the limited sets of circumstances under which those requirements for consent might be waived.

Critical to obtaining valid consent is the process of providing participants with sufficient information to enable them to make an informed choice about whether or not they want to participate in the research. Often, but not always, this will require the researcher to provide potential participants with a participant information sheet, which explains in layperson's language what the researchers propose to do, what the potential benefits and risks of the research are, what will be done with any data they contribute, and what their participation will entail. Participants will often formalise their agreement to participate by signing a written consent form, confirming that they have been provided with this information and that they agree to participate in the research. Any additional variables in the research methodology that the participants agree to—such as being photographed or recorded, or being identified by name, or agreeing to be invited to participate in further research—will usually also be documented on the consent form.

Section 4 of the National Statement also deals specifically with the value of respect for participants, by providing guidance for the conduct of research potentially or directly involving participants whose autonomy may be impaired, potentially affecting their ability to provide free and fully informed consent to participate in research, or are otherwise deemed to be vulnerable, for reasons such as being over-sampled or in particular relationships. Examples of groups of people who attract specific further ethical considerations include: pregnant women and unborn children; children and young people; people in unequal relationships; people whose dependence on medical care may affect their ability to provide consent; people with cognitive impairment, mental illness or disability; people involved in illegal activities; Aboriginal and Torres Strait Islander peoples; and people in other countries. That list is not exhaustive, nor are the examples provided within each of the categories exhaustive. 'People in dependent or unequal relationships', for example, may include domestic or social relationships, but can also include employment relationships, or even relationships with institutions or government service providers.

Generally, the effect of these requirements is not to bar research on these populations, but instead ensure that any research they do participate in is justified in terms of its potential benefits, that any risks they are exposed to as a result of participating in the research are minimised to the fullest extent possible, and that they are treated with respect.

Research will be found to have *merit* if: the potential benefits of the research outweigh the identified risks; if the research is well designed and based on a comprehensive under-standing of the existing literature; is carried out by researchers, or teams of researchers, with appropriate knowledge, skills and experience; and is carried out in appropriate facilities, with appropriate levels of support. Research will have *integrity* if the researchers can demonstrate their commitment: to carrying out the research honestly and in accordance with research governance principles, including, but not limited to, the National Statement; to furthering knowledge on the topic; and to disseminating the results of their research, whether those results are favourable or otherwise, in the interests of allowing scrutiny and further developing knowledge of the field.

Justice in research requires that the risks and benefits of the research be equitably distributed across the community, and that the selection and recruitment of research participants be conducted fairly, avoiding the imposition of an unfairly onerous burden on one category of participant, for example, or restricting access to the benefits of research to particular groups within the community.

Beneficence requires that the benefits of doing the research—whether to the participants themselves or to the community more broadly—should justify any harm or inconvenience imposed on participants as a consequence of the research. In the event that an unforeseen risk emerges, beneficence requires that the researchers stop and reconsider whether the risks are still outweighed by the benefits, and then either proceed—with the approval of the ethics committee—or terminate the research if they do not.

Other considerations outlined in the National Statement include: data storage, reten-tion, access and destruction; privacy and confidentiality; and other matters specific to particular types of research—for example, the biobanking of tissue samples, and genetic research.

The National Statement also provides for the establishment of institutional human research ethics committees. These committees must have a range of members in order to be valid ethics committees, including lay members, pastoral care members, legal members, healthcare or counselling professionals, and researchers. Committees need to be balanced with respect to gender, and need to include at least one-third membership from outside the institution convening the committee. These standards necessitate that committees represent a variety of disciplinary and societal views, and minimise the risk of committees being coerced to make certain decisions by the convening institution. The National State-ment also outlines the reporting requirements for committees, which are required to monitor adverse events, changes to protocols, and progress of approved protocols, as well as undertake the initial approval, and report outlines of their membership back to the NHMRC on an annual basis.

Conclusion

In this chapter, we have considered what research is, and why it is important, as well as who might undertake research. We have briefly examined the stages of the scientific method process, and considered how they relate to activities we might undertake in designing and executing a research protocol. We have considered the ethical obligations attendant on human research in Australia, and briefly examined some of the key features of the National Statement, the document governing all Australian research conducted on humans.

Review Questions

1 What is 'research'?

2 Can you identify three components of the scientific method process? What are they?

3 What are the key values underpinning ethical human research in Australia?

4 How does the National Statement reflect 'respect for humans'? Provide two examples.

5 Identify three categories of people identified as vulnerable according to the National Statement. Why are they vulnerable? What additional considerations apply to their participation in research?

6 What does the code of conduct say about undertaking research?

Endnotes

1 National Health and Medical Research Council, Australian Research Council, and Universities Australia. (2007; updated 2018) *National Statement on Ethical Conduct in Human Research*. Canberra: Commonwealth of Australia. Available: https://nhmrc.gov.au/about-us/publications/national-statement-ethical-conduct-human-research-2007-updated-2018 (accessed February 2019).

2 Australian Research Council (ARC). (2015/2016) *State of Australian University Research Volume 1 ERA National Report*. Available: https://www.arc.gov.au/sites/g/files/net4646/f/minisite/static/4551/ERA2015/downloads/ARC03966_ERA_ACCESS_151130.pdf (accessed March 2019).

3 New South Wales Government, *Research glossary*.

4 Jenner, E. (1801) *On the Origin of the Vaccine Inoculation*. London: D.N. Shury.

5 Harvard University's series The Harvard Classics 1909–1914 included all of Edward Jenner's key works: *An Inquiry into the Causes and Effects of the* Variolæ Vaccinæ, *or Cow-Pox* (1798); *Further Observations on the* Variolæ Vaccinæ, *or Cow-Pox* (1799); *A Continuation of Facts and Observations Relative to the* Variolæ Vaccinæ, *or Cow-Pox* (1800).

6 World Health Organization. (1980). Declaration of global eradication of smallpox / Proclamation de l'éradication de la variole dans le monde entier. *Weekly Epidemiological Record* 55(20), 148. Available: http://www.who.int/iris/handle/10665/223060 (accessed 2 May 2018).

7 Australian Research Council. *Discovery Projects Funding Rules for funding commencing in 2013.* Online. Available: https://www.legislation.gov.au/Details/F2012L01142/Html/Text#_ftnref1 (accessed 2 February 2019).

8   Oxford Dictionaries. *Definition of 'scientific method'.* (British and World English.) Online. Available: https://en.oxforddictionaries.com/definition/scientific_method (accessed 2 May 2018).

9   Crawford, S. and Stucki, L. (1990) Peer review and the changing research record. *Journal of the American Society of Information Science* 41, 223–228.

10 Polgar, S. and Thomas, S.A. (2013) *Introduction to Research in the Health Sciences*, 6th ed. London: Churchill Livingstone, at pp. 4–10.

11 Kidd, C.V. (1959) Basic research: description versus definition. *Science* 129, 368–371.

12 Cohen, I.B. (1948) *Science, Servant of Man*. Boston, Mass.: Little, Brown, at p. 303.

13 Paramedics Australasia. *Code of Conduct.* Melbourne: Paramedics Australasia. Online. Available: https://www.paramedics.org/code-of-conduct/ (accessed 2 May 2018).

14 Australian Health Practitioner Regulation Agency (AHPRA). (2014) *Code of Conduct for Registered Health Practitioners.* Online. Available: https://www.paramedicineboard.gov.au/Professional-standards/Codes-guidelines-and-policies/Code-of-conduct.aspx (accessed 2 February 2019).

15 Wardle, J. (2013) Plagiarism and registered health professionals: navigating the borderlands between scholarly and professional misconduct. *Journal of Law and Medicine* 21(2), 399–414.

16 *USA v Karl Brandt, et al.* (1946–1947). Transcripts and indictment documents of this case, and for other of the Nuremberg Trials, are held at the Harvard Law School Library Nuremberg Trials Project. Online. Available: http://nuremberg.law.harvard.edu/ (accessed 2 May 2018).

17 Office of Special Investigations, Criminal Division. (1992, October) *In the Matter of Josef Mengele: A Report to the Attorney General of the United States.* Washington, DC: United States Department of Justice. Available: https://www.justice.gov/sites/default/files/criminal-hrsp/legacy/2011/02/04/10-01-92mengele-rpt.pdf (accessed 2 May 18).

18 Stein, R. (2010, 1 October) U.S. apologizes for newly revealed syphilis experiments done in Guatemala. *The Washington Post, Friday.* Online. Available: http://www.washingtonpost.com/wp-dyn/content/article/2010/10/01/AR2010100104457.html (accessed 2 May 2018).

19 Tuskegee Syphilis Study Legacy Committee. (1996) *Bad Blood: The Tuskegee Syphilis Study. Final Report of the Tuskegee Syphilis Study Legacy Committee—May 1996.* Available: http://exhibits.hsl.virginia.edu/badblood/report (accessed 2 May 2018).

20 Pernkopf, E. and Platzer, W. (1989) *Pernkopf's Anatomy: Atlas of Topographic and Applied Human Anatomy*, 3rd ed. Baltimore: Urban and Schwarzenberg.

21 Malina, P. and Spann, G. (1999) Studies in anatomical science at the University of Vienna from 1938–1945. *Wien Klin Wochenschr* 111(18), 743–753; Riggs, G. (1998) What should we do about Eduard Pernkopf's atlas? *Academic Medicine* 73(4), 380–386.

22 Rickham, P.P. (1964) Human experimentation. Code of ethics of the World Medical Association. Declaration of Helsinki. *British Medical Journal* 2(5402), 177; World Medical Association. (2013) Declaration of Helsinki: ethical principles for medical research involving human subjects. *Journal of the American Medical Association* 310(20), 2191–2194.

23 National Health and Medical Research Council, Australian Research Council, and Universities Australia, *National Statement on Ethical Conduct in Human Research*.

Glossary

Accident Compensation Act 2001 **(NZ):** Legislation defining the accident compensation system and the treatment of injury.

Act of Parliament: See 'Legislation'.

Actus reus: Latin for 'guilty act'.

Adult: A person who has reached the age of 18 years of age in Australia, and 20 years in New Zealand, and has full legal capacity. In South Australia, an adult is someone 16 years or over for medical purposes.

Advanced care directive: A document that expresses a person's wishes in relation to medical treatment in the event of becoming incapacitated, and must relate to the condition at hand. It must have been signed by the patient.

Age of majority: The age at which a person reaches full legal capacity (18 years in all Australian states and territories, and 20 years in New Zealand).

Alternative argument: The best argument you can conceive of for an alternative course of action.

Assault: A general term to include both a threat of, and the actual infliction of, personal violence.

Attorney: A person who has been appointed by another to make decisions for, and on behalf of, them at a time when they are no longer capable of making decisions.

Beyond reasonable doubt: The standard of proof required to find a person guilty of a criminal offence.

Bullying: According to the *Fair Work Act 2009* (Cth), a worker is bullied at work when 'an individual or group of individuals repeatedly behaves unreasonably towards the worker, or a group of workers of which the worker is a member, and that behaviour creates a risk to health and safety' (s 789FD).

Capacity: The ability to understand the nature, purpose and consequences of a decision. All adults are presumed to have capacity unless demonstrated otherwise. Minors do not have capacity at law, although exceptions can be made based on whether a child can demonstrate sufficient maturity and understanding to grant them the right to choose or refuse proposed healthcare: *Gillick v West Norfolk and Wisbech Area Health Authority* [1987] AC 112; *Secretary, Department of Health and Community Services (NT) v JWB and SMB* (1992) 175 CLR 218 *(Marion's case)*.

Case law: The principles of law arising from the judicial decisions of legal cases.

Child: A child or minor is a person who has not yet reached the age of capacity; however, the definition of a 'child' for the purposes of providing consent for medical treatment may vary between jurisdictions.

Child maltreatment or child abuse and neglect: One or more of the following: physical abuse, sexual abuse, psychological and emotional abuse, and neglect. Exposure to domestic violence (EDV) is also considered an example of child maltreatment.

Code of conduct: The published basis for the guidance of ethical and professional behaviour.

Code of Health and Disability Services Consumers' Rights: Code defining healthcare and disability services consumers' 10 rights.

Common law: The law developed by courts over the ages, and applied in similar cases to provide consistency and certainty in law-making, which forms the doctrine of precedent.

Competence: In the healthcare context, and in particular in end-of-life decision-making, a person is competent or has decision-making capacity if they are able to understand the nature, purpose and consequences of a decision. This is demonstrated when the patient can 'comprehend, retain and weigh up relevant information', make a decision regarding their future healthcare treatment, and then communicate that decision to others. There is a presumption of competence in adults; it is a matter for healthcare staff to demonstrate otherwise.

Confidentiality: A duty not to inappropriately disclose or misuse sensitive corporate or personal information, protected under confidentiality law.

Consequentialist ethics: The view that holds that an action is ethical if, as a consequence of the action, the maximum overall amount of good results (e.g. happiness).

Criminal law: The body of rules and legislation that prohibits certain conduct and imposes a penalty or punishment on those who are found to have committed such conduct.

Defendant: The party who responds to proceedings initiated by another party seeking relief in formal legal proceedings.

Deontological ethics: The view that holds that an action is ethical if it is guided by a set of universal moral rules.

Discrimination: When a person, or a group of people, is treated less favourably than another person or group because of their background or certain personal characteristics. This is known as *direct discrimination*. It is also discrimination when an unreasonable rule or policy applies to everyone but has the effect of disadvantaging some people because of a personal characteristic they share. This is known as *indirect discrimination*.

Drug substitution: Where a drug is replaced by a non-authentic replacement, most commonly with restricted drugs. For example, fentanyl is replaced with water.

Duty of care: A requirement that a person act towards others in a manner that a reasonable person in the circumstances would behave to avoid reasonably foreseeable harm.

Employee: A person directly engaged by a business or undertaking, paid as an individual.

Employment contract: A formal contract between two parties, outlining the terms and conditions of employment.

Ethical dilemma: A case that requires you, in responding, to make a choice between equally unfavourable options.

Ethics: The study of what it means for something to be morally right or wrong.

Euthanasia: A deliberate act or omission undertaken with the intention of causing the death of another person in order to relieve that person's suffering. Euthanasia can be *voluntary*, *involuntary* or *non-voluntary*.

Futile treatment: Treatment that would offer no reasonable benefit to the patient nor achieve a better outcome for the patient.

Guardian: A person appointed, usually by a court or tribunal, to make decisions on behalf of another who has impaired decision-making capacity.

***Health Practitioners Competence Assurance Act 2003* (NZ):** Legislation governing the registration of healthcare practitioners.

Human research: 'Research conducted with or about people, their data, or their tissue.'

Illegal: Describes behaviour that is contrary to criminal law.

In loco parentis: Latin for 'in place of a parent'.

Independent contractor: A person who works for a business or undertaking, but who is engaged and remunerated as a company, partnership, sole trader, or other business structure.

Involuntary euthanasia: When the person concerned may possess the capacity to consent, but their life is terminated against their will.

Judiciary: Those people who adjudicate legal disputes in courts of law.

Jurisdiction: The scope or area the law's authority covers.

Law: 'The system of rules which a particular country or community recognises as regulating the actions of its members and which it may enforce by the imposition of penalties.'

Legislation: A law or body of laws made and enacted by the Parliament (known as a statute or an Act of Parliament).

Life-sustaining treatment: Treatment that includes cardiopulmonary resuscitation (CPR), assisted ventilation, artificial nutrition and hydration, but *does not* include blood transfusions.

Mandatory reporting: The law generally phrases mandatory reporting in this way: if personnel have reasonable grounds for suspecting or believing that a child has been abused, or is at risk of being abused, the person must, as soon as practicable, notify a prescribed child welfare authority of his or her suspicion and the basis for the suspicion. Mandatory reporting also refers to the obligation on registered health practitioners to report any practitioner with an impairment to AHPRA.

Mens rea: Latin for 'guilty mind'.

Mental health emergency: A circumstance in which an individual's mental illness presents an immediate danger to the individual or others, often characterised by delusions, hallucinations, and/or serious disorders of the thought, mood, perception or memory.

Mental illness: A clinically significant disturbance of thought, mood, perception or memory.

Minor: A person who has not yet reached the age of majority—18 years in Australia, and 20 years in New Zealand.

Natural justice: The notion that proceedings are conducted impartially, fairly and without prejudice.

Negligence: The failure to exercise appropriate levels of care, which causes reasonably foreseeable harm.

Non-economic loss: Damage suffered that cannot be directly calculated in monetary terms, and may include pain and suffering, disfigurement and loss of enjoyment of life; while noting that any actual compensation under this head of damages will still be provided in monetary terms.

Non-voluntary euthanasia: When a patient is incapable of forming an opinion on euthanasia, or is unable to communicate any such opinion.

On the balance of probabilities: The standard of proof required to establish liability in a civil matter.

Parens patriae: The jurisdiction of the court to intervene and make decisions to ensure the welfare of those who are vulnerable and unable to care for themselves.

Patient healthcare record (PHCR): A document containing personal, sensitive and healthcare information, including a patient's medical history and the healthcare provided by health professionals to facilitate the ongoing safe care and treatment of a patient. The PHCR does not just relate to a traditional ambulance 'case sheet', but may also include referral letters, plans, forms, 'schedule' or 'section' documents, and transfer-of-care records, and may be on paper, be electronic or be a combination of both (hybrid).

Plaintiff: The party who initiates formal legal proceedings seeking relief against another party.

Poisons Standard: A commonwealth instrument that is designed to promote uniform scheduling of substances and uniform labelling and packaging requirements throughout Australia.

Precedent: A decision that interprets law and acts as a guide for future cases. It is an important doctrine that ensures there is a stable and consistent legal framework on which to consider each new legal case.

Prescription: The authorisation, by an authorised person, to another to be supplied a restricted drug.

Privacy: A human right involving a freedom from inappropriate physical interference or observation, conceptualised in different ways and protected under a range of law.

Profession: 'An occupation whose core element is work, based on the mastery of a complex body of knowledge and skills. It is a vocation in which knowledge of some department of science or learning, or the practice of an art founded on it, is used in the service of others. Its members profess a commitment to competence, integrity, morality, altruism, and the promotion of the public good within their domain. These commitments form the basis of a social contract between a profession and society.'

Reconnaissance: The process of going out into the field to gather salient facts in order to make better informed decisions.

Research: 'The creation of new knowledge and/or the use of existing knowledge in a new and creative way so as to generate new concepts, methodologies, inventions and understandings.'

Research misconduct: 'Includes fabrication, falsification, plagiarism or deception in proposing, performing, or reporting the results of, research.'

Restricted drugs: Schedule 4 and schedule 8 drugs as defined by the Poisons Standard. These are sometimes referred to as *controlled drugs* because they are addictive.

Sexual harassment: An unwelcome sexual advance, unwelcome request for sexual favours or other unwelcome conduct of a sexual nature which makes a person feel offended, humiliated and/or intimidated, where a reasonable person would anticipate that reaction in the circumstances.

Statute: See 'Legislation'.

Strict liability: Where liability is not based on any form of culpability or fault, but only on proof that the act in question occurred.

Substitute decision-maker: A person appointed to make decisions on behalf of another who lacks the requisite mental capacity to make decisions for themselves. A person may be appointed to the role formally through an instrument (e.g. an enduring guardianship form) or by order of a court or a tribunal; or they may be appointed informally via a hierarchy of decision-makers as noted in guardianship legislation (e.g. *Guardianship Act 1987* (NSW), s 33A).

Terminal illness: An illness or condition that is likely to result in death. The 'terminal phase' of such an illness is defined as 'the phase of the illness reached when there is no real prospect of recovery or remission of symptoms (on either a permanent or temporary basis)'.

The four principles of bioethics: The view that holds that an action is ethical if it is the action that best upholds the principles of autonomy, non-maleficence, beneficence and justice.

Tort: A civil wrong or wrongful act, as distinct from a criminal proceeding.

Trespass: The tort of trespass is touching a person without their consent, or a threat or conduct that creates an apprehension that the said conduct will occur.

Unlawful: An action that is in breach of civil law. (It can also be used in reference to breach of criminal law.)

Urgent treatment: Treatment urgently needed by a patient to save that patient's life, or to prevent serious damage to the patient's health, or to prevent the patient from suffering or continuing to suffer significant pain or distress.

VACIS system: A computerised patient healthcare record system designed by Ambulance Victoria that is now used by a number of Australian ambulance services. ('VACIS' is an acronym for 'Victorian Ambulance Clinical Information System'.)

Vicarious liability: The liability imposed on one person or corporation for the wrongful act of another on the basis of the legal relationship between them.

Virtue ethics: The view that holds that an action is ethical if it is motivated by virtue.

Voluntary euthanasia: When euthanasia is carried out at a competent patient's request. For example, a person's life is ended through the withdrawal or withholding of medical treatment at the patient's request (*passive euthanasia*).

Worker: Changes to harmonise the work health and safety (WHS) legislation in 2011 introduced the term 'worker' to describe anyone involved in a workplace. Workers, in this context, include paid employees, contractors, volunteers, students, visitors, and even members of the public.

Index

Page numbers followed by '*f*' indicate figures, '*t*' indicate tables, and '*b*' indicate boxes.

intellectual privacy, 242
interdisciplinary teamwork, 8
internal haemorrhaging, 202*t*
International Covenant on Civil and Political Rights
	(ICCPR), 64–65, 242
international law, 63–65
Intervention Orders (Prevention of Abuse) Act 2009
	(SA), 197*t*
intoxication
	civil liability and, 131
	common law and, 131
	negligence and, 131
	see also alcohol; drugs
involuntary assessment, for mental illness, 222
involuntary euthanasia
	definition of, 156*b*–157*b*
	passive euthanasia and, 167–169
Ipp Report *see Review of the Law of Negligence Report*

J

Jehovah's Witnesses
	blood transfusion and, 18*b*, 62*b*, 89*b*, 96*b*
	car crash, 62*b*, 96*b*
Jenner, Edward, 336
judiciary
	definition of, 54*b*–55*b*
	see also court system
jurisdictions
	consent and, 91
	definition of, 54*b*–55*b*
	guardianship regime in, 99–100
	and mental illness, 222
	negligence and, 124
	PHCR and, 267–268
justice, 348
	PRECARE and, 43
	principle of, 33–35, 34*b*

K

Kantianism *see* deontological ethics
Katelaris, A., 158
knowledge, advantage of, 2

L

Larrey, Dominique Jean, 223–224
laws, 3–4
	from authority, 56
	common
		definition of, 120*b*–121*b*
		intoxication and, 131
		negligence and, 122, 126
		voluntary assumption of risk and, 131

for consent, 9
constitution and, 58
court system and, 65–67
creation of, 57–61
definition of, 1*b*, 56–57
for disputes, 56
ethics and, 16–17, 16*b*
how to read, 67
human rights and, 56, 64
from legislation, 59
of negligence, 122
in place, 294, 309*t*–311*t*
professionalism and, 54–83
from regulations, 56
from rules, 56
types of, 61–65
Law Reform Act 1995 (Qld), 105*t*
lawful correction, 182–183
leave, 296
	annual, 296
	community service, 296
	long-service, 297
	parental, 296
	personal/carer's, 296
legal causation, 128
legal duty, 318
legal standard of care, 9–10
legal system, 56
legislation, 59
	common law and, 60–61
	for contemporary mental healthcare,
		218–220
	definition of, 54*b*–55*b*, 120*b*–121*b*
	delegated, 59
	law from, 59
	mental health, safeguards within, 230–231
	for negligence, 122
	see also specific laws
liability
	with advance care directive, 163–164
	strict
		definition of, 120*b*–121*b*
		torts and, 122
	vicarious
		definition of, 120*b*–121*b*, 128–129
		in employer/employee relationship, 128
	waivers of, 123
liberty, autonomy and, 30
life-sustaining treatment, 156*b*–157*b*
listening devices, privacy and, 246–247
literature survey, 340
local courts, 66
Locke, John, 56–57
long-service leave, 297
lower court, initial finding by, 134

Index

post-modernist theories of research, 339–340
post-positivism, 338
'power imbalance', 294
Powers of Attorney Act 2006 (ACT), 102t–103t
Powers of Attorney Act 1998 (Qld), 164
  substitute decision-makers and, 102t–103t
practice element, 225
'practise as a paramedic', 72–73
Practitioner Regulation National Law Act, 241
PRECARE decision-making model, 40–51
  alternative argument in, 46
  application of, 50t
  case study, 40b
  code of conduct in, 45
  ethics in, 43–45
  evaluation in, 48–51
  problem in, 41–42
  reconnaissance in, 42–43
  regulations in, 47–48
precedent, 60–61
  common law and, 60–61
  definition of, 54b–55b, 120b–121b
  doctrine of, 60–61
preference consequentialism, 23
pregnancy, domestic violence in, 181–182
prescription, drugs, 279b, 285
prescription animal remedy, 282t
prescription-only medicine, 282t
presenting problem, in PHCR, 270
prima facie, 166
principles
  of necessity, 91
  neighbour, 124
  theory, 56–57
  see also four principles of bioethics
prison sentences, 304
privacy, 241–242
  in Australia, 245–246
  case study on, 239b–240b
  definition of, 239b
  employees, 247
  employers, 247
  as freedom from inappropriate interference, 242–244
  inappropriateness, 243
  interference, 243–244
  with mental illness, 231
  in New Zealand, 245–246
  with PHCR, 263–264
  proportionate, 244
  protection, for paramedicine practitioners, 250–253
  rubric of data protection, 242
  technology and, 246–247
Privacy Act 1988 (Cth), 248

Privacy Act 1998 (Cth), 264–265
Privacy Act 1993 (NZ), 264, 320
Privacy Amendment (Private Sector) Act 2000 (Cth), 264–265
privacy law
  Australian, 245–246
  Australian Privacy Principles, 248–250
  Health Practitioner Regulation National Law Act, 251
  information privacy, 247–248
  New Zealand, 245–246
  predates paramedicine, 246
problem, in PRECARE, 41–42
professional
  competence of, 56
  definition of, 1b
  laws and, 54–83
  misconduct, 73
  obligation of, 7
  paramedic as, 68–80
  traits of, 2
professional association, 3–4
professional conduct, issues of, 74–76
professional regulation, 68–80
professional standards, 71
professionalisation, 68–80
professionalism
  defining, 3–6
  as ethical practice, 6–8
  ethics and, 8–10
  law and, 8–10
  patient's interests and, 5
  regulations, 3–4
prohibited substance, in poisons schedules, 282t
prohibition notice, 304
promethazine, 282–283
property rights, of Indigenous Australians, 63
prosecution, 304
Protection of Personal and Property Rights Act 1988 (NZ), 102t–103t
protective jurisdiction, 177–212, 178b–180b, 220
  child abuse and neglect, 182–194
    child in need of protection, 184–185
    child protection history in, 183–184
    mandatory reporting of, 185
    types of, 185–193
  community violence, 180–181
  definitions in, 177b–178b
  domestic violence, 181–182
    attempted strangulation, 182
    exposure to, 190–191
    see also exposure to domestic violence
    in pregnancy, 181–182
  useful websites for, 205t–208t
provisional diagnosis, in PHCR, 270